GRAINGER & ALLISON'S DIAGNOSTIC RADIOLOGY

Paediatric Imaging

SIXTH EDITION

GRAINGER & ALLISON'S DIAGNOSTIC RADIOLOGY

Paediatric Imaging

SIXTH EDITION

EDITED BY

Catherine M. Owens, BSc, MBBS, MRCP, FRCR

Jonathan H. Gillard, BSc, MA, MD, FRCP, FRCR, MBA

ELSEVIER

London   New York   Oxford   Philadelphia   St Louis   Sydney   Toronto

ELSEVIER

ISBN: 978-0-7020-6939-0

Executive Content Strategist: Michael Houston
Content Development Specialist: Louise Cook
Project Manager: Andrew Riley
Design: Christian Bilbow
Marketing Manager: Rachael Pignotti

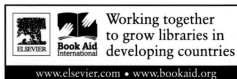

CONTENTS

PREFACE

The 8 chapters in this book have been selected from the contents of the Paediatric Imaging section in *Grainger & Allison's Diagnostic Radiology, Sixth Edition*. These organ-specific chapters provide a succinct up-to-date overview of current imaging techniques and their clinical applications in daily practice and it is hoped that with this concise format the user will quickly grasp the fundamentals they need to know. Throughout these chapters, the relative merits of different imaging investigations are described, variations are discussed and recent imaging advances are detailed.

Grainger & Allison's Diagnostic Radiology has long been recognized as the standard general reference work in the field, and it is hoped that this book, utilizing the content from the latest sixth edition of this classic reference work, will provide radiology trainees and practitioners with ready access to the most current information, written by internationally recognized experts, on what is new and important in the radiological diagnosis of paediatric patients.

List of Contributors

Maria I. Argyropoulou, MD, PhD
Professor of Radiology, Department of Radiology, University of Ioannina, Greece

Owen Arthurs, MB, Bchir, PhD, FRCR
Consultant Paediatric Radiologist, Radiology, Great Ormond Street Hospital, London, UK

Jean-François Chateil, MD, PhD
Professor, CHU de Bordeaux, Service d'imagerie anténatale, de l'enfant et de la femme; University of Bordeaux, Bordeaux, France

W.K. 'Kling' Chong, BMedSci, MBChB, MD, MRCP, FRCR
Specialty Lead for Radiology/Imaging; Consultant Paediatric Neuroradiologist, Department of Radiology, Great Ormond Street Hospital, London, UK

Marina Easty, MBBS, BSc, MRCP, FRCR, PGCert Nuc Med
Consultant Paediatric Radiologist, Radiology Department, Great Ormond Street Hospital, London, UK

Veronica Donoghue, FRCR, FFRRCSI
Consultant Paediatric Radiologist, Radiology Department, Children's University Hospital, Dublin, Ireland

Pilar Garcia-Peña, MD, PhD
Paediatric Radiologist, Hospital Materno-Infantil, Barcelona, Spain

Claudio Granata, MD
Consultant Radiologist, Department of Radiology, IRCCS Giannina Gaslini, Italy

Roxana S. Gunny, MBBS, MRCP, FRCR
Consultant Neuroradiologist, Department of Radiology, Great Ormond Street Hospital, London, UK

Paul Humphries, BSc, MBBS, MRCP, FRCR
Consultant Paediatric Radiologist, University College London Hospital NHS Trust and Great Ormond Street Hospital, London, UK

Karl Johnson, BSc, MB ChB, MRCP, FRCR
Consultant Paediatric Radiologist, Birmingham Children's Hospital, Birmingham, UK

Amaka C. Offiah, BSc, MBBS, MRCP, FRCR, PhD, HEFCE
Clinical Senior Lecturer, Academic Unit of Child Health, University of Sheffield; Consultant Paediatric Radiologist, Academic Unit of Child Health, Sheffield Children's NHS Foundation Trust, Sheffield, UK

Øystein E. Olsen, PhD
Consultant Radiologist, Radiology Department, Great Ormond Street Hospital, London, UK

Lil-Sofie Ording Müller, MD, PhD
Consultant Paediatric Radiologist, Section for Paediatric Radiology, Division of Diagnostics and Intervention, Oslo University Hospital, Ullevål, Oslo, Norway

Catherine M. Owens, BSc, MBBS, MRCP, FRCR
Consultant Radiologist and Honorary Reader, Department of Imaging, Great Ormond Street Hospital, London, UK

Anne Paterson, MBBS, MRCP, FRCR, FFRRCSI
Consultant Paediatric Radiologist, Department of Radiology, Royal Belfast Hospital for Sick Children, Belfast, UK

Michael Riccabona, OA
Professor, Department of Radiology, Division of Pediatric Radiology, Universitätsklinikum-LKH, Graz, Austria

Karen Rosendahl, MD, PhD
Consultant Paediatric Radiologist, Haukeland University Hospital; Professor, Department of Clinical Medicine, University of Bergen, Norway

Andrea Rossi, MD
Head, Pediatric Neuroradiology Unit, Istituto Giannina Gaslini; Contract Professor of Neuroradiology, University of Genoa, Genoa, Italy

Tom A. Watson, MBChB, FRCR
Paediatric Radiology Fellow, Department of Imaging, Great Ormond Street Hospital, London, UK

Carolyn M. Young, HDCR
Radiographer, Radiology Department, Great Ormond Street Hospital, London, UK

CHAPTER 1

CHALLENGES AND OVERVIEW OF SPECIAL FEATURES AND TECHNIQUES

Catherine M. Owens • Carolyn Young • Øystein E. Olsen

CHAPTER OUTLINE

Ultrasound is the primary diagnostic technique for follow-up in paediatric imaging, and its application is described in the organ-specific chapters in this section. This chapter describes general principles for the application of radiography, computed tomography and magnetic resonance imaging in paediatric radiology.

Medical diagnostic imaging has evolved and rapidly improved over the past five decades as a result of novel development in diagnostic digital imaging and interventional techniques. With technical advances in computer processing power, along with high-resolution display monitors/workstations, together with increased computing power and electronic data archive systems, diagnostic imaging departments have transformed, from being labour-intensive analogue film-based imaging units into fully integrated digital environments.

However, with all this new technology readily available, there remains a lack of dedicated purpose-built equipment suitable for use in children and easily available on the market.

Although manufacturers are aware of the more important radiation implications pertaining to children, and have made inroads into lowering medical radiation doses, the ultimate responsibility remains with radiology technicians and radiologists, who control and operate diagnostic equipment, to adapt and adjust the (primarily adult-designed) techniques and protocols to suit the younger, more radiation-vulnerable population.

PROJECTION RADIOGRAPHY

The development of digital imaging in plain film radiography is advantageous within paediatric imaging. First introduced to computed radiography (CR) and later in direct readout radiography (DR) systems (utilising flat-panel detector (FD) technology), this technology helped provide greater efficiency in converting incident X-ray energy into image signal. This, together with its inherent wide dynamic range, greatly improved image quality, when compared with conventional screen-film-based systems, if equivalent exposure parameters were used. This has the potential for lowering radiation dosage for the patient and also reducing the risk of failed, i.e. non-diagnostic, exposure. Using post-processing capabilities, both bone and soft-tissue anatomy can now be optimally displayed on the same image, thus eliminating the need for repeated radiation exposure.[1-3]

However, care must be taken when setting exposure factors, as unlike with film-based techniques, overexposure can easily occur with digital imaging. This happens without adverse effect on image quality, and may not be recognised by the operator, as the image brightness can be freely adjusted, independent of exposure level.[4,5]

In general, FD technology is an efficient method for obtaining high-quality image data and enabling immediate image preview, storage and distribution over local area networks for viewing by clinicians, thus enhancing efficiency and productivity within high workflow departments.

Other applications of FD technology include digital tomosynthesis (or digital tomography), providing quasi 3-dimensional images, adapted for use in chest imaging. As a chest radiograph is a 2-dimensional image, sensitivity may be reduced when detecting underlying pathology because of overlapping anatomy. This can be overcome by CT applications but with an inherent increased radiation dose. Tomosynthesis evolved from conventional geometric tomography and was introduced as a low-dose alternative for chest radiographic examination in monitoring children with cystic fibrosis, and in the detection of pulmonary nodules.[6,7] This technique, involving the acquisition of a number of projection images at different angles during a single vertical motion of the X-ray tube (between a given angular range of −17.5° and +17.5°) directed at a stationary digital flat-panel detector, results in up to 60 coronal sectional images at an arbitrary depth.[6-8] Anatomical structures within each image section are sharply depicted, whilst structures located anteriorly and posteriorly are blurred. Spatial resolution is higher in tomosynthesis than in CT in the acquired imaging plane, but depth resolution is inferior, due to the limited angles used.

Further limitations to this imaging technique include the necessity of a 10-s acquisition time, increasing the likelihood of respiratory motion artefacts in non-compliant patients, which will exclude younger children who are unable to hold their breath. Although the radiation dose for tomosynthesis is much reduced compared with CT, it is three times higher than that for a frontal chest radiograph. This can be offset by a higher nodular detection rate than that seen with the plain radiograph, making this technique a possible alternative to CT examinations in some children.

FLUOROSCOPY

The introduction of digital fluoroscopy with its high-speed digitisation of the analogue video signal has revolutionised real-time fluoroscopy that relied on the use of image intensifier/TV systems to display the diagnostic image. Development of fluoroscopy FD technology with its fast digital readout and dynamic acquisition of image series at high frame rates (up to 60 frames per second) has become a well-established application in cardiac paediatric angiography. The other important application is within minimally invasive interventional procedures, due to their less invasive nature, when compared with conventional surgery. Advantages of FD compared with image intensifier systems that help minimise radiation dose include pulsed fluoroscopy, last-image hold and screen capture, which negate further diagnostic image exposures. Other features that improve image quality include homogeneous image uniformity with lack of geometric distortion across the entire image, reduced veiling glare, and a rectangular or square field-of-view, which utilises the full width of the image monitor. The small compact size of FD mounted on a dedicated C-arm system increases operational flexibility and ease of patient access, both features which are particularly pertinent within paediatric imaging.[2,3]

Modern C-arm angiography systems utilising FD technology are equipped with rotational angiography applications, providing 3-dimensional CT image capture (FD-CT) that is used mainly in interventional procedures. The ability to combine 2-dimensional fluoroscopic and 3-dimensional CT imaging within a single unit is advantageous for providing planning, guidance and monitoring of interventional procedures and intraoperative imaging.[9,10] The image quality is lower in FD-CT than in clinical CT, but in situations where a quick CT control diagnosis is required, an alternative lower spatial resolution image is acceptable. In addition, due to the slow rotation of FD-CT, patient movement and respiratory artefacts in body imaging further reduce spatial resolution. The radiation dose is noted to be higher in FD-CT due to lower detection efficiency, although the milliamperes per second (mAs) per single image acquisition is much lower. It is the cumulative dose of the procedure that is crucial in this instance, with variation seen in each individual investigation/treatment.

COMPUTED TOMOGRAPHY (CT)

CT is a proven essential diagnostic imaging technique and is considered the most sensitive method for evaluating airway diseases in children.

Two CT imaging configurations exist: namely, multi-detector CT (MDCT) with up to 320 detector rows and dual-source CT (DSCT) utilising MDCT technology. The increasing temporal and better spatial resolutions have extended the role of CT applications in young children to include cardiac imaging. Advantages of these systems include subsecond tube rotation times (down to 0.33 s). This increase in acquisition speed has the potential for reducing motion and respiratory artefacts and improving image quality. The overall reduction in examination acquisition time may also obviate the need for sedation in some children. The availability of small detector elements (0.5 mm) combined with thin-slice collimation provides isotropic resolution that allows image data to be manipulated/reformatted in any orthogonal plane and displayed as either 2- or 3-dimensional images that have the same spatial resolution as the base axial data set and with reduced partial volume artefact.

320-Row MDCT

The availability of 320-slice MDCT allows for larger volume coverage of up to 16 cm in the z-axis coverage. The advantage is that this coverage is well within the clinical range of thoracic length in neonates and young children. Therefore, imaging of the entire chest can be accomplished in a single-volume cone beam acquisition during one tube rotation of 0.35 s.[11] This is much faster than either helical MDCT or DSCT acquisition. Axial volumetric acquisitions have the potential of radiation dose saving. Due to the large nominal beam width used, the contribution of the penumbra effect is less prominent. Also, unlike in helical CT, over-ranging in the longitudinal axis is not applicable in this instance, as the exposed range corresponds exactly to the imaged range and therefore more effective usage of the radiation exposure for image formation. Axial volumetric acquisition can be applied to other clinical situations that include cardiac imaging in children, as when using prospective ECG-gating, the entire heart can be imaged within a single tube rotation.[11]

Dual-Source CT

The second-generation DSCT system (Siemens Flash, Forchheim, Germany) is currently the latest in CT technology. It incorporates two X-ray tubes each with corresponding 64-row detector systems (each contributing 128 slices by means of a z flying focal spot), mounted at an angular offset of 90° to each other. Designed for cardiac imaging, the two-tube detector system does not operate simultaneously, but in tandem, whereby data from the second detector system are collected a quarter of a rotation later following the first set of detectors. This allows gapless volume high-pitch CT (up to 3.2 pitch), avoiding overlapping slices with reduced radiation dose.[12,13] Together with a fast gantry rotation time of 0.28 s, a 75-ms temporal resolution is achieved, enabling helical prospective ECG-triggered cardiac imaging for the first time.[14] High heart rates are no longer a limiting factor when imaging children, and DSCT is invaluable for both the pre- and post-surgical assessment of a wide variety of congenital heart diseases, resulting in improved visualisation of the coronary arteries if data are captured in the systolic phase[15] even in younger children. Prospectively gated cardiac imaging is the preferred technique in young children, where often only morphological and proximal coronary artery detail is required. This negates the need for retrospectively gated imaging with its higher radiation burden. The sharp anatomical delineation between adjacent structures seen in prospective gating is superior to that seen in non-gated CTA studies, and with lower radiation dose levels.

Dual-Energy Dual-Source CT

The availability of two X-ray tubes allows simultaneous acquisition of two data sets at different tube potentials (80 and 140 kVp), during the same phase of contrast enhancement and excludes temporal changes and spatial misregistration. This technique takes advantage of differences between tissue and material composition and differences in their photon absorption characteristics. In particular, materials with a high atomic number (like iodine) exhibit a different degree of attenuation between the two tube potentials. By applying specific post-processing algorithms to the acquired data, virtual unenhanced and virtual angiographic data sets can be generated, based on the three-material composition principle;[16–18] e.g. within the abdomen, the materials analysed are soft tissue, fat and iodine, whilst in the chest, soft tissue, air and iodine are analysed. Application of the bone removal algorithm will display an angiographic data set without overlying bony structures, resulting in easier image interpretation. This eliminates the need for pre-intravenous contrast CT examinations imaging, as may be required if using a single tube device, for data subtraction purposes. Thus radiation doses are halved.

Overall radiation dose associated with dual-energy CT (DECT) is noted to be comparable to that of single-source MDCT systems. Other clinical dual-energy applications include characterisation of abdominal masses, chemical composition of renal calculi, myocardial and pulmonary perfusion imaging.

The depiction of iodine distribution for the detection of peripheral lung perfusion defects from suspected pulmonary emboli adds functional information to conventional pulmonary CT angiography. Its application in paediatrics is relevant in the evaluation of subsegmental pulmonary emboli.[17,19] By applying advanced post-processing software to the acquired data set, an iodine distribution map is generated and overlaid onto a grey-scale image. A normal perfusion image will show homogeneous colour distribution extending to the lung periphery and is displayed in a multiplanar format that can be manipulated manually. The presence of a filling or hypoperfusion is indicative of an obstructed vessel supplying the relevant lung segment. Review of the grey-scale image will help determine anatomical detail and location.

Other DECT applications include the use of xenon ventilation in chest imaging, as it is found to be more sensitive in the evaluation of regional and global airway and lung abnormalities in children.[20] Conventional CT investigation requires both inspiratory and expiratory acquisitions to demonstrate whether air-trapping exists. However, the use of xenon with the ability to demonstrate regional ventilation defects on inspiration obviates the need for an additional expiratory phase acquisition, with consequent radiation dose saving. In addition, the quantitative evaluation of lung density on CT is dependent on age and level of respiration. As this varies in young children, the use of xenon with its insensitivity to respiration level will provide more accurate measurements.

Radiation Dose Consideration

The increase in radiation burden associated with CT imaging and the potential risk to children cannot be ignored. CT requests must, therefore, be justified; a robust risk–benefit analysis should always be carried out before undertaking CT examination in children. Imaging techniques and dedicated paediatric protocols must be available to the operators, ensuring adherence to the ALARA principle. Adjustments to the CT parameters could be based on the patient's age, body weight or body diameter.

A list of guidelines for routine imaging are detailed in Tables 1-1 to 1-5. The use of 120 kVp is no longer

TABLE 1-1 Routine Chest Imaging

Indications	Airway disease
	Tumour masses and metastases
	Tracheomalacia
	Tracheobronchial stenosis
	Vascular anomalies
CT mode	Helical
CT parameter	Under 9 kg: 80 kVp, 60 ref mAs
	10 kg and above: 100 kVp, 30-48 ref mAs
Tube rotation	0.5 s
Tube collimation	0.6 mm
Pitch	1
CT slice width	0.6 mm
Recon slice width	1 mm
Recon kernel	Medium-soft B30 and high-resolution B60
Contrast media	Omnipaque 300 2 mL per kg to a maximum of 100 mL
CT delay	Using pressure injector, 25 s from start of injection

TABLE 1-2 Routine Abdominal Imaging

Indications	Tumour masses
	Vascular anomalies
CT mode	Helical
CT parameter	100 kVp, 60–75 ref mAs
Tube rotation	0.5 s
Tube collimation	Under 15 kg: 0.6 mm
	16 kg and above: 1.2 mm
Pitch	1
Tube current modulation	On
CT slice width	0.6 mm
Recon slice width	1 mm
Recon kernel	Medium-soft B30
Contrast media	Omnipaque 300 2 mL per kg to a maximum of 150 mL
CT delay	Using pressure injector, 45 s from start of injection

TABLE 1-3   Routine Head Imaging

Indications	Postoperative for tumour removal
	NAI
	Bleed/subdural
	Infection
CT mode	Sequential
CT parameter	120 kVp, 160–300 ref mAs
Tube rotation	1 s
Tube collimation	1.2 mm
Tube current modulation	On
CT slice width	1.2 mm
Recon slice width	5 mm, 2 mm if reformat required
Recon kernel	Medium-soft C30
Contrast media	Omnipaque 300 1 mL per kg to a maximum of 100 mL
CT delay	Hand injection, 3 min post-injection

TABLE 1-4   Hydrocephalus Assessment

Indications	Hydrocephalus
	Blocked shunt
CT mode	Sequential
CT parameter	Under 6 years: 100 kVp, 180–230 ref mAs
	7 years and above: 120 kVp, 220 ref mAs
Tube rotation	1 s
Tube collimation	10 mm
Tube current modulation	On
CT slice width	10 mm
Recon slice width	10 mm
Recon kernel	Medium-soft C30
Contrast media	Not required

TABLE 1-5   Low-dose 3-Dimensional Head Imaging

Indications	Maxillofacial assessment
CT mode	Helical
CT parameter	Under 6 years: 100 kVp, 50 ref mAs
	7 years and above: 120 kVp, 50 ref mAs
Tube rotation	1 s
Tube collimation	0.6 mm
Pitch	0.9
Tube current modulation	On
CT slice width	0.6 mm
Recon slice width	1 mm
Recon kernel	Soft C20
Contrast media	Not required

advocated in paediatric body imaging, and can be reduced to 80 or 100 kVp[21] without detriment to image quality, and, indeed, improves contrast resolution, thus allowing a smaller concentration of contrast medium to be administered. The tube current can also be reduced but at the detriment of increased image noise and reduced spatial resolution.[22] The degree of reduction is dependent on the level of 'tolerable' image noise deemed acceptable by the reporting radiologists. In general, image noise is less well tolerated in small children, due to the lack of inherent soft-tissue contrast (i.e. less fat), compared with adults, resulting in the necessity for proportional increase in milliamperes per second when imaging younger children. Utilisation of automatic tube current modulation (ATCM) with real-time ('on the fly') adaptation of tube current ensures that a constant image noise level is maintained across the area of interest, with the potential for reducing radiation dose. The disadvantage of this is that the tube current will increase, e.g. at the level of the shoulders, and at the lung base/diaphragm regions in thoracic imaging and across the pelvis in abdominal imaging. ATCM effectiveness is also debatable in younger children as they are more rounded in body shape, rendering angular tube current modulation futile.

More recent developments in radiation dose reduction strategies include exposure modulation over sensitive organs, where the radiation output is reduced when the X-ray tube is in the AP position over the breast and thyroid region. This eliminates the need for bismuth shielding that can increase tube current especially if ACTM is employed. The issue with over-ranging in the longitudinal axis, associated with helical imaging, has been overcome in modern devices by deployment of dynamic collimators at the start and end of the helical range, to block unnecessary radiation and reduce dose to the patient.

Iterative reconstruction is also widely available on modern CT systems. It allows use of lower exposure factors with significant reduction in image noise, without loss of diagnostic information, with a reported dose reduction of 35% noted in chest CT[23] and 23–66% in abdominal CT.[24]

Patient Care

Due to the speed of present-day CT machines, children over 3 years of age are usually compliant for their procedure, provided they are properly prepared through play therapy beforehand, using a mock-up toy of the machine to take the child and their parents through the imaging process. It is also a good opportunity to assess the child's ability to respond to breath-holding instructions; otherwise, gentle respiration is encouraged. A range of suitable sedatives may be prescribed to younger children, which include the light-acting sedative chloral hydrate at a dose of 50 mg/kg, or the short-acting midazolam hydrochloride at 0.1 mg/kg body weight.

Some centres prefer the more quick-acting sedative proprofol but this must be administered in the presence of an anaesthetist. The use of general anaesthesia is reserved only for non-compliant patients, or in cases where sedation had not been successful.

Dental Cone Beam CT

Diagnostic imaging is essential in clinical dental assessment and for those receiving orthodontic treatment.[25] This is accomplished by intra-oral projection radiography, and with rotational panoramic radiography (RPR) providing 2-dimensional images of what is really a 3-dimensional object, and often with inaccurate measurement due to inherent magnification and geometric distortion of the image. The development of low-dose cone beam computed tomography (CBCT) is a significant advancement in dental imaging, providing accurate high-resolution volumetric visualisation of the osseous structures in the maxillofacial region, and this has extended applications to treatment planning and image guidance for surgical procedures.[26]

There are various CBCT designs based on the available vertical height or field-of-view (FOV), ranging between 5 and 13 cm with coverage from a localised region to include the facial skeleton. It is important to select the correct equipment for the intended diagnostic task.

The systems operate in a similar fashion to RPR, utilising a divergent pyramidal-shaped source of radiation; the system rotates around the patient in a single 180° to 360° arc, acquiring multiple sequential planar projections directed onto the detector. The resultant number of base images is dependent on the frame rate, speed of rotation and completeness of the trajectory arc. These base images, similar in appearance to cephalometric radiographic images, are then integrated and displayed as a 3-dimensional volumetric data set.[26,27] Image quality is dependent to a certain extent on the acquired number of image projections, and can be improved by increasing the tube rotation from 180° to 360°, but with an increase in radiation dose. By way of limiting radiation dose and exposure to radiosensitive tissues (salivary gland and thyroid), the FOV should be adjusted in height and width to cover the area of interest only.

Using a large FOV, the base of skull and spinal anatomy is included in the resultant image. Thes images will require interpretation and reporting, and this in turn may not be within the remit of the dental practitioner, and will need to be coreported by a radiologist. This increases workload on reporting radiologists and needs to be reflected in optimal practice.

CBCT is comparable to conventional CT, and may be better at delineating bony details of the jaw and skull, but the system is unable to display soft-tissue structures. It is unsuitable for dental caries diagnosis in some cases, due to streak artefacts and dark bands across the image caused by beam hardening from data acquisition and from restored dentition. Radiation dose is much lower in CBCT than in CT, but higher than in conventional dental radiography.[28,29] A low-dose technique with 50% tube current reduction without loss of diagnostic quality can be applied for the purposes of orthodontic treatment and pre-surgical implant planning.[30] It is therefore important that exposure parameters used should be appropriate to the diagnostic task and to the size of the patient.

MAGNETIC RESONANCE IMAGING (MRI)

Apart from imaging of lung parenchyma and cortical bone, and in some cases of cardiovascular malformations and in trauma cases, MRI is the preferred cross-sectional imaging technique in children. This is due to the multitude of tissue contrasts inherent to this technique, and because there is no exposure to ionising radiation. Paediatric MRI is, in practice, somewhat different from the adult equivalent in that it requires particular attention to preparing the child, optimising the signal-to-noise ratio (SNR), handling motion artefacts and adjusting for differences in tissue contrast.

Patient Preparation

It may seem appealing to opt for the fastest pulse sequences in a potentially moving child; however, such a strategy may compromise the diagnostic performance of MRI. For example, whereas steady-state free-precession-type pulse sequences may be very useful for bowel imaging and for certain types of non-contrast-enhanced vascular imaging, they are in general not a good option for imaging tissues. Some of the best anatomical imaging sequences available, e.g. volumetric T2-weighted spin-echo, require a long acquisition time (in excess of 10 min). Since long acquisitions are usually required and because movement during the MR data acquisition is detrimental to the diagnostic quality of the resulting images, careful preparation is necessary.

A developmental age of less than 6–8 years in general means that sedation or general anaesthesia is required. General anaesthesia is considered safe, with reported fatal complications at 10 in 101,885 anaesthetic episodes (about 0.001%)—all related to pre-existing medical conditions.[31] Sufficient sedation is usually possible in children with bodyweight less than 15 kg; however, there are important contraindications such as airways being compromised.[32] Compared with general anaesthesia, sedation may be considered less safe (no airways protection), but this depends on the medical condition of the child and on local procedures for the safe selection of children for sedation. For the imager, sedation is less reliable (about 75% success rate in one study[33]) than general anaesthesia, and it does not allow breath-holding during the procedure. Sedation is hence often suboptimal for MRI of the chest and abdomen, but may suffice for neuro- and musculoskeletal MRI.

Postprandial sleep may sufficiently immobilise the young infant. The child is fed and gently swaddled (feed-and-wrap) to induce sleep. Acoustic shielding is then applied. Success is more likely if the feed follows 4 hours of fasting.[34]

In the older child, previous introduction to the imaging environment by means of a mock machine may improve compliance during the MRI examination.[35] Thorough briefing appropriate for the developmental stage of the child and availability of in-built entertainment systems are helpful.

Radiofrequency Coils

The coil is the single most important determinant of SNR. Multi-channel coils result in higher SNR.[36] A coil or coil combination that gives optimal coverage is essential.[37] The coverage should be about 1.5 times the size of the region of interest. A coil coverage that is too small would give insufficient signal reception, whereas a larger-than-required coverage would add noise. Therefore, a wide spectrum of coils needs to be available to allow selection of a coil combination that most appropriately fits the region of interest. This might, for example, mean using an adult knee coil for abdominal or chest MRI in a neonate.[38]

Motion Artefact Reduction

The amount of gross motion is managed by adequate patient preparation. Attenuation of peristalsis is important for T2-weighted spin-echo acquisitions, and is achieved with intravenous administration of glucagon or hyoscine-*N*-butylbromide. Physiological gating freezes periodic motion by only allowing readout during well-defined event-driven time windows. This window may be end-diastole for ECG-gated acquisitions and around end-expiration for ventilatory-gated acquisitions.

In chest imaging, a combination of ECG- and ventilation-gating is possible. Fast imaging techniques make dual gating practically more feasible. Physiological gating is less feasible for T1-weighted spin-echo sequences, but good fat suppression may partly compensate for this deficiency. Gating is not required for diffusion-weighted acquisitions.[39] When gating is impossible, one may consider: (1) targeted saturation and (2) advanced *k*-space trajectories.

Manipulation of *k* space may be as simple as changing the phase-encoding direction to direct any artefact away from an area of interest. For example, axial images of the thymus may be improved with a right-to-left phase-encoding direction. Some pulse sequences have *k*-space trajectories designed to reduce the impact of motion artefact. One example is a trajectory that uses several different readout directions (PROPELLER, BLADE, MultiVane, RADAR, JET). The result is that motion artefact is distributed over several radial directions and, hence, becomes less perceivable in the final image.

Tissue Contrast

Poor SNR is more tolerable if the image contrast is optimised. The principles for good image contrast are: (1) to always use a combination of different image weightings and (2) to use intravenous contrast media.

Most childhood tumours have restricted water diffusion,[40] so diffusion-weighted imaging is mandatory for imaging mass lesions in children. Fat suppression at T1-weighted imaging is useful for depicting the pancreas, and fat suppression also accentuates the enhancement following gadolinium administration. Non-fat-suppressed sequences need to be part of any MR protocol for two reasons: (1) for the detection of fat-containing lesions (e.g. teratoma, lipoblastoma) and (2) for the definition of anatomical planes.

Hyaline cartilage of epiphyses, epiphyseal equivalents and apophyses constitute a large and important portion of the skeleton in young patients. Cartilaginous defects may be constitutional (e.g. proximal focal femoral deficiency) or acquired (e.g. secondary to juvenile idiopathic arthritis). Cartilage has intermediate signal intensity on fat-suppressed T1-weighted images, on proton density spin-echo and on fat-suppressed (double-echo) balanced steady-state free-precession images.[37]

Intravenous gadolinium-based contrast media generally improve the diagnostic efficacy of MRI. In childhood tumours this is sometimes due to the negative contrast of a poorly enhancing tumour against normally enhancing surrounding tissues. Arterial or early portal venous phase volumetric spoiled gradient-echo acquisitions often show the perimeter of the lesion, and demonstrate important vascular (arterial, portal venous, renal venous) relations. As for adults, gadolinium should be used with caution in children with reduced renal function. Young infants (less than 6 months of age) have physiologically low renal function, and it may be recommended to routinely estimate GFR in these. There are also licensing restrictions to using gadolinium in children (as for many other pharmaceuticals), so institutional policies need to be in place.

Image Resolution

MRI measures signal intensity voxel by voxel. A voxel cannot be depicted if its signal intensity is lower than that of the background noise. Since a small voxel contains fewer hydrogen nuclei, it will have a lower MRI signal than a larger voxel. SNR is therefore proportional to the voxel volume. Hence, if decreasing the size of the field of view, one needs to revise the acquisition matrix or else risk suboptimal SNR. However, due to the finer anatomical landscape in children, it is often desirable to maintain a voxel size somewhat smaller than that in adult imaging. Either one must then accept a lower SNR (which may be tolerable if the contrast is good and if there is only minimal motion artefact) or one needs to compensate for the loss in SNR. Compensation may be achieved by averaging a higher number of acquisitions, decreasing the receiver bandwidth, reducing the parallel imaging factor and/or by oversampling *k* space.

Imaging Planes

Imaging planes are fundamentally arbitrary and may be ignored in volumetric imaging, where optimal planar reconstruction is left to the post-processing stage. Isotropic imaging has in the past been restricted to gradient-echo sequences, and to spin-echo sequences with very long echo times. The problem with intermediate echo times has been degradation from blurring of the contrast due to long echo trains. This problem is solved with the implementation of volumetric proton density and T2-weighted spin-echo sequences (SPACE, VISTA, CUBE) that use a scheme of variable flip-angle evolutions to assign different weights to readouts depending on their order.

However, 2-dimensional acquisitions may still be required, and for these the imaging planes need to be perpendicular to the most important anatomical planes, and at least two different planes need to be acquired. Generally, in the abdomen, axial imaging is most useful because the axial plane is perpendicular to the largest portions of the peritoneum and body wall, the aorta and inferior vena cava and the renal fossae, and perpendicular to the planes between most of the major organs. In the pelvis, the sagittal plane is most useful because it transects

TABLE 1-6   Suggested Basic Protocol for Abdominal MRI in a Child with an Abdominal Mass Lesion

Pulse Sequence or Event, Key Parameters	Image Volume	Voxel Size, mm (approx.)
Localisers		
Intravenous Administration of Hyoscine		
STIR coronal, ventilatory gated	Abdomen and pelvis	1.1 × 1.1 × 5.0
Volumetric T2-weighted spin-echo with variable flip-angles, ventilatory gated	Region of lesion	0.9 × 0.9 × 0.9
Diffusion-weighted imaging (*b* values, at least 0 and 1000) axial	Lesion	2.7 × 2.7 × 6.0
Fat-suppressed T1-weighted spin-echo axial	Region of lesion	1.0 × 1.0 × 6.0
Fat-suppressed volumetric spoiled gradient-echo, breath-hold	Abdomen	0.9 × 1.0 × 1.1
Administration of Gadolinium-Based Contrast Agent via Power Injector		
Fat-suppressed volumetric spoiled gradient-echo, breath-hold, early portal venous phase using bolus tracking	Abdomen	0.9 × 1.0 × 1.1
Fat-suppressed T1-weighted spin-echo axial	Region of lesion	1.0 × 1.0 × 5.0

the planes between the bladder, internal genital organs, the rectum and the anterior/posterior body walls. The sagittal image plane is also chosen for other midline structures, such as the thymus.

Practical Consequences

One protocol for abdominal MRI in a child with an abdominal mass lesion is suggested in Table 1-6. This protocol incorporates several image contrasts: water-sensitive sequences (STIR), diffusion-weighted imaging, non-fat-suppressed imaging (2-D or 3-D T2-weighted spin-echo) and contrast-enhanced acquisitions. Dynamic contrast-enhanced volumetric gradient-echo sequences are optional but improve the definition of vascular relations. A large FOV coronal STIR acquisition is included for lesion detection over a large anatomical region. Motion artefact is reduced by mostly using fat-suppressed sequences, by administration of hyoscine and by using respiratory gating whenever possible.

REFERENCES

1. Korner M, Weber CH, Wirth S, et al. Advances in digital radiography: physical principles and system overview. Radiographics 2007;27:675–86.
2. Spahn M. Flat detectors and their clinical applications. Eur Radiol 2005;15:1934–47.
3. Seibert JA. Flat-panel detectors: how much better are they? Pediatr Radiol 2006;36(2):173–81.
4. Willis CE. Strategies for dose reduction in ordinary radiographic examinations using CR and DR. Pediatr Radiol 2004;34(3):S196–200.
5. Managing patient dose in digital radiology, ICRP publication 93.
6. Vult von Steyern K, Bjorkman-Burtscher I, Geijer M. Tomosynthesis in pulmonary CF with comparison to radiography and CT: a pictorial review. Insights Imaging 2012;3:81–9.
7. Vikgren J, Zachrisson S, Svalkvist A, et al. Tomosynthesis and chest radiography for the detection of pulmonary nodules: human observer of clinical cases. Radiology 2008;249:1034–41.
8. Dobbins JT 3rd, Godfrey DJ. Digital x-ray tomosynthesis: current state of the art and clinical potential. Phys Med Biol 2003;48(19):R65–106.
9. Kalander WA, Kyriakou Y. Flat-detector computed tomography. Eur Radiol 2007;17:2767–79.
10. Hausegger KA, Furstner M, Hauser M, et al. Clinical application of flat-panel CT in the angio suite. Rofo 2011;183(12):1116–22.
11. Kroft LJM, Roelofs JJH, Geleijns J. Scan time and patient dose for thoracic imaging in neonates and small children using axial volumetric 320-detector row CT compared to helical 64, 32, and 16 detector row CT acquisition. Pediatr Radiol 2010;40:294–300.
12. Lell M, Marwan M, Schepis T, et al. Prospectively ECG-triggered high-pitch spiral acquisition for coronary CT angiography using dual source CT: technique and initial experience. Eur Radiol 2009;19:2576–83.
13. Goetti R, Feuchtner G, Stolzmann P, et al. High-pitch DSCT coronary angiography: systolic data acquisition at high heart rates. Eur Radiol 2010;20:2565–71.
14. Alkadhi H, Stolzman P, Desbiolles L, et al. Low dose, 128-slice, dual-source CT coronary angiography: accuracy and radiation dose of the high-pitch and the step-and-shoot mode. Heart 2010;96:933–8.
15. Ben Saad M, Rohnean A, Sigal-Cinqualbre A, et al. Evaluation of image quality and radiation dose of thoracic and coronary dual-source CT in 110 infants with CHD. Pediatr Radiol 2009;39:668–76.
16. Graser A, Johnson TRC, Chandarana H, Macari M. Duel energy CT: preliminary observations and potential clinical applications in the abdomen. Eur Radiol 2009;19:13–23.
17. Hoey ETD, Gopalan D, Ganesh V, et al. Dual-energy CT pulmonary angiography: a novel technique for assessing acute and chronic pulmonary thromboembolism. Clin Radiol 2009;64:414–19.
18. Johnson TRC, Kraub B, Sedlmair M, et al. Material differentiation by DECT: initial experience. Eur Radiol 2007;17:1510–17.
19. Goo HW. Initial experience of dual-energy lung perfusion CT using a DSCT system in children. Pediatr Radiol 2010;40:1536–44.
20. Goo HW, Yang DH, Hong SJ, et al. Xenon ventilation CT using dual-source and dual-energy technique in children with bronchiolitis obliterans: correlation of xenon and CT density values with pulmonary function test results. Pediatr Radiol 2010;40:1490–7.
21. Kim JE, Newman B. Evaluation of a radiation dose reduction strategy for pediatric chest CT. AJR Am J Roentgenol 2010;194:1188–93.
22. Paterson A, Frush DP. Dose reduction in paediatric MDCT: general principle. Clin Radiol 2007;62:507–17.
23. Pontana F, Duhamel A, Pagniez J, et al. Chest CT using IR vs FBP: image quality of low-dose CT examinations in 80 patients. Eur Radiol 2011;21:636–43.
24. Sagara Y, Hara AK, Pavlicek W, et al. Abdominal CT: comparison of low-dose CT with ASIR and routine-dose CT with FBP in 53 patients. AJR Am J Roentgenol 2010;195:713–19.
25. Mah JK, Huang JC, Choo HR. Practical applications of cone-beam computed tomography in orthodontics. J Am Dent Assoc 2012;141(Suppl. 3):S7–13.
26. Scarfe WC, Li Z, Aboelmaaty W, et al. Maxillofacial cone beam computed tomography: essence, elements and steps to interpretation. Aust Dent J 2012;57:46–60.
27. Dawood A, Patel S, Brown J. Cone beam CT in dental practice. Br Dent J 2009;207:23–8.

28. Roberts JA, Drage NA, Davies J, Thomas DW. Effective dose from cone-beam CT examinations in dentistry. Br J Radiol 2009;82: 35–40.

29. Lorenzoni DC, Bolognese AM, Garib DG, et al. Cone-beam computed tomography and radiographs in dentistry: aspects related to radiation dose. Int J Dent 2012;2012:813768. doi:10.1155/2012/813768. Epub 2012 Apr 4.

30. Kwong JC, Paloma JM, Landers MA, et al. Image quality produced by different CBCT settings. Am J Orthod Dentofacial Orthop 2008;133:317–27.

31. van der Griend BF, Lister NA, McKenzie IM, et al. Postoperative mortality in children after 101,885 anesthetics at a tertiary pediatric hospital. Anesth Analg 2011;112:1440–7.

32. Sury MR, Smith JH. Deep sedation and minimal anesthesia. Paediatr Anaesth 2008;18:18–24.

33. Heng Vong C, Bajard A, Thiesse P, et al. Deep sedation in pediatric imaging: efficacy and safety of intravenous chlorpromazine. Pediatr Radiol 2012;42:552–61.

34. Windram J, Grosse-Wortmann L, Shariat M, et al. Cardiovascular MRI without sedation or general anesthesia using a feed-and-sleep technique in neonates and infants. Pediatr Radiol 2012;42: 183–7.

35. Carter AJ, Greer ML, Gray SE, et al. Mock MRI: Reducing the need for anaesthesia in children. Pediatr Radiol 2010;40: 1368–74.

36. Vasanawala SS, Lustig M. Advances in pediatric body MRI. Pediatr Radiol 2011;41(Suppl. 2):549–54.

37. Jaramillo D, Laor T. Pediatric musculoskeletal MRI: basic principles to optimize success. Pediatr Radiol 2008;38:379–91.

38. Helle M, Jerosch-Herold M, Voges I, et al. Improved MRI of the neonatal heart: feasibility study using a knee coil. Pediatr Radiol 2011;41:1429–32.

39. Olsen OE, Sebire NJ. Apparent diffusion coefficient maps of pediatric mass lesions with free-breathing diffusion-weighted magnetic resonance: feasibility study. Acta Radiol 2006;47:198–204.

40. Humphries PD, Sebire NJ, Siegel MJ, et al. Tumors in pediatric patients at diffusion-weighted MR imaging: apparent diffusion coefficient and tumor cellularity. Radiology 2007;245:848–54.

CHAPTER 2

THE NEONATAL AND PAEDIATRIC CHEST

Veronica Donoghue • Tom A. Watson • Pilar Garcia-Peña • Catherine M. Owens

THE NEONATAL CHEST

NORMAL ANATOMY AND ARTEFACTS

The anteroposterior (AP) diameter of the neonatal chest is almost as great as its transverse diameter, giving the chest a cylindrical configuration. The degree of rotation is best assessed by comparing the length of the anterior ribs visible on both sides. As newborn chest radiographs are taken in the AP plane, the normal cardiothoracic ratio can be as large as 60%.

The thymic size is variable and may alter with the degree of lung inflation. It may blend with the cardiac silhouette, it may have an undulating boarder due to underlying rib indentation (Fig. 2-1) or it may exhibit the classic 'sail sign' more commonly seen on the right side. It may involute rapidly with prenatal or postnatal stress, for example in severe illnesses such as hyaline membrane disease or infections, or following corticosteroid treatment.

There are some well-recognised artefacts on a newborn chest radiograph. The hole in the incubator top may be confused with a pneumatocele or lung cyst. Skin folds may be visible over the chest wall and may mimic a pneumothorax. These can usually be seen to extend beyond the lung.

NORMAL LUNG DEVELOPMENT

The normal lung development is well described by Agrons et al.[1] During the embryonic phase of gestation (from 26 days to 6 weeks) the lung bud develops from the primitive foregut and divides to form the early tracheobronchial tree. During the pseudoglandular phase (6–16 weeks) there is airway development to the level of the terminal bronchioles, with a deficient number of alveolar saccules. Multiple alveolar ducts develop from the respiratory bronchioles during the cannicular or acinar phase (16–28 weeks). These ducts are lined by type II alveolar cells which can produce surfactant, and which differentiate into thin type I alveolar lining cells. At the end of this phase primitive alveoli form. Progressive thinning of the pulmonary interstitium allows gas exchange with approximation of the proliferating capillaries and the type I cells.

During the saccular phase (28–34 weeks) there is an increase in the number of terminal sacs, further thinning of the interstitium, continuing proliferation of the capillary bed and early development of the true alveoli.

The alveolar phase extends from approximately 36 weeks' gestation until 18 month of age, with most alveoli formed at 5–6 months of age.

IDIOPATHIC RESPIRATORY DISTRESS SYNDROME

Idiopathic respiratory distress syndrome (IRDS) or hyaline membrane disease (HMD) mainly affects the premature infant less than 36 weeks' gestational age. The primary problem in HMD is a deficiency of the lipoprotein pulmonary surfactant in association with structural immaturity of the lungs. The lipoproteins are produced in the type II pneumocytes, are concentrated in the cell lamellar bodies and then transported to the cell surface and expressed onto the alveolar luminal surface. These lipoproteins then combine with surface surfactant

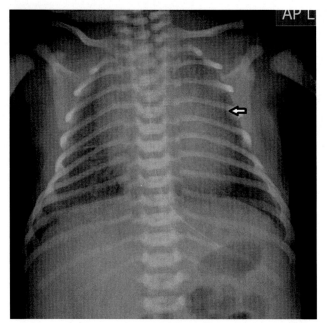

FIGURE 2-1 ■ **There is mediastinal widening, due to normal thymic tissue.** The undulated appearance of the left thymic border is due to rib indentation (arrow).

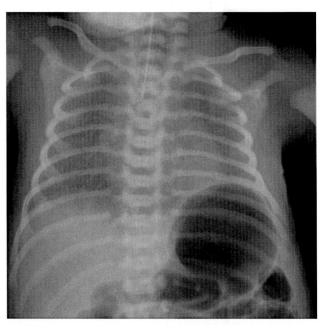

FIGURE 2-2 ■ **Infant born at 26 weeks' gestation.** There is poor lung inflation and aeration with mild diffuse granular opacification in keeping with IRDS.

proteins (A, B, C, D), which are also produced by the type II pneumocytes to form tubular myelin. This is the principal contributor at the alveolar air–fluid interface which lowers alveolar surface tension and prevents acinar collapse on expiration.[1] Without this, there is alveolar collapse and, as a result, poor gas exchange, hypoxia, hypercarbia and acidosis. The alveolar ducts and terminal bronchioles are distended and lined by hyaline membranes which contain fibrin, cellular debris and fluid, thought to arise from a combination of ischaemia, barotrauma and the increased oxygen concentrations used in assisted ventilation.[2] Hyaline membrane formation can also occur in other neonatal chest conditions requiring ventilation.

Clinically these premature infants are usually symptomatic within minutes of birth with grunting, retractions, cyanosis and tachypnoea. Chest radiographic findings may be present shortly after birth but occasionally the maximum features may not be present until 6–24 hours of life.

Before the commencement of treatment, the typical radiographic features include underaeration of the lungs, fine granular opacification, which is diffuse and symmetrical, and air bronchograms (Fig. 2-2), due to collapsed alveoli interspersed with distended bronchioles and alveolar ducts. When there is less distension, the granularity is replaced by more generalised opacification or complete white-out of the lungs (Fig. 2-3). Atelectasis is the main cause of this opacification, but in the very premature infant in particular, oedema, haemorrhage and occasionally superimposed pneumonia contribute.

Very premature infants, less than 26 weeks' gestation, may have clear lungs or mild pulmonary haziness initially. Their lungs are structurally and biochemically immature and require prolonged ventilatory support. Prenatal

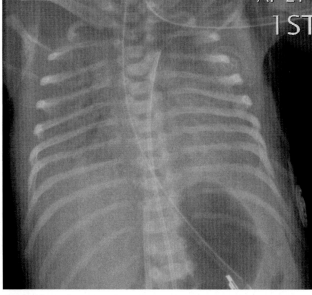

FIGURE 2-3 ■ **Premature infant with severe IRDS.** There is almost complete 'white-out' of the lungs with air bronchograms.

corticosteroid administration during the 2 days prior to delivery significantly reduces the incidence of IRDS in premature infants.

The clinical use of artificial surfactant, given as a liquid bolus through the endotracheal (ET) tube, has been a major therapeutic advance. It may not be evenly distributed throughout the lungs, leading to areas of atelectasis interspersed with areas of good aeration, and may produce radiographic findings similar to neonatal pneumonia or pulmonary interstitial emphysema (PIE) (Fig. 2-4).

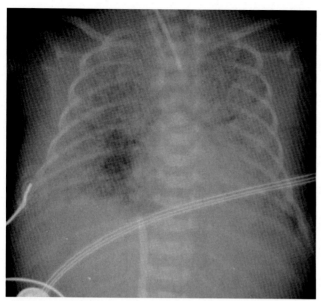

FIGURE 2-4 ■ **Uneven aeration following surfactant administration.** The appearances in some areas mimic those of PIE.

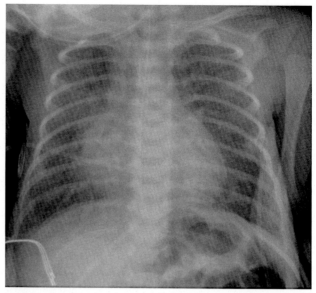

FIGURE 2-6 ■ There is cardiac enlargement, splaying of the carina indicating left atrial enlargement, prominent pulmonary vasculature and hazy opacification centrally, suggestive of a left-to-right shunt at PDA level.

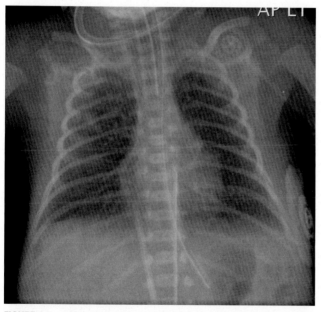

FIGURE 2-5 ■ **Very premature infant born at 24 weeks' gestation.** The chest radiograph at 24 hours demonstrates some hyperinflation, hazy and streaky opacification, similar to the changes seen in bronchopulmonary dysplasia.

Correlation with the clinical picture is, therefore, very important.

In general, infants greater than 27 weeks' gestation respond best to surfactant therapy. In the very premature infant, less than 27 weeks' gestation, the lungs become clear following surfactant administration, but they are still immature with fewer alveoli than normal. This results in inadequate gas exchange, leads to prolonged ventilation, hazy lung opacification and occasionally a picture similar to that seen in bronchopulmonary dysplasia (Fig. 2-5).

A patent ductus arteriosus is frequent in the premature infant and contributes to the disease. The rigid lungs caused by IRDS and the associated hypoxia and hypercarbia may lead to right-to-left shunting through the ductus. With surfactant therapy and improved oxygenation there is reduced pulmonary resistance and as a result there may be left-to-right shunting. Initial treatment if required is with ibuprofen, which inhibits prostaglandin production, but surgery may occasionally be required.

The chest radiograph may demonstrate sudden cardiac enlargement, left atrial enlargement causing elevation of the left main bronchus and varying degrees of pulmonary oedema (Fig. 2-6). There is an increasing use of prophylactic continuous positive airway pressure (CPAP) ventilation in infants suspected of developing IRDS, which helps reduce the incidence of complications in these infants. High-frequency ventilation is also used to reduce the incidence of barotrauma, particularly in the very premature infant. In these infants the radiographs do not differ significantly from those infants receiving conventional ventilation. The chest radiograph is used to assess the degree of lung inflation. The dome of the diaphragm should project at the level of the 8th–10th posterior ribs if the mean airway pressure is appropriately adjusted.

The use of positive pressure ventilation in the newborn is the most common cause of pneumothorax, pneumomediastinum, pulmonary interstitial emphysema (Fig. 2-7) and pneumopericardium (Fig. 2-8). These complications have become much less common in infants who have been treated with surfactant and high-frequency ventilation. Areas of atelectasis can occur in surfactant deficiency and are frequently due to poor clearance of secretions (Fig. 2-9). Premature infants are at an increased risk of pneumonia, which may coexist with IRDS. Pulmonary haemorrhage resulting in airspace

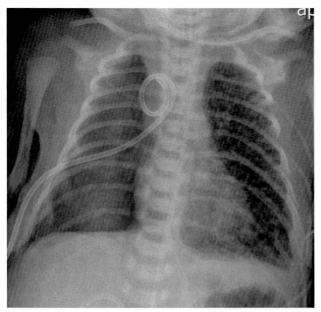

FIGURE 2-7 ■ **Left pulmonary interstitial emphysema.** On the right there is hyperlucency with a sharp mediastinal edge, a sharp right heart border and right hemidiaphragm indicating a right pneumothorax. There is a pigtail drainage catheter in situ.

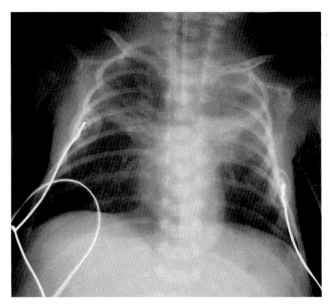

FIGURE 2-9 ■ **Bilateral upper lobe segmental atelectasis.**

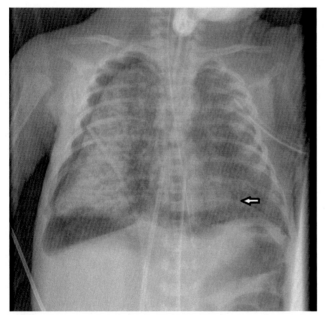

FIGURE 2-8 ■ There is a lucency surrounding the heart and the pericardial sac is visible as a white line (arrow), indicating a pneumopericardium. There is also a right pneumothorax.

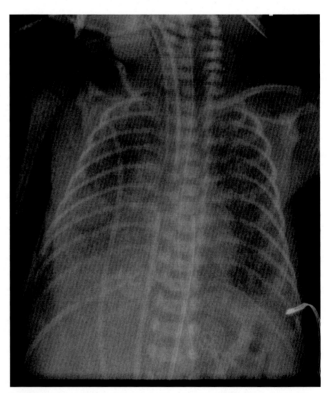

FIGURE 2-10 ■ **Infant born at 24 weeks' gestation.** The chest radiograph at 24 hours demonstrates airspace opacification in the right middle and both lower lobes due to intrapulmonary haemorrhage. Blood was seen to ooze from the ET tube prior to obtaining the radiograph.

opacification may also be a superimposed problem, and is usually due to severe hypoxia and capillary damage (Fig. 2-10). Bronchopulmonary dysplasia (BPD) or chronic lung disease is a significant long-term complication of IRDS. Because of the many advances in neonatal care, its incidence and severity have reduced significantly in infants born at 28 weeks' gestation or older. The unchanged overall incidence is due to the increased survival of the infants of extreme prematurity as they require more prolonged ventilation. Air leaks, patent ductus arteriosus and infection are contributing factors as they also prolong ventilation. A higher incidence of BPD has been demonstrated in infants with previous culture-proven *Ureaplasma urealyticum* pneumonitis.[3]

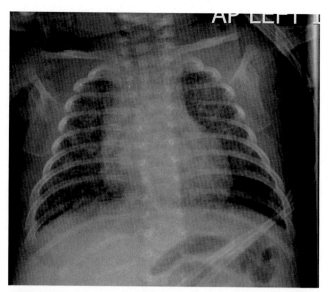

FIGURE 2-11 ■ **Premature infant ventilated for IRDS.** Chest radiograph at 4 weeks of age demonstrates hyperinflation, interstitial and alveolar opacification throughout both lungs in keeping with BPD.

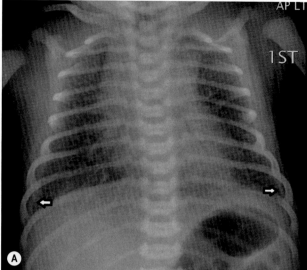

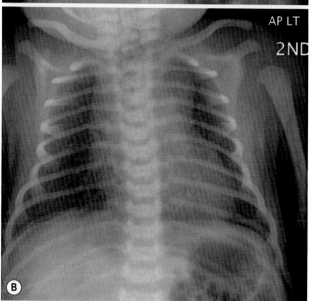

FIGURE 2-12 ■ (A) Term infant. Radiograph shows mild hyperinflation, prominent vasculature, interstitial opacification most marked in the lower lobes and small pleural effusions (arrows) suggestive of TTN. (B) There is almost complete resolution at 24 hours.

The four classic stages of BPD described by Northway[4] are now very rarely seen. Nowadays the most common radiographic appearance is diffuse interstitial shadowing with mild-to-moderate hyperinflation of gradual onset (Fig. 2-11). A new type of BPD was described by Jobe in 1999[5] in immature infants with minimal lung disease at birth, and who become symptomatic during the first week of life. This entity seems inseparable from the condition described previously as Wilson–Mikity syndrome.

TRANSIENT TACHYPNOEA OF THE NEWBORN (TTN)

This condition is also referred to as retained fetal lung fluid or wet-lung syndrome. Normally fluid is cleared from the lungs at, or shortly after, birth by the pulmonary lymphatics and capillaries. In TTN the normal physiological clearance is delayed. The incidence is greater in infants delivered by Caesarean section, in hypoproteinaemia, hyponatraemia and maternal fluid overload. There is also an increased incidence in small, hypotonic and sedated infants who have had a precipitous delivery.

Typically the infants have mild-to-moderate respiratory distress without cyanosis in the first couple of hours. The process resolves rapidly with almost complete resolution in 48 hours. Treatment consists of supportive oxygen and maintenance of body temperature. Radiographically, the most common appearances are mild overinflation, prominent blood vessels, perihilar interstitial shadowing and fluid in the transverse fissure with occasional small pleural effusions (Fig. 2-12). There may be mild associated cardiomegaly. The appearances may be asymmetrical with right-sided predominance, which remains unexplained. The features may simulate

meconium aspiration syndrome and congenital neonatal pneumonia, particularly when severe.

MECONIUM ASPIRATION SYNDROME

The definition of meconium aspiration syndrome is an infant born through meconium-stained amniotic fluid where the symptoms cannot be otherwise explained.[6] It is thought that fetal hypoxia causes fetal intestinal hyperperistalsis and passage of meconium, which is aspirated by a gasping fetus. It is most common in infants who are post-mature. It is diagnosed by the presence of meconium below the level of the vocal cords.

The radiographic features may, in part, be due to the inhalation of meconium itself in utero or during birth.

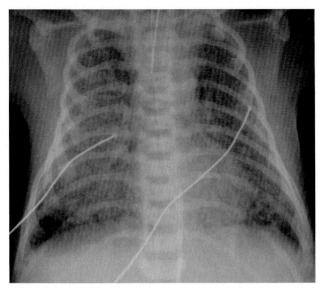

FIGURE 2-13 ■ **Infant born at 42 weeks' gestation.** There is bilateral asymmetrical coarse opacification in the lungs in keeping with meconium aspiration.

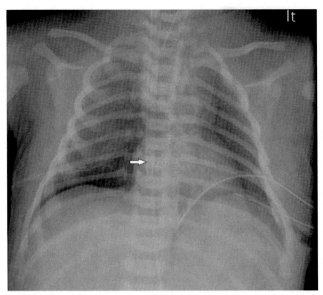

FIGURE 2-14 ■ **Term infant with meconium aspiration undergoing ECMO.** Radiograph obtained immediately following insertion of a veno-venous catheter in the right atrium (arrow). There are bilateral pneumothoraces with chest drains in situ bilaterally.

It is a thick viscous substance and may lead to areas of atelectasis and overinflation. It may migrate to the distal airways, causing complete or partial obstruction and lead to a 'ball-valve' effect. It may also cause a chemical pneumonitis (Fig. 2-13). There may be associated alterations in the pulmonary vasculature, leading to pulmonary arterial hypertension. Air leaks are common and small associated pleural effusions may be seen.

Approximately 30% of infants will require mechanical ventilation. The mortality rate has been improved by the use of inhaled nitric oxide, to treat severe pulmonary hypertension and also by extracorporeal membrane oxygenation (ECMO), which is used only in those infants where the conventional treatments have failed. The ECMO technique can be used either with the veno-arterial method, where one catheter is placed in the internal jugular vein and one in the carotid artery, or the veno-venous method, where a double lumen catheter is placed in the internal jugular vein, superior vena cava or right atrium (Fig. 2-14). The circulation bypasses the lungs, which are minimally inflated, and allows physiologic levels of oxygen saturation.

NEONATAL PNEUMONIA

Neonatal infections acquired transplacentally, such as TORCH (toxoplasmosis, rubella, cytomegalovirus, herpes), are rare and seldom develop pulmonary abnormalities. Infections acquired perinatally can occur via ascending infection from the vagina, transvaginally during birth or as a hospital-acquired infection in the neonatal period. Prolonged rupture of membranes prior to delivery is a major risk factor. It is thought that most cases of neonatal pneumonia occur during birth, when the infant may swallow and/or aspirate infected amniotic fluid or vaginal tract secretions. Group B streptococcus

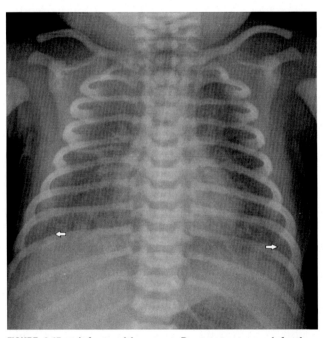

FIGURE 2-15 ■ **Infant with group B streptococcus infection.** There is bilateral asymmetrical coarse pulmonary opacification and small bilateral pleural effusions (arrows). The appearances are similar to those seen in meconium aspiration syndrome.

is the most common organism identified. The radiological features are non-specific.

The most common features seen on the chest radiograph in term infants who present with severe acute symptoms in the first 24–48 h are coarse bilateral asymmetrical alveolar opacification with or without associated interstitial change (Fig. 2-15). In these infants the

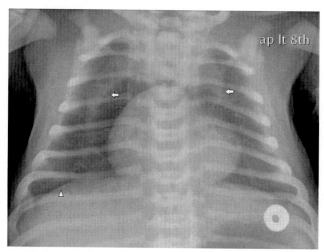

FIGURE 2-16 ■ Spontaneous pneumomediastinum outlining the thymus (arrows) and right pneumothorax (arrowhead).

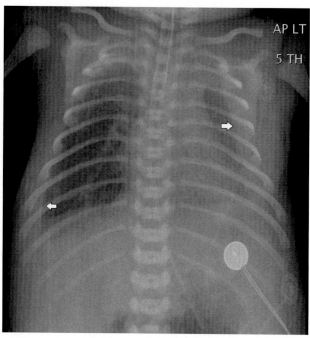

FIGURE 2-17 ■ **Newborn with bilateral chylothoraces.** Radiograph demonstrates bilateral pleural effusions (arrows).

radiographic changes may mimic meconium aspiration syndrome or severe transient tachypnoea. The presence of pleural effusions, pulmonary hyperinflation and mild cardiomegaly may not be helpful in differentiating pneumonia from these other conditions.

In the premature infant there maybe diffuse fine granular opacification, similar to the appearances seen in IRDS.[7] Some infants may have both IRDS and group B streptococcus pneumonia. Chlamydial infection classically presents first with conjunctivitis at 1–2 weeks after birth and the lung infection does not usually become evident until 4–12 weeks of age. Typically the radiograph demonstrates interstitial opacification with some hyperinflation.

The association of *Ureaplasma urealyticum* with neonatal pneumonia is increasingly recognised. These infants have a mild early course and develop features of BPD at an earlier age than would be expected in a premature infant.[8]

AIR LEAKS

Spontaneous pneumothorax and pneumomediastinum causes respiratory distress in the newborn infant. Many are transient and do not require intervention. A pneumothorax may be radiographically subtle in sick infants as supine radiographs are usually performed and free air accumulates over the lung surface, producing a hyperlucent lung and increased sharpness of the mediastinum (Figs. 2-7 and 2-14). A pneumomediastinum usually outlines the thymus (Fig. 2-16) and when there is a pneumopericardium the air surrounds the heart (Fig. 2-8).

PLEURAL EFFUSIONS

In infants who do not have hydrops, the most common cause of a congenital pleural effusion is chylothorax. The

cause is unknown, and late maturation of the thoracic duct has been suggested as an aetiology. The abnormality is usually detected on antenatal ultrasound (US) and in utero drainage may be performed to prevent pulmonary hypoplasia. Postnatally, the chest radiograph demonstrates the pleural effusions (Fig. 2-17). Aspirated fluid will have a high lymphocyte count but will not have a milky appearance until such time as the infant is fed with fat. Resolution is usually complete but often after multiple aspirations.

SURFACTANT DYSFUNCTION DISORDERS

Disorders of surfactant deficiency due to a genetic abnormality in the surfactant protein B (SpB)[9] and C (SpC)[10] and the ATP-binding cassette transporter protein A3 (ABCA3) can lead to interstitial lung disease. Inherited mutations in the SpB and ABCA3 are autosomal recessive and may present immediately after birth with respiratory symptoms. Mutations in the SpC are autosomal dominant and may present later in infancy. The chest radiograph may show diffuse hazy opacification initially, with the later development of interstitial shadowing which may be progressive (Fig. 2-18A). Computed tomography (CT) demonstrates diffuse ground-glass opacification with septal thickening[11] and cystic change (Figs. 2-18B and C).

Pulmonary interstitial glycogenosis (PIG) may present in the preterm or term infant very soon after birth. It has been reported in isolation but is frequently associated

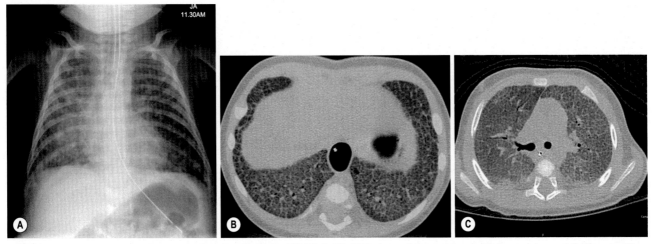

FIGURE 2-18 ■ **Infant with surfactant dysfunction disorder (ABCA3).** (A) CXR shows bilateral interstitial, granular and fluffy opacification. (B, C) Two axial CT slices demonstrate ground-glass opacification and septal thickening, giving a 'crazy paving' appearance similar to the pattern typically described in alveolar proteinosis.

with conditions that affect lung growth and the diagnosis is made by the pathological examination of lung tissue. The imaging features may be similar to those seen in the other disorders of surfactant deficiency.

LINES AND TUBES

The tip of an ET tube may vary considerably with head and neck movement and the correct position must therefore be assessed by taking the patient's head position and the tip of the tube into consideration.

The umbilical arterial line courses inferiorly in the umbilical artery, into the internal and common iliac arteries and then into the aorta. The tip should be positioned to avoid the origins of the major vessels, which are usually between T6 and T9 (Fig. 2-19) or in some institutions inferior to L3 vertebral bodies.

The umbilical venous line courses superiorly towards the liver. It enters the left portal vein, through the ductusvenosus and into the inferior vena cava (IVC). The ideal position is at the junction of the IVC and the right atrium (Fig. 2-19).

The correct position of central venous lines or peripherally inserted central catheters (PICC) is controversial. The position of PICC line tips inserted through the upper limbs is usually in the superior vena cava. The tips of those inserted through the lower limbs are usually positioned at the junction of the IVC and the right atrium. US may be particularly helpful in assessing a catheter's position and injection of very small amounts of intravenous water-soluble, low osmolar contrast medium may also be useful in checking the position of the tip.

Nasogastric tube tip positions should always be reported on, in order to avoid misplacement of nasogastric feeds.

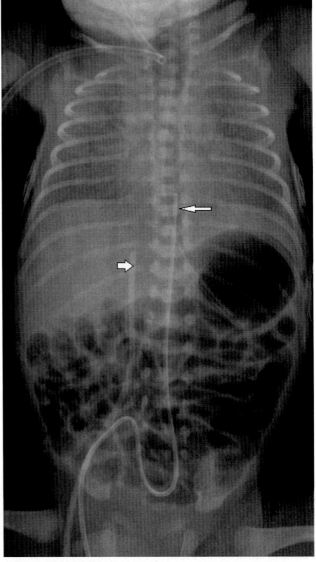

FIGURE 2-19 ■ **Umbilical arterial and venous catheters.** The tip of the umbilical arterial catheter is at T7 level (long arrow). The tip of the umbilical venous catheter is in the IVC (short arrow) and should ideally be placed more distally in the IVC close to the right atrium.

THE CHEST IN OLDER CHILDREN

Diseases of the respiratory tract occur frequently in children. These will range from the presentation of congenital abnormalities, infections through to complex immunodeficiency syndromes and malignancy.

The chest radiograph is the most frequently requested radiological investigation encountered within paediatric practice, and although pathological manifestations may mimic that seen in adults, a thorough knowledge of the variations within paediatric practice is vital to the general radiologist. In this section, we will cover some of the unique aspects of chest disease in the older child.

THE CHEST RADIOGRAPH

The plain chest radiograph remains the first radiological examination in use for the evaluation of the chest in children. Frontal chest radiographs are widely performed. Lateral views tend only to be performed after review of the frontal radiograph, when there are unanswered clinical questions.

A PA erect radiograph taken at full inspiration is optimal but difficult to obtain in uncooperative children; hence, an AP supine view is usually obtained in infants and small children. An inspiratory plain chest radiograph is considered adequate when the right hemidiaphragm is at the level of the eighth rib posteriorly. Poor inspiration may cause significant misinterpretation of the chest radiograph (Fig. 2-20). Radiographs obtained in expiration frequently show a rightward kink in the trachea, owing to the soft cartilage, relatively long trachea and the presence of a left aortic arch in the majority of children. Other features of an expiratory radiograph include some degree of ground-glass opacification of the lungs and relative enlargement of the heart. Rotation of the patient causes problems with interpretation, including apparent mediastinal shift/distortion of vasculature, the thymus and vessels mimicking a 'mass' (Fig. 2-21) and relative lucency of one lung compared to the other, simulating oligaemia/air trapping.

NORMAL VARIANTS

The normal thymus is a frequent cause of physiological widening of the anterior mediastinum occurring during the early years of life.

Normal thymic tissue is soft, malleable and compliant; hence, it often undulates beneath the overlying ribs, giving it a lobulated appearance known as the 'thymic wave'. The right thymic margin can often have a sharp 'sail-like' configuration (Fig. 2-1). The thymus may involute during periods of illness, severe stress or whilst on steroids or other chemotherapy. Rebound hyperplasia of the thymus may then occur following recovery or cessation of therapy, and this should not be confused with the development of a pathological mediastinal mass. If chest radiographic differentiation between normal thymus and pathology proves difficult on the radiograph,

US can help distinguish intrathymic or adjacent masses within the anterior mediastinum from a normal isoechoic homogeneous thymus. Pathological tissue is heterogeneous, and may cause compression or indeed occlusion of adjacent airway or vasculature, something which never occurs with a normal thymus. In some cases where US is inconclusive, magnetic resonance imaging (MRI) is performed to differentiate a normal thymus from mediastinal pathology. On T2-weighted spin-echo sequences, the normal thymus has an intermediate signal similar to that of the spleen. On gadolinium-enhanced T1-weighted spin-echo sequences, the thymus should show only minimal enhancement.[12] Care should be taken to avoid confusing overlying plaits or braids of hair superimposed over the upper chest film as intraparenchymal lung pathology.

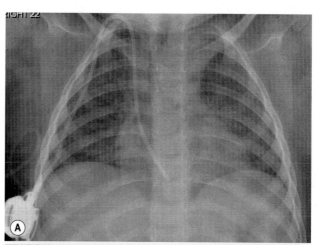
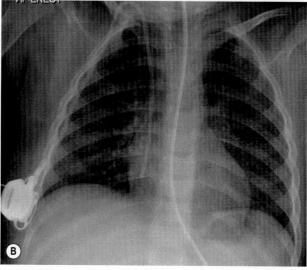

FIGURE 2-20 ■ The effect of inspiration. Two radiographs of the same patient highlight the problems in interpreting radiographs taken in poor inspiration. (A) The child's trachea is buckled and the heart appears enlarged; both phenomena are not shown on a subsequent radiograph (B) taken in good inspiration.

TABLE 2-1   **Asymmetric Lung Densities**

Respiratory Causes with Contralateral Mediastinal Shift	Respiratory Causes without Mediastinal Shift	Cardiac Causes
Foreign body aspiration—may be normal on inspiratory image, fluoroscopy can help	Unilateral hypoplastic lung	Pulmonary embolism—rare
Mucous plugging—asthmatics and ventilated patients	Congenital venolobar syndrome	Post-cardiac surgery—e.g. Blalock–Taussig shunt
Congenital lobar emphysema	Constrictive bronchiolitis—formerly known as Sywer–James syndrome	
External mass compression—mediastinal mass compressing a bronchus		
Bronchomalacia		
Endobronchial lesion—e.g. bronchial carcinoid		

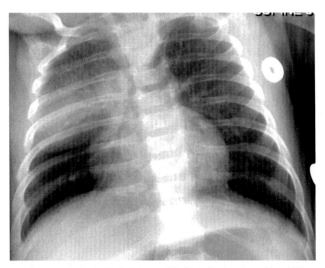

FIGURE 2-21 ■ **The effect of rotation.** A rotated patient showing a normal thymus (proven on subsequent radiograph) masquerading as a mediastinal mass.

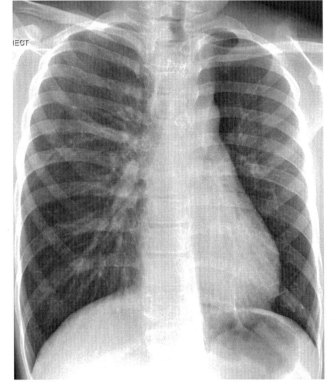

FIGURE 2-22 ■ **Assymmetric lung density.** The left lung is more hyperlucent than the right and there is a paucity of left-sided vascular markings. Tracheal and left main bronchus stents can be seen in this patient with known tracheobronchomalacia.

CARDIAC OR RESPIRATORY?

When the chest radiograph shows asymmetrical lung volumes, the lung with fewer vessels per unit area is usually the abnormal lung. The lack of, or reduction in, vascular markings is usually due to the presence of primary airways disease in children and the resultant homeostatic reflex vasoconstriction (Table 2-1) (Fig. 2-22). The presence of reduced vascularity in the hyperlucent areas resulting from a primary vascular pathological process, such as thromboembolism or pulmonary hypertension, is rare in children, although various congenital cardiac disorders can result in pulmonary oligaemia.

Prominent/enlarged generalised lung parenchymal vessels could indicate the presence of a left-to-right shunt at either intracardiac or great vessel level. Cardiac failure as a primary cause of pleural effusion in children is not common. In children, fluid overload tends to cause peribronchovascular oedema, which then results in overinflation of the lungs due to air trapping, along with perihilar infiltrate and upper lobe venous diversion.

THE LUNGS

Pulmonary Infection

Respiratory infections in children are the most frequent disorders encountered by paediatricians.[13] Chest radiography is the primary imaging technique used to evaluate acute lung disease.

Chest CT has, however, an important role in evaluating immunocompromised patients and both the acute and chronic complications of respiratory tract infection, such as empyema and bronchiectasis.[14] A frontal radiograph is usually adequate to confirm or exclude pulmonary infection/pneumonia.

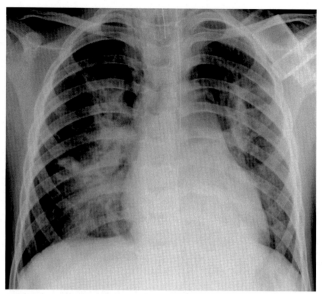

FIGURE 2-23 ■ **Perihilar consolidation.** This child was admitted to intensive care with severe respiratory distress due to influenza infection. The initial CXR shows extensive perihilar opacities with numerous air bronchograms, in keeping with severe influenza pneumonia.

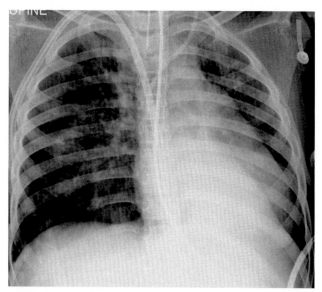

FIGURE 2-24 ■ **Lobar consolidation.** Left lower lobe consolidation/collapse in an intubated child.

Bacterial vs Viral

Within all age groups, viral infection is more common than bacterial. Viral infection usually affects the respiratory mucosa and airways, causing bronchial and bronchiolar oedema. This results in hyperinflation (due to air trapping as a result of partial bronchial obstruction as a result of peribronchial thickening), segmental and subsegmental atelectasis and small patches of consolidation frequently occurring in a perihilar location (Fig. 2-23).[16] *Streptococcus pneumoniae* is the causative pathogen in >90% of normal hosts. Radiographs shows a rounded or spherical opacity with poorly defined margins, unlike a primary or metastatic chest tumour (which are usually very well circumscribed).[17]

Bacterial pneumonia, in general, causes inflammation within the acini, resulting in oedema and intra-alveolar exudate. This causes consolidation within the air spaces and results in the presence of 'air bronchograms' seen on radiographs. The typical location is lobar or segmental, and associated pleural (parapneumonic) effusions are not uncommon (Fig. 2-24). Although these patterns have traditionally been associated with viral and bacterial pathogens, studies indicate that prediction of causative pathogen using radiographic patterns is notoriously inaccurate.[15] In addition viral and bacterial infection may be present simultaneously, so these 'classic' radiographic patterns are not always accurate.

Features of Infection

Round Pneumonia

Round pneumonias occur frequently in young children, usually under 8 years of age, due to the presence of immature collateral ventilation pathways between the small airways (Fig. 2-25).[16] *Streptococcus pneumoniae* is the causative pathogen in >90% of normal hosts. Radiographs shows a rounded or spherical opacity with poorly defined margins, unlike a primary or metastatic chest tumour (which are usually very well circumscribed).[17]

Follow-up chest radiography to ensure resolution of pneumonia is not routinely necessary, in an otherwise previously healthy child. Follow-up should be reserved for those children who have persistent or recurrent symptoms, or have an underlying condition such as immunodeficiency. Causes of recurrent/persistent pneumonia include infection within a pre-existing lung abnormality, bronchial obstruction, aspiration associated with gastro-oesophageal reflux and rarely an H-type congenital trachea-oesophageal fistula (Fig. 2-26).

Necrotising/Cavitatory Pneumonia

Necrotising pneumonia with ensuing cavitatory necrosis has been described in association with staphylococcal pneumonias, and less frequently with *Klebsiella* infection. Areas of decreased or absent enhancement on contrast-enhanced CT indicate the presence of necrotising pneumonia with parenchymal ischaemia or infarction. Unlike the adult population, this is not such a poor prognostic indicator in children and good recovery of lung occurs with non-surgical therapy. Infected congenital bronchopulmonary foregut (cystic) malformations may sometimes have appearances very similar to that of cavity necrosis, and evaluation with CT may be helpful.[18] Thin-walled pneumatoceles are classic sequelae of staphylococcal infection (Fig. 2-27).[12] These commonly occurring lesions can be differentiated from lung abscesses by a lack of wall enhancement and their anatomical location within the interstitial spaces of the lungs.

Specific Infections

Tuberculosis

Tuberculosis remains an enormous worldwide public health issue. Within the traditionally 'low-risk' industrialised countries of western Europe, as a result of the

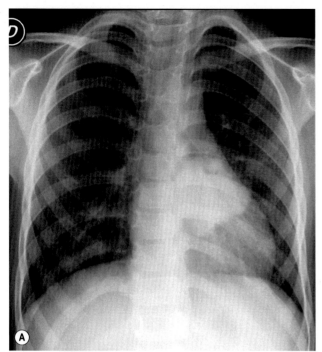

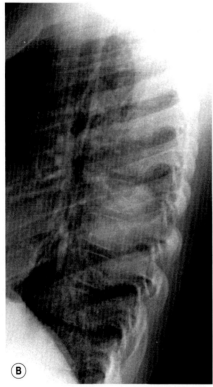

FIGURE 2-25 ■ **Round pneumonia.** This child presented with cough and pyrexia. (A) The CXR shows a rounded opacity behind the left heart adjacent to the mediastinum. (B) The lateral view confirms its position posteriorly within the lung parenchyma. The lesion resolved on a follow-up radiograph following antibiotic treatment.

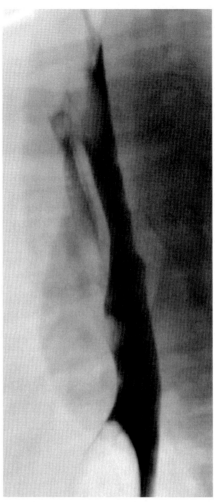

FIGURE 2-26 ■ **H-type fistula.** Tube oesophagram in a child with a history of recurrent unexplained chest infections. There is a mid-oesophageal fistula with abnormal passage of contrast medium into the trachea.

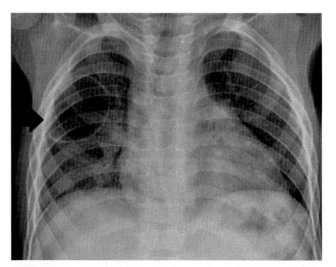

FIGURE 2-27 ■ **Pneumatocele.** Post-severe staphylococcal pneumonia. A thin-walled cyst in the right upper zone is in keeping with a pneumatocele.

increase in world travel, immigration (and in particular the HIV epidemic), infection rates have increased to such an extent that areas of inner city London now have similar TB disease prevalence (according to WHO) as parts of the Third World.

Children, and in particular, infants infected with TB, are at much greater risk of severe (invasive) disease, extra-pulmonary dissemination and death, than adults. Many cases of primary TB infection in children do not become symptomatic. Young age (infants are at increased risk) and compromised immune status (HIV, primary immunodeficiency) carry an increased risk.[19,20]

Most cases of paediatric tuberculosis are due to primary infection, and therefore presentation and radiographic appearances are different to the adult-type disease. Early chest X-ray findings are of alveolar consolidation, which has a predilection for the lower lobes. The infection then progresses onto regional and hilar lymph nodes (Fig. 2-28); the combination is referred to as a Ranke complex. The process may spontaneously regress at this point, but can progress onto enlarging and often caeseating lymphadenopathy particularly in those high-risk groups already described. CT is superior to the chest radiograph in the diagnosis and assessment of mediastinal lymphadenopathy.[21] In children the smaller-calibre airways are more easily compressed by enlarged tuberculous lymph nodes and, as a result, lung hyperinflation and air trapping (due to partial airway obstruction and obstructive over-inflation) are commonly seen on CT. Caeseating nodes completely obstruct regional bronchi, causing inflammation and lobar consolidation, with ensuing collapse–consolidation. Mediastinal lymphadenopathy is the hallmark of primary infection.[22] Table 2-2 lists other causes of hilar enlargement in children. Children are also at increased risk of developing disseminated disease; again this is particularly true in infants. Features of disseminated tuberculous disease include multiple lung parenchymal nodules of variable size and distribution, and this has led to the term 'acute disseminated tuberculosis', which is preferred to 'miliary' tuberculosis (Fig. 2-29).[23] The presence of either a sympathetic pleural effusion or cavitations is a rare complication in primary tuberculosis (Fig. 2-30).[24] True tuberculous empyema is exceptionally rare.

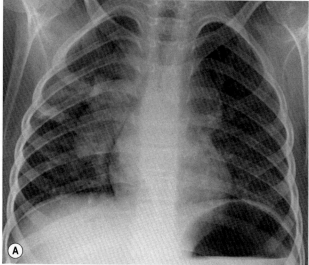

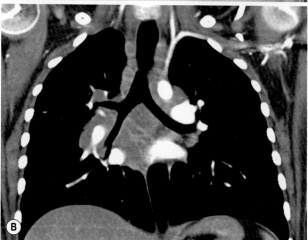

FIGURE 2-28 ■ **Primary tuberculosis.** (A) CXR and (B) coronal CT reformat in a child presenting with tuberculosis infection. Extensive right paratracheal, subcarinal and bilateral hilar adenopathy is demonstrated and is causing tracheal compression.

TABLE 2-2   Causes of Bilateral Hilar Enlargement

Bilateral	Unilateral
Lymphadenopathy	
Viral and bacterial infection—common	Tuberculosis
Lymphoma/leukaemia—paratracheal enlargement is frequent	Pulmonary metastases—usually well-defined
Tuberculosis—bilateral involvement is rare	Lymphoma/leukaemia—rarely unilateral
Sarcoidosis—normally presents with extrathoracic symptoms in children	Viral/bacterial/fungal infection—the most common cause
Metastases—lobulated and well-defined	
Vascular Enlargement	
Left–right shunt—ASD/VSD/PDA	Post-stenotic dilatation—enlarged main pulmonary trunk and proximal left pulmonary trunk
Pulmonary hypertension—central enlarged vessels and peripheral pruning	Pulmonary hypertension with absent contralateral pulmonary artery—e.g. in unilateral pulmonary hypoplasia
Cardiac failure—increased vessel calibre with an ill-defined outline	

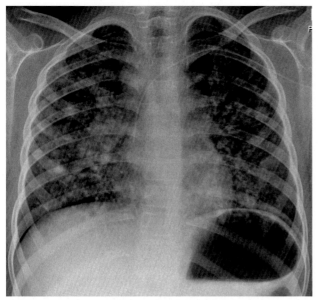

FIGURE 2-29 ■ Acute disseminated (haematogenous/miliary) tuberculosis. Frontal CXR shows widespread ill-defined nodules of varying sizes in a random distribution throughout the lung parenchyma. More confluent areas of consolidation indicate coalescence of the nodules. Appearances of 'miliary' TB in children are more diverse than in adults.

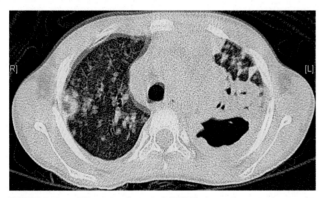

FIGURE 2-30 ■ TB cavitation. Axial CT image shows a large air-filled cavity in an area of consolidation in the left upper lobe. Several nodules throughout the remainder of the lungs are related to endobronchial seeding of TB. Images are degraded due to respiratory motion artefact as the patient was tachypnoeic.

Resolution of radiographic findings is a slow process and may take in excess of 6 months and it is not essential for complete resolution to have occurred prior to cessation of antituberculous therapy.[25]

Mycoplasma pneumoniae

Mycoplasma pneumoniae is a common and important cause of atypical community-acquired pneumonia usually in children of school age. The predominant symptom is often a dry persistent cough. Radiographic findings are non-specific but may range from diffuse interstitial change or perihilar bronchial wall thickening and dilatation through to segmental or lobar consolidation. There is often a discrepancy between the severity of

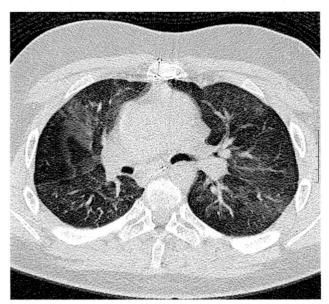

FIGURE 2-31 ■ Constrictive (obliterative) bronchiolitis. Axial expiratory CT slice shows a classic mosaic pattern indicating widespread severe small airways disease.

radiographic findings and the relatively minor clinical picture. Though the majority of cases respond well to medical therapy, *M. pneumoniae* is an important cause of constrictive obliterative bronchiolitis in a minority of those infected, particularly if not treated promptly or effectively.[26]

Late Complications of Infection

The most common chronic complications of pneumonia are bronchiectasis (large airways disease) and constrictive (obliterative) bronchiolitis (i.e. small airways disease), previously known as obliterative bronchiolitis or Swyer–James–Macleod syndrome.

Bronchiectasis is the most frequent chronic complication, and is defined as irreversible dilatation and wall thickening of the bronchi. On high-resolution CT (HRCT) the bronchus is considered dilated if the lumen is larger than the associated adjacent pulmonary artery. Hyperlucent lung, with decreased pulmonary (pruned) vasculature, which persists on expiratory scans, indicates air trapping and is the hallmark of small airways disease (analogous with constrictive obliterative bronchiolitis) (Fig. 2-31), which often coexists with bronchiectasis. Common causative infectious causes include *M. pneumoniae* and adenovirus.[27,28]

Pleural Effusion

There are many causes of pleural effusion in children (Table 2-3) but the most common is due to infection. Parapneumonic effusions are more commonly associated with bacterial infections, usually pneumococcus, but other infections (such as tuberculosis) should be considered, particularly if unresponsive to routine antibacterial therapy. Pleural effusions should be evaluated with US, and can be categorised as low grade (anechoic fluid

TABLE 2-3   Causes of Pleural Effusion

Cause	Diagnosis
Infection	• Parapneumonic*
	• Empyema—commonly secondary to streptococcal or staphylococcal infection
	• Tuberculosis*—rare in children
Neoplasm	• Common: leukaemia/lymphoma Metastatic—especially Wilms' tumour
	• Less common—primary lesions such as PNET* or mesothelioma
Inflammatory	• Pancreatitis—small and left-sided
Fluid overload	• Low albumin states
	• Cardiac failure
	• Severe sepsis
Trauma	• Haemothorax*—hyperdense on CT (>30 HU)
Congenital	• Diaphragmatic hernia*—opaque hemithorax rather than effusion
	• Chylothorax—may reflect lymphangiectasia

*Common causes of opaque hemithorax.

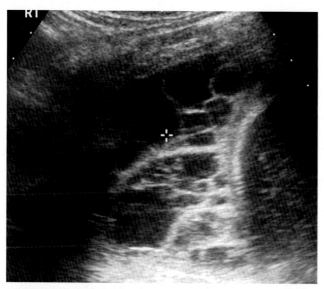

FIGURE 2-32 ■ **High-grade parapneumonic effusion.** Longitudinal US image shows a complex multiseptated loculated pleural effusion in a child with a known chest infection.

without internal echoes) or high grade (fibropurulent organisation with presence of fronds, septations or loculi) (Fig. 2-32). This is important for further management, as high-grade effusions may require thoracoscopy and surgical debridement, whereas low-grade effusions may be treated more conservatively.[29]

The Acutely Wheezing Child

Asthma[30]

Asthma (reactive airways disease) is a common cause of childhood wheeze, but the diagnosis is clinical and should not normally require radiological intervention unless there are atypical features or complications. However, most children diagnosed with asthma will, at some point in their diagnostic pathway, have a chest radiograph performed. This is useful for excluding other causes of wheeze, such as congenital tracheobronchial/vascular anomalies, lung parenchymal disease or, very importantly, radiographic sequelae of an inhaled foreign body.

In children requiring hospitalisation for an acute asthmatic attack, imaging is useful for assessing complications, such as consolidation related to either mucous plugging or secondary bacterial infection. The chest radiograph commonly shows overinflated lungs, often with peribronchial thickening that is often more marked in the middle lobe. Lobar collapse is frequent, particularly in children with concomitant infections, and is usually due to mucous plugging. Pneumothorax and pneumomediastinum are less frequently observed but important findings.

Inhaled Foreign Bodies

It is important to bear in mind that toddlers are inquisitive and may ingest or inhale foreign bodies, with or without the knowledge of their carer; i.e. the episode may not be witnessed by an adult and may result in acute respiratory distress causing immediate airway compromise, and the need for urgent investigation. Alternatively, the episode may not result in acute symptoms until the child presents at a later stage with a chronic wheeze or recurrent/persistent infections. If there is an unexplained acute respiratory deterioration in a toddler with lung collapse or overinflation, there should be rapid recourse to bronchoscopic assessment, with timely removal of the foreign body to ensure a good short- and long-term prognosis.

A plain radiograph should be the initial investigation of choice in less emergent cases. Findings may include a radio-opaque foreign body (although most are radiolucent, such as nuts and plastic toys), lobar collapse or air trapping. The radiograph should be scrutinised for hypertransradiancy, which may be localised, or diffuse, and occurs due to a ball–valve mechanism in larger airways, causing distal air trapping. A quick fluoroscopic examination using pulsed fluoroscopy can be extremely useful when evaluating differing lung radiolucencies in suspected foreign body aspiration, and in stridor.[31] The obstructed (overinflated) lung will not change in volume with respiration, and the mediastinum will swing contralaterally on expiration.

Certain organic matter, e.g. peanuts, are particularly irritant and cause a severe local inflammatory reaction within the adjacent airway, which may make complete extraction difficult, and they often fragment thence embolise into more distal airways, causing increased consolidation post-bronchoscopy.

Stridor

Stridor may arise secondary to infection in children. Lateral-view fluoroscopy can be useful for dynamic evaluation of tracheomalacia, where the trachea collapses completely during expiration. Barium swallow, with the child in the true lateral position, and good distension of the oesophagus, is still the primary study in patients with a suspected vascular ring or sling. The rings/slings will abnormally indent the contrast column within the

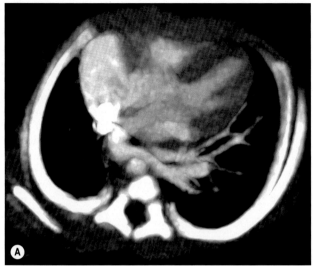

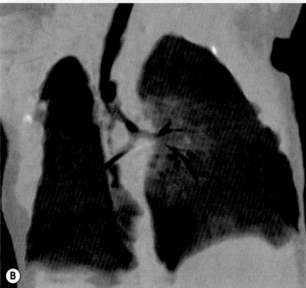

FIGURE 2-33 ■ **Left pulmonary arterial sling.** (A) CTA maximum intensity projection (MIP)—the large left pulmonary artery arises from the right pulmonary artery and passes posterior to the trachea and anterior to the oesophagus. Note the marked narrowing of the trachea at this level. (B) CT minimum intensity projection (MinIP) demonstrates the long-segment tracheal stenosis and wide/splayed carinal angle.

oesophagus. This test may also be valuable for assessing the presence of other extrinsic masses. Thin-section CT with volume rendering and multiplanar reconstruction techniques has almost eliminated the need for contrast bronchography in children being assessed for vascular rings and slings (Fig. 2-33); however, the technique is still used in functional studies for assessing the dynamics of intermittent airway obstruction.

Congenital Chest Abnormalities

Bronchopulmonary Foregut Malformations

Bronchopulmonary foregut malformations (BPFM) are now considered as part of a spectrum of anomalies of lung development ranging from tracheobronchial anomalies such as congenital cystic hamartomatous (adenomatoid) malformations and bronchogenic cysts, to anomalies with abnormal vascularity such as pulmonary sequestration and the hypogenetic lung (or scimitar) syndrome. There is considerable overlap between these groups, with a significant percentage of lesions being of mixed type, i.e. hybrid lesion: for example a 'cystic' malformation with systemic arterial supply (i.e. sequestration). Multidetector CT (MDCT) can offer excellent imaging for this range of anomalies, being able to simultaneously depict detail of lung parenchyma and the systemic arterial vascular supply, and the pattern of venous drainage (either conventional into the pulmonary veins in intralobar types or into the systemic venous systems in extralobar sequestrations).

Congenital Thoracic Cysts

These can occur in the mediastinum (mediastinal bronchogenic cysts, enteric duplication cysts and pleuropericardial cysts) and within lung parenchyma (intrapulmonary bronchogenic cysts). Bronchogenic cysts are more frequently located within the mediastinum (85%), typically in the subcarinal position. Ten to 15% are intrapulmonary, most frequently in the lower lobes, but usually within the proximal third of the lung (Fig. 2-34).[32] Rarely, they can also be located within the diaphragmatic leaflets, or below the diaphragm, and even within the liver or in the neck. These congenital lesions are lined with bronchial epithelium and often communicate with the tracheobronchial tree. The cysts generally contain mucinous or serous fluid, but blood (related to haemorrhage within), or air, can also be contained. Associated congenital malformations include congenital lobar overinflation (emphysema), bronchial atresia and pulmonary (intra- or extralobar) sequestration.[33,34] Mediastinal cysts are often asymptomatic and incidentally found on imaging later in life. They can, however, cause mass effect, resulting in tracheal/bronchial or oesophageal compression, presenting with wheeze, stridor or dysphagia. The cysts can become infected and cause repeated pneumonias. The lesions are often seen as mediastinal masses on plain radiographs, but CT allows better evaluation of the relationships with adjacent structures. The cyst content is usually water attenuation on CT, but may appear iso- or hyperdense due to intracystic haemorrhage or high protein (mucinous) content. MRI, which has a better contrast resolution than CT, can better evaluate the nature of the cyst contents. The cysts are typically hyperintense on T2-weighted spin-echo images. T1-weighted images show different signal intensity, depending on the cyst content.[35] Air within the cyst could be due to infection, instrumentation or communication with the airway or gastrointestinal tract. Surgical treatment is indicated in symptomatic lesions.

The differential diagnosis should include oesophageal duplication (usually located within the posterior mediastinum) and with neurenteric cysts (located in posterior mediastinum and associated with vertebral defects) (Fig. 2-35).

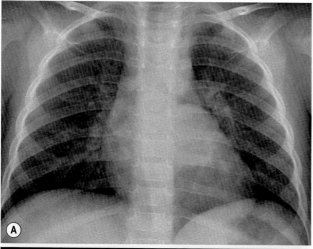

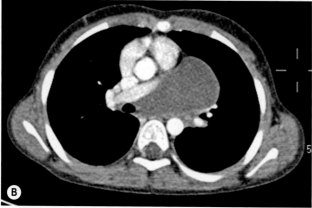

FIGURE 2-34 ■ **Bronchogenic cyst.** (A) CXR in a child showing a smooth round opacity elevating the LMB and splaying the carina. (B) CECT shows an intermediate-density homogeneous mass in a subcarinal position with a classical appearance of a mediastinal bronchogenic cyst.

Congenital Pulmonary Airway Malformations

Congenital pulmonary airway malformations (CPAM) are a group of cystic and non-cystic lung lesions resulting from early airway maldevelopment. It is preferable to use this term instead of the previous nomenclature of congenital cystic adenomatoid malformation (CCAM), as only one type (i.e. type 3) is a true adenomatoid lesion[36] (Table 2-4).[37]

CPAMs can communicate with the airways and are relatively frequently infected (30%).[38] Blood supply is from the pulmonary artery with drainage via pulmonary veins. Hybrid lesions with histological and imaging features of both a CPAM and bronchopulmonary sequestration will have, by definition, a systemic arterial supply.

Fetal US may show an echogenic soft-tissue mass, with multiple variable-size anechoic cysts or a homogeneous echogenic solid mass. Large lesions may cause mediastinal shift, resulting in lung hypoplasia, polyhydramnios and hydrops fetalis.[39,40] Fetal MRI may be carried out to further delineate the mass prior to delivery, and to calculate the overall functional lung volumes. The lesions are hyperintense on T2-weighted sequences and

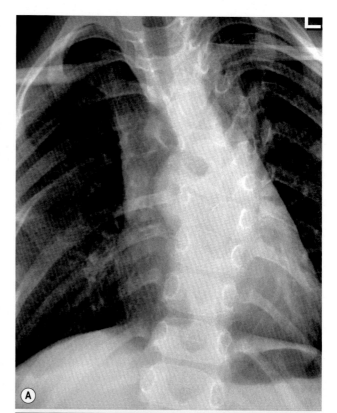

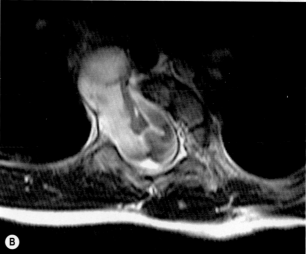

FIGURE 2-35 ■ **Neurenteric cyst.** (A) Thoracic spine radiograph highlights a right-sided paravertebral mass with an associated developmental vertebral anomaly. (B) Axial T2-weighted SE image demonstrates intradural communication.

can be uni-/multilocular or solid.[41] Postnatal radiographs demonstrate variable density, depending on the fluid contents of the cysts, and mediastinal shift, depending on the size of the lesion. In the early neonatal period the mass may be completely opaque, as the cysts are still full of fluid. With time, this fluid is gradually replaced with air and prominent air–fluid levels are seen. Approximately 40% of antenatally diagnosed lesions are not detected on plain chest radiography.[37] Spiral CT allows better evaluation, demonstrating a mass made up of multiple cysts of different sizes (Figs. 2-36 and 2-37).[42] Chest

TABLE 2-4 Modified Stocker CPAM Classification[37]

Type	Description
0	Incompatible with life
1	Commonest type (>65%)
	Several large intercommunicating cysts (up to 10 cm)
	Mediastinal shift is common
2	10–15% of cases
	Smaller than other types
	Small evenly sized cysts (up to 2 cm)
	Often associated with other congenital abnormalities
3	~8% of cases
	Large solid lesion with small cysts (1.5 cm)
	Nearly always causes mediastinal shift
	Poor prognosis
4	10–15% of cases
	Large cysts (up to 7 cm)
	May be associated with, or a precursor of, pleuropulmonary blastoma

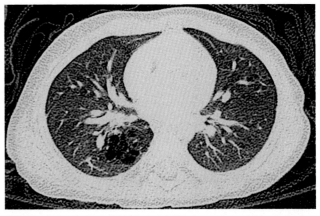

FIGURE 2-37 ■ **Type 2 CPAM.** Axial CT shows a multicystic lesion in the right lower lobe. No significant mediastinal shift is present and the lesion was subsequently excised.

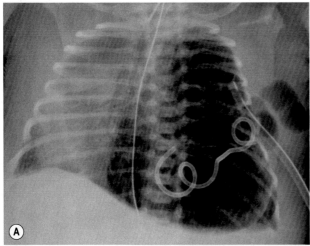

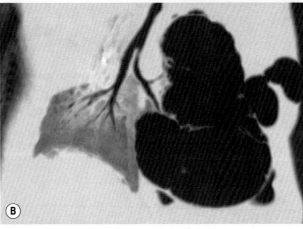

FIGURE 2-36 ■ **Type 1 CPAM.** (A) CXR shows a large air-filled abnormality in the left lung causing marked contralateral mediastinal shift. Attempts have been made to insert intercostal drains. (B) Coronal CT reformat confirms the presence of a large multicystic mass. Note the narrowed and displaced left main bronchus.

radiography and CT can demonstrate surrounding lung consolidation in cases complicated by infection. Large lesions are usually surgically managed, due to mass effect, but smaller lesions may also be resected owing to frequent infections.

Congenital Diaphragmatic Hernia

One of the differential diagnoses for a large cystic thoracic mass is the congenital diaphragmatic hernia, or Bochdalek hernia, which occurs in approximately 1 in 3000 live births. In 40–50% of cases there are associated congenital abnormalities, most commonly of the central nervous system (CNS). Associated cardiac abnormalities affecting the ventricular outflow tracts (i.e. tetralogy of Fallot and hypoplastic left heart syndrome) are the most important associations, with important impact in terms of prognostic outcome.[43]

In isolated hernias, the most important prognostic factor is the degree of associated lung hypoplasia. The hernia arises from a defect in the posterolateral diaphragmatic leaflet, usually on the left. The lesion is usually detected on antenatal US. These lesions tend to have a worse prognosis owing to associated complications or the degree of lung hypoplasia. Herniation, which occurs later in fetal development, is associated with less severe lung hypoplasia.[44] Fetal MRI can supplement antenatal US, and is particularly useful if prenatal intervention is being considered.[45]

Postnatal chest radiographs are usually sufficient for diagnosis of new presentations, usually demonstrating a large cystic or solid mass, containing bowel loops within the chest (Fig. 2-38). In the minority of cases where there is confusion, contrast studies can demonstrate intrathoracic bowel.

Pulmonary Sequestration

Pulmonary sequestration is a mass of lung tissue, disconnected from the bronchial tree, which derives its blood supply from one or more systemic vessels, commonly the thoracic or abdominal aorta.[46] There are two types, intra- and extralobar sequestration.

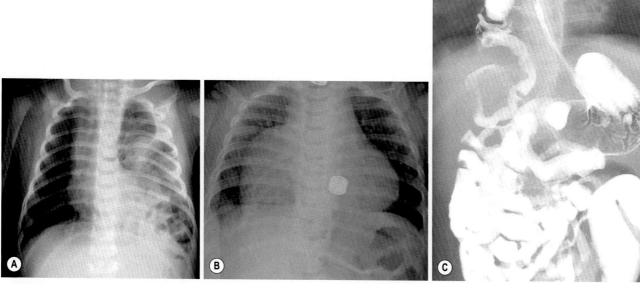

FIGURE 2-38 ■ Diaphragmatic hernia. (A) Bochdalek-type hernia with multiple loops of bowel in the left hemithorax. (B) On this frontal CXR, a mass is present at the right cardiophrenic angle in keeping with a Morgagni-type diaphragmatic hernia. These occur through an anterolateral diaphragm defect and typically present later in life. (C) Bowel loops passing into a Morgagni hernia on a contrast study.

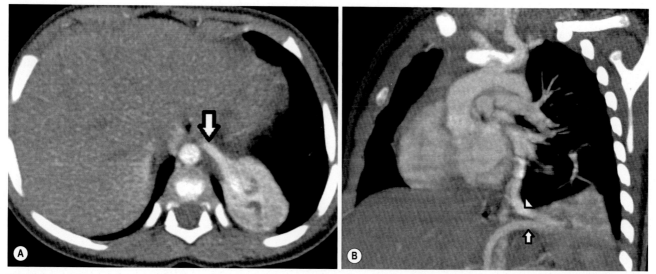

FIGURE 2-39 ■ Pulmonary sequestration. (A) Axial CT shows an enhancing mass in the posterior left lower lobe with a large (enhancing) feeding vessel (arrow). (B) Oblique coronal reformat highlights the mass receiving arterial supply from a branch of the coeliac artery (arrow) with venous drainage occurring via a left pulmonary vein (arrowhead).

Intralobar sequestration (ILS) is more common (75%) than extralobar sequestration (ELS) (Fig. 2-39). ILS is surrounded by normal lung, i.e. shares the pleural investment with the surrounding normal lung, and usually drains into the pulmonary venous system. Sixty per cent of the cases are located in the left lower lobe and they relatively frequently become infected.[47] Extralobar sequestration usually has its own pleural covering, and systemic venous drainage to the azygos or portal venous systems.[48] The ELS are usually located at the left base in 77% of cases.[49] Extralobar sequestration can be located below the diaphragm and mimic a neuroblastoma or adrenal haemorrhage.[50] ELS are associated with multiple congenital malformations in 65% of cases, including other types of bronchopulmonary foregut malformation.[51]

A homogeneous opacity at the lung base may be seen on plain chest radiographs. US will show a homogeneous hyperechoic mass, with a systemic feeding artery. CT depicts the feeding artery and the venous drainage, and may show a homogeneous soft-tissue mass, or a mass containing air or fluid cysts. MDCT is more sensitive in detecting small systemic vessels than MRI, due to the superior spatial resolution in CT, especially in small children, and can evaluate lung parenchyma at the same time.

CT is the technique of choice for evaluating pulmonary sequestrations.[52]

MRI demonstrates a solid, well-defined and hyperintense mass on T2-weighted images, with a systemic feeding artery. Hybrid lesions show imaging findings of both sequestration and CPAM.[53] Symptomatic patients require surgical resection.[54]

Congenital Lobar Overinflation[55]

This bronchial abnormality results in a check–valve mechanism, causing progressive hyperinflation of the affected lobe. The left upper lobe is the most frequently affected (42%), followed by the middle lobe (35%). Radiographs in the immediate postnatal period may show a radio-density as the affected lobe is still full of fluid. Later radiographs will demonstrate hyperlucency and overexpansion of the affected lobe with variable degree of mediastinal shift (Fig. 2-40). CT will exclude other causes of secondary lobar overinflation; for example, vascular anomalies, compression of the bronchi or mediastinal masses. In asymptomatic patients, conservative treatment and follow-up can show a reduction in overinflation. Excision of the affected lobe is necessary in symptomatic children.

Bronchial Atresia

Bronchial atresia is a congenital malformation characteristically located within the left upper lobe, characterised by obliteration of a segmental, subsegmental or lobar bronchus. Air enters the affected lobe or segment by collateral channels, producing overinflation and air trapping. Mucous secretions accumulate in the atretic bronchus, forming a mucocele.[56] Chest X-ray (CXR) and CT demonstrate pulmonary overinflation with air trapping during expiration, and a tubular, branched or spherical opacity (mucocele) in a central position (Fig. 2-41). Significant mediastinal shift and collapse of the ipsilateral lobes is more frequent in congenital lobar overinflation. Symptoms may be absent and radiological features may progressively improve. Infection of the unconnected lung is rare.

Lung Agenesis-Hypoplasia Complex

Three categories of pulmonary underdevelopment are grouped under the term of 'agenesis and hypoplasia complex', as they have similar radiologic findings on chest radiograph. Pulmonary agenesis is a complete absence of lung parenchyma, bronchus and pulmonary vasculature; pulmonary aplasia is a blind-ending rudimentary bronchus, without lung parenchyma or pulmonary vasculature; and pulmonary hypoplasia is a rudimentary lung and bronchus, with airways, alveoli and pulmonary vessels decreased in number and size.

They appear on a chest radiograph as a diffuse opacity of one hemithorax, with mediastinal shift and contralateral lung hyperinflation, simulating collapsed lung.[57] Lung agenesis, aplasia and hypoplasia can be differentiated with use of CT or MRI (Fig. 2-42). This lung complex can be associated with other congenital malformations of the cardiovascular, gastrointestinal, genitourinary and skeletal systems.

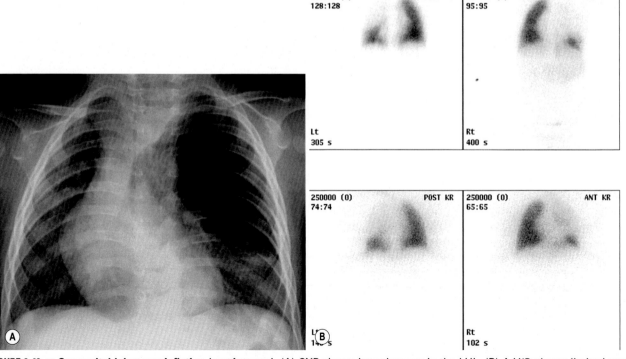

FIGURE 2-40 ■ **Congenital lobar overinflation (emphysema).** (A) CXR shows hyperlucency in the LUL. (B) A V/Q shows limited ventilation but no perfusion within the overinflated segment.

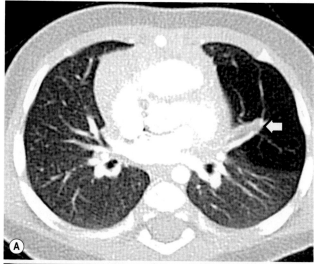

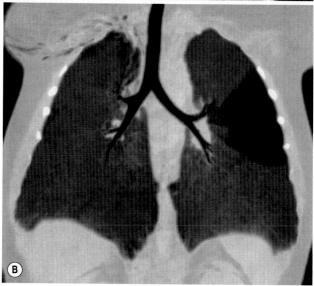

FIGURE 2-41 ■ **Bronchial atresia with mucocele.** (A) Axial CT on lung windows shows segmental hyperlucency in LUL with a soft-tissue density at the left hilum in keeping with an atretic LUL segmental bronchus containing a mucocele. (B) Coronal MinIP confirms the segmental hyperlucency.

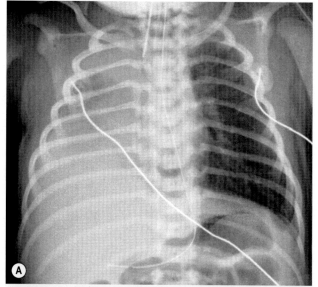

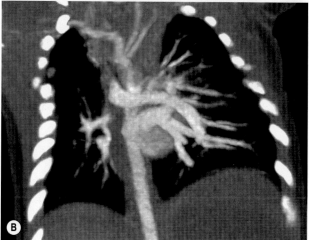

FIGURE 2-42 ■ **Lung hypoplasia.** (A) Right lung hypoplasia in a child with complex congenital cardiac abnormalities. CXR shows complete white-out of the right lung with ipsilateral mediastinal shift. (B) Coronal CT reformat highlights the hypoplastic right pulmonary vein and paucity of pulmonary vessels on the right with a relatively normal left lung.

Pulmonary hypoplasia can also be secondary to lung compression during lung development. The most common intrathoracic cause of hypoplasia is congenital diaphragmatic hernia, but other intrathoracic causes include CPAM and pulmonary sequestration. Extrathoracic causes include severe oligohydramnios secondary to genitourinary anomalies, also known as the Potter sequence, and skeletal dysplasias with a small dysmorphic thoracic cage such as in thanatophoric dysplasia.

Congenital Venolobar Syndrome—Scimitar Syndrome

This is a congenital abnormality comprising lung hypoplasia and ipsilateral anomalous systemic venous drainage. An anomalous pulmonary vein, usually on the right, drains into the inferior vena cava, portal vein, coronary sinus or right atrium. Most patients are

asymptomatic but the anomalous venous return constitutes a left-to-right shunt and can lead to pulmonary hypertension.

Radiographic appearances are similar to those of isolated lung hypoplasia. The differential finding is the anomalous (scimitar) vein that may be seen as a tubular shadow, running towards the base of the lung, resembling a curved sword (scimitar), though the vein is not seen in half of the cases on the chest radiograph. CT is the best technique for evaluating the lung, the abnormal vein and to where it drains (Fig. 2-43).

Malignancy
Mediastinal Masses

The mediastinum may be divided into three compartments, anterior, middle and posterior. The most common

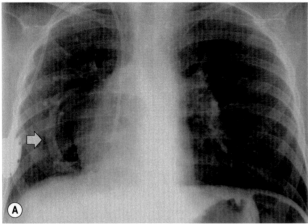

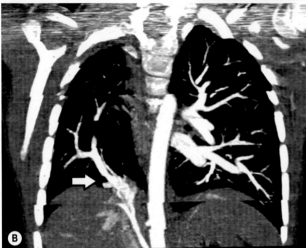

FIGURE 2-43 ■ Congenital venolobar syndrome (scimitar syndrome). (A) CXR showing (1) shift of the heart into the right hemithorax, (2) a small right lung with an abnormal vessel (arrow) paralleling the right heart border and (3) overinflation (compensatory) of left lung. (B) Coronal CT reformat highlights the abnormal 'scimitar vein' (arrow) draining below the diaphragm into the systemic venous system bypassing the pulmonary veins.

anterior mediastinal masses are normal thymus and thymic disorders (abnormalities in thymic size, shape or location), lymphoma or leukaemia (relatively frequent), germ-cell tumours (teratoma, hamartomas, teratocarcinomas, seminomas, dysgerminomas, embryonal cell carcinomas, endodermal sinus tumour, choriocarcinomas) and thymoma. In middle mediastinum, congenital cysts (bronchogenic cyst, duplication, neurenteric cyst) and lymph nodes (infectious and malignant nodes) are usually located. Neurogenic tumours are located in posterior mediastinum (neuroblastomas, ganglioneuromas) (Table 2-5).

The chest radiograph is usually the primary radiologic investigation for a suspected mediastinal mass. US, contrast-enhanced CT or MRI will give further information on the mass itself and its location and anatomical relationships. Bone scintigraphy or PET-CT can be used for staging. Imaging guides the approach for potential biopsy by defining the extent of disease and its relation to major vascular, airway and spinal structures. Involvement of trachea, pericardium, major vessels or spine may necessitate cardiothoracic or neurosurgical input.

Anterior Mediastinum. The most common malignant tumours in children are lymphoma and leukaemia. Abnormal thymic masses appear nodular and lobulated and frequently compress adjacent vascular structures.

Germ-cell tumours are commonly located in the anterior mediastinum (94%). The most common is mature teratoma, with usually well-defined margins, thick walls, some fatty tissue and frequently internal calcification (25%).[58] CT and MRI are superior to US in analysing these anterior mediastinal masses and detecting compression of adjacent structures, tumour extension and invasion of pericardium or pleura.

Middle Mediastinum. The most common mass found in the middle mediastinum is lymphadenopathy, most commonly secondary to infection (TB),[59] but as in the anterior mediastinum, malignancies, in particular, lymphoma and leukaemia, are frequently seen. Other masses encountered in the middle mediastinum are usually congenital, i.e. bronchopulmonary foregut malformations. Middle mediastinal masses, due to their location,

TABLE 2-5   Mediastinal Masses

Anterior	Middle	Posterior
Normal thymus	Lymphadenopathy (see Table 2-1)	Neurogenic tumours—neuroblastoma/ganglioneuroblastoma/ganglioneuroma
Lymphadenopathy (see Table 2-1)	Bronchopulmonary foregut malformations—bronchogenic cyst, oesophageal duplication	Spinal abscess—*Staphylococcus*/TB
Teratoma	Congenital vascular rings	Spinal tumours—PNET/Ewing's
Thymic infiltration—leukaemia/lymphoma/histiocytosis	Hiatus hernia	Trauma—vertebral haematoma
Thymoma/thymic cyst		Bochdalek hernia
Morgagni hernia		Bronchopulmonary foregut malformations—neurenteric cyst
Cervicomediastinal soft-tissue vascular malformation—lymphangioma/haemangioma		

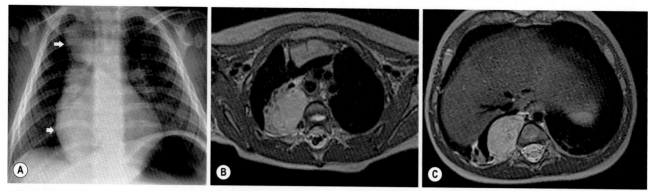

FIGURE 2-44 ■ **Neuroblastoma.** (A) CXR shows two nodular masses in the right posterior mediastinum with mild splaying of the intercostal space at the right 10th and 11th ribs posteriorly. (B, C) Two axial T2-weighted volumetric acquisition MRI studies confirming the presence of the two right-sided thoracic paraspinal masses in keeping with neuroblastoma.

frequently cause airway or oesophageal compression. Contrast-enhanced CT or MRI is the best technique for evaluation.

Posterior Mediastinum. The majority of lesions located in the posterior mediastinum are neurogenic tumours; calcification and extradural spinal extension are commonly demonstrated. Neuroblastoma and ganglio-neuroblastoma usually occur in the first decade of life, with the more benign ganglioneuroma seen in older children. Fifteen per cent of neuroblastomas are of a thoracic origin, which is less malignant than a primary abdominal neuroblastoma. They are solid masses which are calcified in up to 40% of cases (Fig. 2-44).

A posterior mediastinal mass is indicated on a chest radiograph, by posterior rib erosion and widening of the intercostal spaces. CT and MRI can both be used for cross-sectional evaluation but MRI is more accurate for detection of extradural mass invasion. Fifty per cent of children with intraspinal extension can be asymptomatic at presentation.[60]

Pulmonary and Endobronchial Tumours

The most common malignant intraparenchymal tumour is pulmonary metastatic disease (Fig. 2-45), usually from an extrapulmonary location, such as Wilms' tumour or osteosarcoma.

In children, particular care and experience with CT imaging techniques are necessary to allow minimisation of the exaggerated dependent atelectasis present, which may mimic or obscure peripheral pulmonary nodules. Prone or decubitus imaging may help to enable detailed scrutiny of problematic cases, helping to aerate lung within the posterobasal segments which may show atelectasis in the conventional (supine) position.

Primary lung malignancies are exceedingly rare in children, with an incidence of approximately 0.05 per 100,000.[61] The most common tumours are pleuropulmonary blastoma, bronchogenic carcinoma and bronchial adenoma.[62]

Pleuropulmonary blastoma usually occurs below 5 years of age. It can be cystic (type I), cystic and solid (type II) and mainly solid (type III).[63] These tumours tend to

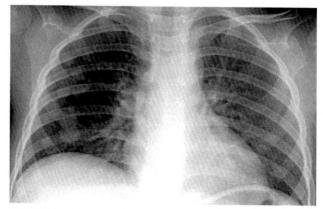

FIGURE 2-45 ■ **Multiple lung metastases.** Child with a primary Wilms' tumour. CXR shows multifocal bilateral soft-tissue density lesions in keeping with metastases.

occur as mixed cystic/solid masses adjacent to the pleura in the lower lobes. They can be confused with the benign lesions, CPAM. Larger lesions often occupy the whole hemithorax and displace mediastinal structures and the contralateral lung.

Bronchogenic carcinoma is very rare in children, representing 17% of primary malignant lung tumours in children. It tends to present in adolescence and is a very aggressive tumour, often with disseminated disease at diagnosis. Radiologically it behaves similarly to the adult tumour.

One-half of all bronchial adenomas, are bronchial carcinoid tumours. Carcinoid syndrome as a cause of Cushing's syndrome (adrenocorticotrophic hormone secretion) is rare in children. Instead, paediatric bronchial carcinoid tumours present with wheezing, lobar collapse or haemoptysis. They usually occur in the central airways, and radiographs may only detect the complications, such as emphysema or collapse. Lung lymphatic metastasis can occur in 5–20% of patients.[64]

Chest Wall Tumours

Chest wall tumours are more frequent than primary lung tumours and they account for 1.8% of all solid tumours in children.[65] The most common are Ewing's sarcoma/ primitive neuroectodermal tumours (PNETs), rhabdomyosarcoma and rarely mesothelioma.

PNETs manifest as peripheral chest wall masses, with or without rib destruction and pleural fluid on CXR.[66] Rib destruction is usually the result of a malignant lesion. Rib osteomyelitis, *Aspergillus* or actinomycosis infection can also destroy ribs, but in a different clinical context. US is the first radiological examination in patients where there is complete opacification of the hemithorax, as US can differentiate a solid mass from pleural fluid.

CT or MRI is required for cross-sectional evaluation. CT shows a solid heterogeneous, occasionally calcified mass, lymphadenopathy and pleural fluid. CT is important for determining rib involvement and evaluating the lung parenchyma for metastases. MRI is superior in determining the extent and local invasion of the mass.[67] Bony scintigraphy/PET-CT can be used for detection of distant skeletal metastases.

Rhabdomyosarcoma represents 10% of the solid tumours in paediatrics and it is the most frequent soft-tissue sarcoma in children.[68] Other primary locations of the tumour are more frequent than the thoracic locations. They usually present as a large chest mass with rapid growth. Pleural effusions are relatively uncommon.

Cystic Fibrosis[69]

Chest radiography is the primary imaging technique and the most widely used diagnostic method for assessing and following progression of cystic fibrosis (CF) lung disease. The current Cystic Fibrosis Trust guidelines recommend annual chest radiographs to assess serial lung parenchymal change in all CF patients.[70]

In children with CF large airways disease, bronchiectasis develops, which is the hallmark feature of established CF. Bronchial wall thickening is universal as the child grows and may precede bronchial dilatation. It is this abnormal wall thickening which allows visualisation of the pathologically thickened airways in the periphery of the lung beyond the level of the segmental bronchi, which are not normally visible.

With further progression of bronchiectasis, large cystic bronchiectatic airways form. Mucoid impaction of the bronchi appears as rounded or band-like opacities of increased density following the course of the dilated bronchi. Lobar and segmental atelectasis may result, most frequently seen in the upper and middle lobes. Interestingly, unlike in the normal host where infection manifests as lobar pneumonia, this pattern is unusual in CF, where patchy nodular areas representing peribronchial consolidation occur (Fig. 2-46).

Immunodeficiency

The immunodeficiency states in children may be subdivided into two major groups: congenital (primary) and acquired (secondary). The spectrum of illness and imaging appearances are similar, regardless of the underlying cause of immunodeficiency. Primary disorders include conditions such as congenital/inherited deficiencies, i.e.

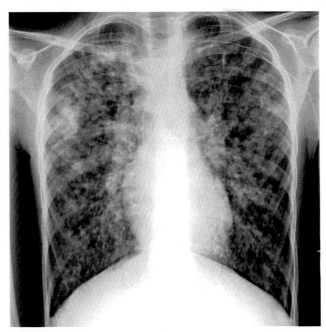

FIGURE 2-46 ■ **Cystic fibrosis.** CXR showing typical features of extensive bilateral bronchial wall thickening in overinflated lungs in a thin patient with advanced bronchiectasis related to CF. There is nodular consolidation in the RUL just above the thickened and elevated (right) horizontal fissure in keeping with an acute infectious exacerbation.

SCID (severe combined immunodeficiency). Secondary causes include chemotherapy, bone marrow and solid organ transplantation, and infectious causes such as AIDS. Both primary and secondary immunodeficiency states result in an increased susceptibility to infection, with the respiratory tract being the most common disease site. All immunodeficiency states are also associated with an increased incidence of malignancy, the lymphoproliferative disorders accounting for the majority of tumours.[71]

The low sensitivity of radiographs in detecting incipient pneumonia in these children may promote the use of CT for detection or exclusion of pulmonary infection in an acute clinical deterioration. Multiple agents can cause aggressive infections, in particular fungal (*Aspergillus*, *Candida albicans*, *Pneumocystis jiroveci*) and viral (cytomegalovirus).[72,73]

Human Immunodeficiency Virus (HIV). HIV infection is an important cause of acquired immunodeficiency worldwide. Though it is relatively uncommon in the Western world, in certain groups, particularly those in deprived inner city areas, antenatal testing indicates a prevalence of 1 in 125 to 1 in 200.[74] It is therefore important to be aware of the major complications demonstrated by imaging. Vertical transmission remains the commonest cause of paediatric infection, though the risk is considerably reduced with maternal treatment with antiretroviral therapy. HIV progression is much faster in children than in adults. HIV-associated respiratory disease is the cause of death in 50% of affected children.

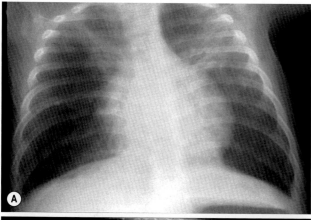

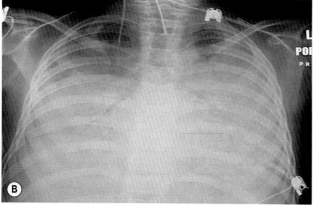

FIGURE 2-47 ■ *Pneumocystis jiroveci (carinii)* **pneumonia.** (A) CXR shows diffuse perihilar granular shadowing in a non-specific pattern. (B) Severe infection; widespread opacification indicates an ARDS-type pattern.

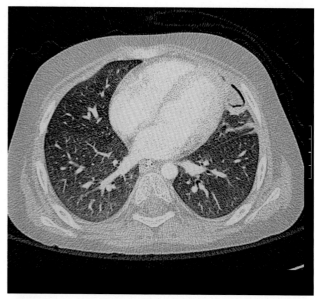

FIGURE 2-48 ■ **Air-crescent sign.** Axial CT image showing a parenchymal cavity partially filled with a soft-tissue mass and a thin rim of air superiorly.

Infectious Pulmonary Complications of Immunodeficiency

Pneumocystis jiroveci (carinii) Pneumonia. This is an opportunistic infection, common in children with HIV/AIDS, particularly within the first year post-diagnosis. Peak incidence is at 3–6 months of age when the protective effect of transplacental maternal IgG begins to wane.

Classical radiographic appearances include hyperinflation with diffuse bilateral interstitial or nodular infiltrates, which may be subtle initially, progressing rapidly to widespread alveolar shadowing, which may eventually progress to adult respiratory distress syndrome (ARDS) (Fig. 2-47). Following treatment, there may be a significant lag in radiographic resolution compared to the clinical improvement.

Invasive Pulmonary Aspergillosis (IPA). IPA typically manifests as multifocal areas of triangular or nodular parenchymal consolidation caused by haematogenous dissemination of the angioinvasive fungus. Haemorrhagic infarction of the lungs occurs as a result of lung necrosis secondary to vascular obstruction.

Classical radiographic features include either solitary or multiple nodules or masses, with or without cavitation. In some cases, however, the chest radiograph appears normal or may demonstrate a focal infiltrate indistinguishable from a pyogenic pneumonia. Specific HRCT features have been described, probably the most characteristic being a 'halo' of ground-glass attenuation representing perilesional necrosis and haemorrhage, surrounding a central focal fungal nodule or infarct. A second commonly described characteristic feature of IPA is lesional cavitation with the formation of an air crescent (Fig. 2-48). Occasionally IPA may manifest as a necrotising pneumonia with infiltration of local structures or organs. Although these classical features have been described, in many cases, imaging appearances are often non-specific.[75,76]

Non-infectious Pulmonary Complications

Lymphoproliferative Disease (LPD) and Lymphocytic Interstitial Pneumonia (LIP). LPD is the most frequent type of neoplasia in immunodeficiency and may involve the chest, abdomen, CNS and soft tissues. Imaging appearances within the thorax are variable and include focal or diffuse infiltrates, solitary or multiple parenchymal nodules or masses and mediastinal lymphadenopathy, which may be large in volume.[77] LIP is a frequent manifestation of LPD and is characterised by a diffuse interstitial infiltrate of lymphocytes and plasma cells, which may be polyclonal or monoclonal. Radiographic features are variable and include either a predominantly interstitial infiltrate, affecting primarily the perihilar regions and lung bases, or discrete parenchymal nodules and/or patchy ground-glass opacity (Fig. 2-49).[78] Appearances are relatively non-specific and may be indistinguishable from infection with opportunistic organisms.

Diffuse Alveolar Haemorrhage (DAH). DAH occurs in approximately 10% of patients undergoing allogeneic bone marrow transplantation (BMT) and usually occurs at the time of engraftment. DAH is usually associated with other pulmonary complications, particularly (fungal) infection, and is associated with a high mortality.

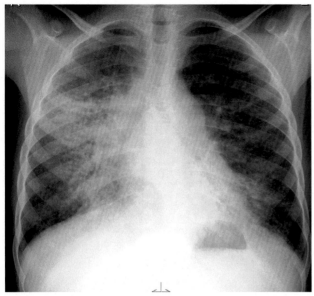

FIGURE 2-49 ■ Lymphocytic interstitial pneumonitis. CXR shows perihilar reticulonodular opacification in a child with known HIV infection. Increased airspace consolidation in the right lower zone indicates an acute infective exacerbation.

Classical radiographic features are those of airspace shadowing, which may be patchy and multifocal or more confluent consolidation with air bronchograms. Cessation of bleeding typically results in rapid clearing over a few days.

Idiopathic Pneumonia Syndrome (IPS). IPS is defined as diffuse lung injury for which no cause has been identified.[79] Both graft-versus-host disease (GVHD) and pre-transplant total body irradiation (TBI) are contributing factors. It usually occurs 6–8 weeks following BMT. Radiographic features are non-specific and variable; they include diffuse airspace shadowing and/or interstitial infiltrates, often with a nodular component. They may be indistinguishable from ARDS.

SUMMARY

In summary chest disease in children is not uncommon. Knowledge of the important categories of disease will help define a diagnostic pathway. Prudent use of chest CT to enable more specific diagnoses may be indicated in selected and complex cases.

REFERENCES

1. Agrons GA, Courtney SE, Stocker JT, et al. Lung disease in premature neonates: radiologic-pathologic correlation. Radiographics 2005;25:1047–73.
2. Wood BP, Davitt MA, Metlay LA. Lung disease in the very immature neonate: radiographic and microscopic correlation. Pediatr Radiol 1989;20:33–40.
3. Wang EEL, Matlow AG, Ohlsson A. *Ureaplasma urealyticum* infections in the perinatal period. Clin Perinatol 1997;24: 91–105.
4. Northway WH Jr, Rosan RC, Porter D. Pulmonary disease following respirator therapy of hyaline membrane disease: bronchopulmonary dysplasia. N Engl J Med 1967;276:357–68.
5. Jobe AH. The new BPD: an arrest of lung development. Pediatr Res 1999;66:641–3.
6. Cleary GM, Wiswell TE. Meconium-stained amniotic fluid and the meconium aspiration syndrome. An update (review). Pediatr Clin North Am 1999;45:511–29.
7. Ablow RC, Driscoll SG, Effmann EL, et al. A comparison of early-onset group B streptococcal neonatal infection and the respiratory-distress syndrome of the newborn. N Engl J Med 1976;295: 65–70.
8. Theilen U, Lyon AJ, Fitzgerald T, et al. Infection with *Ureaplasma urealyticum*: is there a specific clinical and radiological course in the premature infant? Arch Dis Child Fetal Neonatal Ed 2004;89:F163–7.
9. Cole FS, Hamvas A, Rubinstein P, et al. Population-based estimates of surfactant protein B deficiency. Pediatrics 2000;105:538–41.
10. Garmany TH, Wambach JA, Heins HB, et al. Population and disease-based prevalence of the common mutations associated with surfactant deficiency. Pediatr Res 2008;63:645–9.
11. Doan ML, Guillerman RP, Dishop MK, et al. Clinical, radiological and pathological features of ABCA3 mutations in children. Thorax 2008;63:366–73.
12. Wilmott RW, Boat TF, Bush A, et al. Kendig and Chernick's Disorders of the Respiratory Tract in Children: Expert Consult 8th edn. New York: Elsevier; 2012. pp. 145–68.
13. Reynolds JH, McDonald G, Alton H, et al. Pneumonia in the immunocompetent patient. Br J Radiol 2010;83:998–1009.
14. Markowitz RI, Ruchelli E. Pneumonia in infant and children: radiological-pathological correlation. Semin Roengenol 1998;33: 151–62.
15. Wahlgren H, Mortensson W, Eriksson M, et al. Radiological findings in children with acute pneumonias—age more important than infectious agent. Acta Radiol 2005;46:431–6.
16. Bramson RT, Griscom NT, Cleveland RH. Interpretation of chest radiographs in infants with cough and fever. Radiology 2005;236: 22–9.
17. Donnelly LF. Maximizing the usefulness of imaging in children with community-acquired pneumonia. Am J Roentgenol 1999;172: 505–12.
18. Donnelly LF, Klosterman LA. Cavitary necrosis complicating pneumonia in children: sequential findings on chest radiography. Am J Roentgenol 1998;171:253–6.
19. Newton SM, Brent AJ, Andreson S, et al. Paediatric tuberculosis. Lancet Infect Dis 2008;8(8):498–510.
20. Marais BJ, Gie RP, Schaaf HS, et al. The clinical epidemiology of childhood pulmonary tuberculosis: a critical review of literature from the pre-chemotherapy era. Int J Tuberc Lung Dis 2004; 8:278–85.
21. Bosch-Marcet J, Serres-Creixams X, Zuasnabar-Cotro A, et al. Comparison of ultrasound with plain radiography and CT for the detection of the mediastinal lymphadenopathy in children with tuberculosis. Pediatr Radiol 2004;34:895–900.
22. Kim WS, Choi J, Cheon JE, et al. Pulmonary tuberculosis in infants: radiographic and CT findings. Am J Roentgenol 2006;187:1024–31.
23. Jamieson DH, Cremin BJ. High resolution CT of the lungs in acute disseminated tuberculosis and a pediatric radiology perspective of the term 'miliary'. Pediatr Radiol 1993;23:380–3.
24. Leung AN, Muller NL, Pineda PR, Fitzgerald JM. Primary tuberculosis in childhood: radiographic manifestations. Radiology 1992;182:87–91.
25. Correa AG. Tuberculosis: unique aspects of tuberculosis in the paediatric population. Clin Chest Med 1997;18:89–98.
26. John SD, Ramanathan J, Swischuk LE. Spectrum of clinical and radiographic findings in pediatric mycoplasma pneumonia. Radiographics 2001;21:121–31.
27. Lucaya J, Gartner S, Garcia-Peña P, et al. Spectrum of manifestations of Swyer-James-MacLeod syndrome. J Comput Assist Tomogr 1998;22:592–7.
28. Van Rijn RR, Blickman JG. Differential Diagnosis in Pediatric Imaging. Stuttgart: Thieme; 2011. Chapter 1.
29. Rammath RR, Heller RM, Ben-Ami T. Implications of early sonographic evaluation of parapneumonic effusions in children with pneumonia. Pediatrics 1998;101:68–71.
30. Wilmott RW, Boat TF, Bush A, et al. Kendig and Chernick's Disorders of the Respiratory Tract in Children: Expert Consult. 8th ed. New York: Elsevier; 2012. p. 699–735.

31. Rudman DT, Elmaraghy CA, Shiels WE, et al. The role of airway fluoroscopy in the evaluation of stridor in children. Arch Otolaryngol Head Neck Surg 2003;129:305–9.

32. McAdams HP, Kirejczyk WM, Rosado-de-Christenson ML, Matsumoto S. Bronchogenic cysts: imaging features with clinical and histopathologic correlation. Radiology 2000;217:441–6.

33. Kuhn C, Kuhn JP. Coexistence of bronchial atresia and bronchogenic cyst: diagnostic criteria and embryologic considerations. Pediatr Radiol 1992;22:568–70.

34. Grewal RG, Yip CK. Intralobar pulmonary sequestration and mediastinal bronchogenic cyst. Thorax 1994;49:615–16.

35. Lyon RD, McAdams HP. Mediastinal bronchogenic cyst demonstration of fluid-fluid level at MR imaging. Radiology 1993;186:427–8.

36. Stocker JT. Congenital pulmonary airway malformation: a new name for and an expanded classification of congenital cystic adenomatoid malformation of the lung. Symposium 24: non-neoplastic lung disease. Histopathology 2002;41:424–30.

37. Stocker JT. Congenital and developmental diseases. In: Tomashefski JF, Cagle PT, Farver C, Fraire C, editors. Dail and Hammar's Pulmonary Pathology: Nonneoplastic Lung Disease, vol. 1. New York: Springer; 2008. pp. 132–75.

38. Enriquez G, Garcia-Peña P. Pitfalls in chest imaging. Pediatr Radiol 2009;39(3):356–68.

39. Davenport M, Warne SA, Cacciaguerra S, et al. Current outcome of antenatally diagnosed cystic lung disease. J Pediatr Surg 2004;39:549–56.

40. Azizkhan RG, Crombleholme TM. Congenital cystic lung disease: contemporary antenatal and postnatal management. Pediatr Surg Int 2008;24:643–57.

41. Daltro P, Werner H, Gasparetto TD, et al. Congenital chest malformations: a multimodality approach with emphasis on fetal MR imaging. Radiographics 2010;30:385–95.

42. Kim WS, Lee KS, Kim IO, et al. Congenital cystic adenomatoid malformation of the lung. CT-pathologic correlation. Am J Roentgenol 1997;168:47–53.

43. Bohn D. Congenital diaphragmatic hernia. Am J Respir Crit Care Med 2002;166(7):911–15.

44. Lander A. Congenital diaphragmatic hernia. Surgery 2007;25(7):298–300.

45. Leung JWT, Coakley FV, Hricak H, et al. Prenatal MR imaging of congenital diaphragmatic hernia. Am J Roentgenol 2000;174:1607–11.

46. Newman B. Congenital bronchopulmonary foregut malformations: concepts and controversies. Pediatr Radiol 2006;36:773–91.

47. Laurin S, Hägerstrand I. Intralobar bronchopulmonary sequestration in the newborn: a congenital malformation. Pediatr Radiol 1999;29:174–8.

48. Winters WD, Effmann EL. Congenital masses of the lung: prenatal and postnatal imaging evaluation. J Thorac Imaging 2001;16:196–206.

49. Savic B, Birtel FJ, Tholen W, et al. Lung sequestration: report of seven cases and review of 540 published cases. Thorax 1979;34:96–101.

50. Lager DJ, Kuper KA, Haake GK. Sub-diaphragmatic extralobar pulmonary sequestration. Arch Pathol Lab Med 1991;115:536–8.

51. Conran RM, Stoker JT. Extralobar sequestration with frequently associated congenital cystic adenomatoid malformation, type 2: report of 50 cases. Pediatr Dev Pathol 1999;2:454–63.

52. Lee EY, Siegel MJ, Sierra LM, Forglia RP. Evaluation of angioarchitecture of pulmonary sequestration in pediatric patients using 3D MDCT angiography. Am J Roentgenol 2004;183:183–8.

53. Ko SF, Ng SH, Lee TZ, et al. Noninvasive imaging of bronchopulmonary sequestration. Am J Roentgenol 2000;175:1005–12.

54. Garcia-Peña P, Lucaya J, Hendry GMA, et al. Spontaneous involution of pulmonary sequestrations in children: a report of two cases and review of the literature. Pediatr Radiol 1998;28:266–70.

55. Castellote A, Enriquez G, Lucaya J. Congenital malformations of the chest beyond the neonatal period. In: Carty H, Brunelle F, Stringer DA, Kao SCS, editors. Imaging Children. Elsevier; 2005. pp. 1049–74.

56. Ward S, Morcos SK. Congenital bronchial atresia. Presentation of three cases and pictorial review. Clin Radiol 1999;54:144–8.

57. Mata JM, Caceres J. The dysmorphic lung: imaging findings. Eur Radiol 1996;6:403–14.

58. Choi S-J, Lee JS, Song KS, et al. Mediastinal teratoma: CT differentiation of ruptured and unruptured tumors. Am J Roentgenol 1998;171:591–4.

59. Kim WS, Moon WK, Kim IO, et al. Pulmonary tuberculosis in children: evaluation with CT. Am J Roentgenol 1997;168:1005–9.

60. Siegel MJ, Ishwaran HI, Fletcher BD, et al. Staging of neuroblastomas at imaging: report of the radiology diagnostic oncology group. Radiology 2002;223:168–75.

61. Neville HL, Hogan AR, Zhuge Y, et al. Incidence and outcomes of malignant pediatric lung neoplasms. J Surg Res 2009;156(2):224–30.

62. Mc Hugh K. Chest tumours other than lymphomas. In: Lucaya J, Strife JL, editors. Pediatric Chest Imaging: Chest Imaging in Infants and Children. 2nd ed. Berlin: Springer-Verlag; 2008. pp. 263–87.

63. Priest JR, Hill AD, Williams GM, et al. Type 1 pleuropulmonary blastoma registry. J Clin Oncol 2006;24:4492–8.

64. Wang LT, Wilkins EW Jr, Bode HH. Bronchial carcinoid in pediatric patients. Chest 1993;103:1426–8.

65. Soyer T, Karnak I, Ciftci AO, et al. Result of surgical treatment of chest wall tumors in childhood. Pediatr Surg Int 2006;22:135–9.

66. Sallustio G, Pironti T, Lasorella A, et al. Diagnostic imaging of primitive neuroectodermal tumour of the chest wall (Askin tumour). Pediatr Radiol 1998;28:697–702.

67. Dick EA, McHugh K, Kimber C, et al. Radiology of non-central nervous system primitive neuroectodermal tumours: diagnostic features and correlation with outcome. Clin Radiol 2001;56:206–15.

68. McHugh K, Boothroyd AE. The role of radiology in childhood rhabdomyosarcoma. Clin Radiol 1999;54:2–10.

69. Hodson M, Gedes DM, Bush A. Cystic Fibrosis. 3rd ed. London: Hodder Arnold; 2007.

70. The Clinical Standards and Accreditation Group. Standards of Care: Standards for the Clinical Care of Children and Adults with Cystic Fibrosis in the UK 2001. Bromley, Kent: Cystic Fibrosis Trust; Available at: http://www.cfcarepathway.com/docs/Standards_of_Care_2001.pdf. 2001.

71. Pennington DJ, Lonergan GJ, Benya EC. Pulmonary disease in the immunocompromised child. J Thorac Imaging 1999;14:37–50.

72. Mori M, Galvin JR, Barloon TJ, et al. Fungal pulmonary infections after bone marrow transplantation: evaluation with radiograph and CT. Radiology 1995;178:721–6.

73. Marks MJ, Haley PJ, McDermott MP, et al. Thoracic diseases in children with AIDS. Radiographics 1996;349–62.

74. Poznansky MC, Walters J, Cruikshank A, et al. The rising prevalence of HIV-1 infection in patients attending an inner city accident and emergency department. J Accid Emerg Med 1996;13:424–5.

75. Kuhlman JE, Fishman EK, Burch PA, et al. CT of invasive pulmonary aspergillosis. Am J Roentgenol 1988;150:1015–20.

76. Brown MJ, Miller RR, Muller NL. Acute lung disease in the immunocompromised host: CT and pathologic examination findings. Radiology 1994;190:247–54.

77. Bragg DG, Chor PJ, Murray KA, Kjeldserg CR. Lymphoproliferative disorders of the lung: histopathology, clinical manifestations, and imaging features. Am J Roentgenol 1994;163:273–81.

78. Gibson M, Hansell DM. Lymphocytic disorders of the chest: pathology and imaging. Clin Radiol 1998;53:469–80.

79. Clark JG, Hansen JA, Hertz MI, et al. NHLBI workshop summary. Idiopathic pneumonia syndrome after bone marrow transplantation. Am Rev Resp Dis 1993;147:1601–6.

CHAPTER 3

PAEDIATRIC ABDOMINAL IMAGING

Anne Paterson • Øystein E. Olsen • Lil-Sofie Ording Müller

INTRODUCTION

Paediatric gastrointestinal (GI) radiology is most appropriately thought of according to the age of the patient, and for this reason the chapter has been subdivided into sections; the first details neonatal pathology, the latter relates to older children. The clinical presentation of the conditions remains as before. In this latest edition, newer embryological theories, imaging techniques, management details and updated references have been incorporated. As most children with neonatal GI problems now survive to adolescence or adulthood, data have emerged about adult cohorts and some of the longer-term health problems they face. Information detailing some of these issues has also been included.

THE NEONATE

Visible Abnormalities of the Anterior Abdominal Wall

The ventral wall of the embryo is formed during the fourth week of intrauterine development as the cephalic, caudal and lateral edges of the flat, trilaminar embryonal disc fold in upon themselves and the layers fuse together. The resultant embryo is cylindrical in shape, and protruding centrally from its ventral surface are the remains of the yolk sac connected to the midgut via the omphalomesenteric duct, a structure, which normally regresses in the fifth gestational month.[1,2]

If this complex process is incomplete, then several types of anterior abdominal wall defect may result: ectopia cordis and pentalogy of Cantrell, gastroschisis, bladder and cloacal exstrophy, and omphalocele.

Gastroschisis

In patients with gastroschisis, there is a small defect or split in the ventral abdominal wall, classically to the right side of a normally positioned umbilicus. Gastroschisis typically occurs in the absence of other anomalies and is thought to be due either to a localised intrauterine vascular accident or to asymmetry in the lateral body wall folds with failure of fusion.[1]

The incidence of gastroschisis has increased worldwide over the past two decades and it has been documented to occur in clusters in some geographic regions.[2,3] Mothers under the age of 20 years are at greater risk of having a child with the condition.[4]

Antenatal ultrasound shows bowel loops floating freely in the amniotic fluid, with the diagnosis being possible early in the second trimester. There is no covering membrane. 'Complex gastroschisis' as determined by the presence of intestinal atresia or stenosis, bowel perforation, volvulus or necrosis is found in 10–20% of infants.[3,5,6] Exposure to amniotic fluid causes damage to the bowel; postnatally, this can result in a thick, fibrous 'peel' coating the loops of bowel. Short bowel syndrome, liver disease secondary to intestinal failure and intestinal dysmotility are serious consequences of gastroschisis. Necrotising enterocolitis (NEC) is reported in up to 20% of patients with gastroschisis.[7]

Upper GI contrast studies in infants with repaired gastroschisis will often demonstrate gastro-oesophageal reflux (GOR), malrotation, dilatation of small bowel loops and a markedly prolonged transit time.

Repair of the defect may be possible soon after delivery. If not, the bowel is protected in a silo to prevent fluid loss, and gradually returned to the abdominal cavity.

Omphalocele

An omphalocele (*syn.* exomphalos) is a midline anterior abdominal wall defect through which the solid abdominal viscera and/or bowel may herniate. The extruded abdominal contents are covered in a sac. Larger omphaloceles containing liver tissue may be due to failure of fusion of the lateral body folds. Omphaloceles containing only bowel are thought to arise due to persistence of the physiological herniation of gut after the tenth week of fetal development. The umbilical cord inserts at the tip of the defect. A giant omphalocele is said to be present when the liver is contained within the herniated membranes or when the defect measures more than 5 cm in diameter.[8]

Antenatal ultrasound can detect an omphalocele from the second trimester onwards. The prognosis of the infant is dependent upon associated anomalies. Chromosomal and structural abnormalities are seen in more than 50% of patients.[3] The Beckwith–Wiedemann syndrome has an omphalocele (exomphalos), macroglossia and gigantism as its primary components (the 'EMG' syndrome).

The method of surgical closure of the defect is in part driven by its size. Immediate closure, staged procedures or delayed repair following epithelialisation are all surgical possibilities.

Bladder Exstrophy—Epispadias—Cloacal Exstrophy Complex

The terminology of this spectrum of complex disorders is confusing, with many texts using the term OEIS complex (omphalocele, exstrophy, imperforate anus and spinal abnormality) and cloacal exstrophy, interchangeably. In reality, they probably represent different entities of the same spectrum. The epispadias–exstrophy spectrum is rare and complex, extending from epispadias, where males have a urethral meatus opening on the dorsum of the penis, and affected females a cleft urethra, to bladder exstrophy, where the bladder is exposed on the lower abdominal wall and drips urine constantly.

At the far end of the spectrum is cloacal exstrophy, one of the most severe congenital anomalies compatible with life, and which encompasses abnormalities of the genitourinary (GU) and GI tracts, the central nervous and musculoskeletal systems. This condition is thought to arise due to abnormal development of the cloacal membrane[9] and its premature rupture prior to the fifth week of gestation.[10] The cloaca opens onto the lower abdominal wall, where it is seen as an open caecum and prolapsing terminal ileum between two hemibladders. There is an omphalocele of varying size and a blind-ending short gut. The external genitalia are ambiguous. Bilateral inguinal herniae are common to both sexes. There is spinal dysraphism and there is an 'open book' pelvis.[11] Associated renal and lower limb anomalies (club foot and reduction defects) are well described.[9]

Antenatally, the 'elephant's trunk' sign of the prolapsed terminal ileum is said to be pathognomonic for the condition on ultrasound.[9] Non-visualisation of the bladder in association with an omphalocele and myelomeningocele would also be strong predictors of cloacal exstrophy.

Early postnatal imaging includes the extensive use of ultrasound to evaluate the spine and brain, the GU tract and the hips. CT with 3D-VR images is helpful in planning pelvic surgery.[11] Upper GI contrast studies document GI tract anatomy. Magnetic resonance imaging (MRI) of both the pelvis—assessing the genital tract and pelvic floor—and the spine are also required.

Surgery in the immediate postnatal period includes diversion of the faecal stream and colostomy formation, bladder closure ± vesicostomy fashioning, omphalocele reduction and repair, and closure of any open neural tube defects. Genital tract surgeries are often postponed until later in childhood.

Respiratory Distress and Choking

The neonate with disease affecting the proximal GI tract often presents with respiratory symptoms. These symptoms include excess salivation, choking with feeds, coughing, cyanosis and respiratory distress. Conditions that present in this way include oesophageal atresia (OA) with or without tracheo-oesophageal fistula (TOF), laryngeal clefts, swallowing disorders, diaphragmatic hernias, vascular rings and GOR; the latter is by far the most common. The chest radiograph may show airspace disease and atelectasis, should aspiration have already occurred.

Oesophageal Atresia and Tracheo-Oesophageal Fistula

OA with or without a fistulous connection to the trachea is one of the more common congenital anomalies of the GI tract. It is caused by abnormal partitioning of the foregut into separate respiratory (ventral) and GI (dorsal) components early on in the first trimester of fetal life. Five different major anomalies result (Fig. 3-1). The atretic segment of the oesophagus tends to be at the junction of its proximal and middle thirds. Occasionally an isolated TOF occurs without OA; this is the H-type fistula.

Half of all children with OA and TOF have associated congenital anomalies. Features of the VACTERL spectrum (*v*ertebral anomalies, *a*norectal malformation, *c*ardiovascular malformation, *t*racheo-oesophageal fistula with oesophageal atresia, *r*enal anomalies and *l*imb defects) are especially common, with other GI malformations—notably duodenal atresia, small bowel malrotation and volvulus and a more distal congenital oesophageal stenosis often reported.[12]

OA is usually suspected on an antenatal ultrasound. The cardinal findings of maternal polyhydramnios and an absent stomach bubble have a positive predictive value of 50%.[13] A false-negative exam may be as a result of fluid passing via a lower pouch fistula into the stomach. However, OA can be diagnosed with greater certainty by visualising the dilated, blind-ending upper oesophageal pouch and the use of cine-mode fetal MRI.[13,14]

The remaining group of infants present almost immediately in the postnatal period with choking, coughing, cyanosis and drooling, symptoms which are exacerbated during attempts to feed the infant. Patients with an H-type fistula are usually symptomatic from birth.

Postnatally, the diagnosis is usually made on a chest radiograph, which shows an orogastric tube curled in the proximal oesophageal pouch (Fig. 3-2). The lungs may show features of an aspiration pneumonitis. The presence of gas in the abdomen implies a distal fistula. A gasless abdomen is seen with isolated OA or rarely OA with a proximal fistula.

In those infants in whom a primary repair is not possible, the gap between the proximal and distal

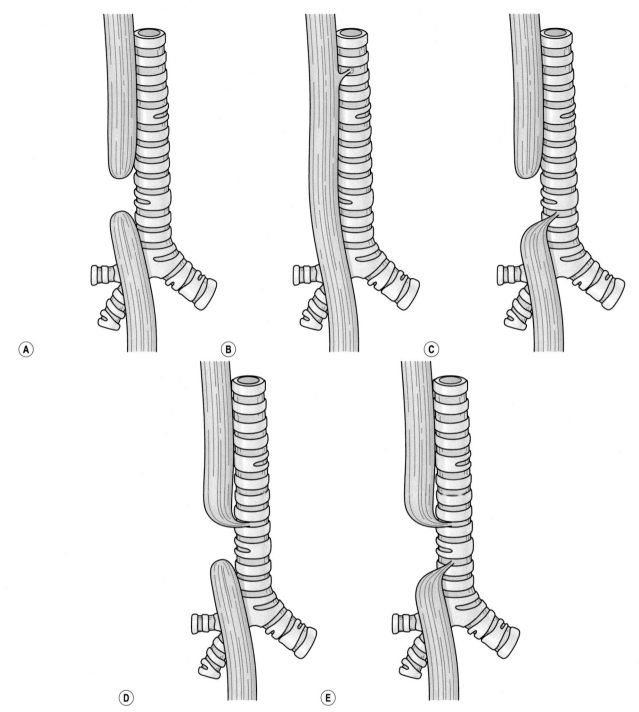

FIGURE 3-1 ■ **Oesophageal atresia and tracheo-oesophageal fistula.** Diagrammatic representation of (A) isolated OA (9%), (B) H-type fistula (6%), (C) OA with distal TOF (82%), (D) OA with proximal TOF (1%) and (E) OA with TOF from both proximal and distal oesophageal remnants (2%).

oesophageal pouches can be assessed following the formation of a feeding gastrostomy. Under fluoroscopic guidance, a Hegar dilator is inserted though the gastrostomy and passed retrogradely into the distal oesophagus. A Replogle tube is simultaneously used to delineate the superior pouch. As both tubes are radiopaque, the degree of separation between the pouches is easily visualised. Thoracic CT imaging, following simultaneous injection of air into the upper pouch, via the indwelling Replogle tube, and also via the gastrostomy, can alternatively be used.[15,16]

The standard, long-established diagnostic technique for an H-type fistula in most institutions remains the 'withdrawal oesophagram', obtained with the infant in the prone position, with a horizontal X-ray beam (or a steep oblique position with a vertical X-ray beam). The contrast is injected under pressure, via a nasogastric tube (NGT) with its tip in the distal oesophagus, as the tube

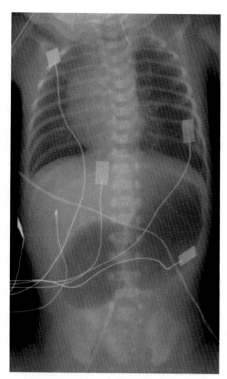

FIGURE 3-2 ■ **Oesophageal atresia with distal pouch tracheo-oesophageal fistula and duodenal atresia.** Supine chest and abdominal radiograph shows a Replogle tube in the proximal oesophageal pouch, with gas outlining the classical 'double bubble' of duodenal atresia in the abdomen.

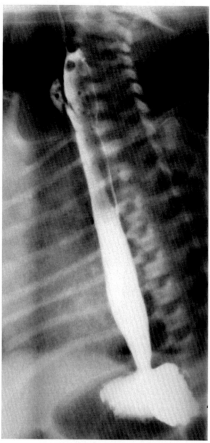

FIGURE 3-3 ■ **H-type TOF.** Upper GI contrast study shows the fistula running obliquely at the level of the thoracic inlet.

is gradually pulled back under fluoroscopic guidance (Fig. 3-3). Care must be taken not to spill barium via the vocal cords into the trachea, or water-soluble contrast medium can be used. Combined bronchoscopy and oesophagoscopy should be performed if there is a high clinical index of suspicion with negative imaging.

A positive contrast medium injection to outline the proximal oesophageal pouch is rarely necessary, but occasionally required to exclude a proximal pouch fistula. Small quantities (1–2 mL) of isotonic, non-ionic contrast medium should be used under fluoroscopic guidance. A proximal fistula can also be demonstrated if air is injected into the Replogle tube during a multidetector CT (MDCT) imaging.[17]

Given the frequent combination of OA/TOF with VACTERL components, a preoperative work-up should involve assessment of the cardiovascular system and GU tract.

Early Post-Surgical Radiology. The immediate complications following OA and TOF repair are recurrence of the TOF, which occurs in up to 10% of patients, and anastomotic breakdown in a further 10–20% of patients. Major leaks will present early with a tension pneumothorax and require repeat surgery.[18] Presentation of a recurrent fistula may be delayed for months after surgery, and the child can suffer recurrent aspiration pneumonitis and pneumonia. A transanastomotic feeding tube is positioned by most surgeons, who will request a postoperative oesophagram (water-soluble contrast media) prior to the recommencement of enteral feeds.

Anastomotic strictures develop in up to 80% of patients,[19] and are more likely in long gap OA, and in those who have marked postoperative GOR. Oesophageal strictures can easily, safely and repeatedly be treated by balloon catheter dilatation using fluoroscopic guidance.

Longer-Term Problems. As many of the early repair cohorts are now in adulthood, data have emerged regarding the long-term problems patients face following OA/TOF surgery.

Dysphagia of varying degrees is experienced in up to 60%; this can be severe enough to cause food impaction.[19] Almost half of patients report GOR or regurgitation. Biopsy-proven Barrett's oesophagus has been reported in patients' following OA repair.[19]

Respiratory problems lasting into adulthood are common. These are generally mild, but include wheezing and reactive airways disease in 25%, choking sensations in 10% and recurrent infections in up to 30%.[20,21]

Non-bilious Vomiting

Vomiting is a common problem in children of all ages and its presence as a symptom does not necessarily indicate GI disease. Vomiting is common with infections in any body system, in metabolic disease, disorders of the central nervous system, and as a side effect of drugs and poisons. Neonatal non-bilious vomiting due to GI causes implies a lesion proximal to the ampulla of Vater, and is most frequently due to GOR. A full clinical history and physical examination are the most important factors in determining what imaging investigations (if any) are required.

Obstruction of the Stomach

Congenital gastric obstruction is rare. It is usually due to a web or diaphragm in the antrum or pylorus. Occasionally a true atresia is present, with a fibrous cord uniting the two blind ends. Pyloric atresia is associated with epidermolysis bullosa simplex.[22] The diagnosis may be suspected antenatally due to maternal polyhydramnios and a large fetal gastric bubble. Postnatally, non-bilious vomiting and upper abdominal distension are found.

A plain radiograph will show a dilated stomach with no distal air. At ultrasound, webs appear as persistent, linear, echogenic structures arising from the antral or pyloric walls and extending centrally.

Enteric Duplication Cysts

Enteric duplication cysts are uncommon congenital anomalies of obscure aetiology. They can occur anywhere along the length of the gut but are most frequently found in the ileum. Gastric duplications account for less than 5% of cases,[23,24] and are usually found on the greater curve. When located in the antropyloric region they may cause gastric outlet obstruction and present in the neonatal period with non-bilious vomiting and a palpable mass. Confirmation of the diagnosis is by ultrasound. The cysts have a layered wall, with an inner echogenic layer corresponding to the mucosa/submucosa and an outer hypoechoic layer that represents a smooth muscle layer (Fig. 3-4). This appearance is referred to as

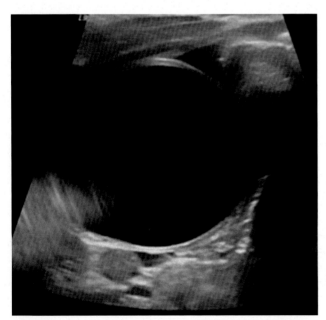

FIGURE 3-4 ■ Ileal duplication cyst. Sonogram showing echogenic mucosal layer and hypoechoic outer muscular layer.

the 'gut signature'. The contents of the cyst are usually hypoechoic, but debris is seen if there has been haemorrhage or infection has developed. Gastric mucosa takes up ^{99m}Tc-pertechnetate, which is helpful to identify the cysts when children present with GI bleeding (see the section 'Enteric Duplication Cysts' under 'Abdominal Distension').

Microgastria

This is a rare abnormality characterised by a small, tubular, midline stomach, severe GOR and a megaoesophagus. The patients present with recurrent vomiting, failure to thrive, signs of malnutrition and recurrent episodes of aspiration pneumonia. Associated anomalies are found in nearly all cases, and include components of the VACTERL sequence, small bowel malrotation, upper limb reduction defects and asplenia. An upper GI contrast study confirms the diagnosis.

Gastric Perforation

Gastric perforation is uncommon but accounts for a significant proportion of cases of neonatal pneumoperitoneum, and is a life-threatening condition. The underlying cause is unclear, but the rate of enteral feed introduction, ischaemia and increased mechanical pressure have been suggested.[25,26] Iatrogenic gastric perforation is recognised after insertion of orogastric tubes. A massive pneumoperitoneum is seen on a plain radiograph of the abdomen.

Bilious Vomiting

Bilious vomiting in the neonate may be the presenting feature of many different conditions. Sepsis, metabolic upset and gastroenteritis are examples requiring 'medical management', whereas, from a surgical perspective, bilious emesis indicates bowel obstruction distal to the ampulla of Vater. The most urgent of all emergencies in a neonate with bilious vomiting is small bowel malrotation complicated by volvulus.

A plain abdominal radiograph alone will not distinguish between the plethora of underlying conditions causing bilious vomiting. However, a complete high intestinal obstruction (mid-ileal level and above), denoted by a few dilated bowel loops only, requires operative intervention irrespective of the cause, and no further imaging is necessary. If there is a low intestinal obstruction (distal ileum and beyond), as demonstrated by the presence of multiple dilated bowel loops on the plain radiograph, a single-contrast enema will generally be performed prior to any definitive treatment.

Small Bowel Malrotation and Volvulus

Malrotation is a generic term used to describe any variation in the normal position of the intestines. In itself, it is not necessarily symptomatic, but the resultant abnormal position of the duodenojejunal flexure (DJF) ± caecum, mean these two organs lie closer together, shortening the base of the small bowel mesentery (Fig. 3-5). The midgut has a propensity to twist around this

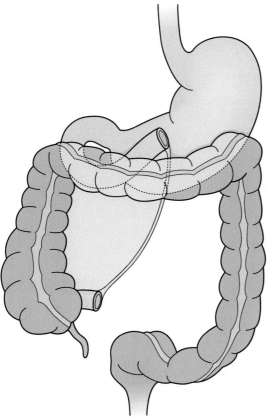

FIGURE 3-5 ■ **The base of the normal small bowel mesentery.** Diagramatic representation demonstrating the normal small bowel mesentery, which runs from the level of the duodenoje- junal flexure (DJF) to the ileocaecal valve.

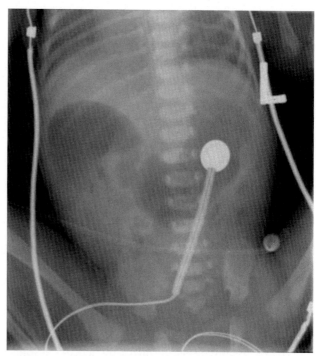

FIGURE 3-6 ■ **Surgically proven small bowel malrotation and volvulus.** Abdominal radiograph with appearances mimicking the double bubble of duodenal atresia.

narrowed pedicle (volvulus), compromising the arterial inflow and venous drainage of the superior mesenteric vessels, which can lead to ischaemic necrosis of the small bowel. Untreated small bowel volvulus has a high mortality rate.

In fetal life, the gut begins as a straight, midline tube, which, as it elongates and develops, herniates into the base of the umbilical cord. Traditional embryological teaching is based upon the theory that between the sixth and tenth weeks of fetal development, the midgut loop undergoes a complex three-stage anticlockwise rotation process centred around the axis of the superior mesenteric artery (SMA). This is said to explain the position of the DJF in the left upper, and the ileocaecal junction in the right lower quadrants of the abdomen. The mesentery of the small bowel extends between these two fixed points, giving it a broad base. More recent work by Metzger et al.[27] proposes that the anatomical position of the gut relies critically upon localised growth and lengthening of the duodenal loop, which pushes it beneath the mesenteric root.

Should the embryological development of the bowel be interrupted, then a variety of abnormal gut positions can occur; infants with congenital diaphragmatic herniae, gastroschisis and omphalocele by definition all have malrotated, malfixated bowel, although volvulus in these patients is rare after repair of the primary abnormality.[28] In general, small bowel malrotation is an isolated

abnormality, though it has been reported in association with pyloric stenosis, duodenal stenosis, web and atresia, preduodenal portal vein, annular pancreas and jejuno-ileal atresias. The heterotaxy syndromes, Hirschsprung's disease and megacystis–microcolon–intestinal hypoperi-stalsis syndrome are also associated with malrotation and volvulus, as are cloacal exstrophy, prune-belly syndrome and intestinal neuronal dysplasia.

Symptomatic babies with malrotation commonly present within the first month of life, with bilious vomit-ing. Older children may present with non-specific symp-toms of chronic or intermittent abdominal pain, emesis, diarrhoea or failure to thrive. Volvulus, though less common in the older child, still occurs. It is important to suspect malrotation and volvulus in a child of *any* age with bilious vomiting, and to investigate accordingly in an emergent fashion.

There are no specific plain radiographic findings in malrotation, even with volvulus. The radiograph may be completely normal if the volvulus is intermittent or if there is incomplete duodenal obstruction, due to a loose twisting of the bowel. If the volvulus is tight, then com-plete duodenal obstruction results, with gaseous disten-sion of the stomach and proximal duodenum. The classical picture is of a partial duodenal obstruction, with distension of the stomach and proximal duodenum, with some distal gas (Fig. 3-6).

A pattern of distal small bowel obstruction is seen in a closed loop obstruction and represents a more ominous finding; the small bowel loops may be thick-walled and oedematous, with pneumatosis being evident. These findings represent small bowel necrosis. A gasless abdomen is seen if vomiting has been prolonged, and in both closed loop obstruction with viable small bowel or massive midgut necrosis. In the neonate with bilious vomiting and a complete duodenal obstruction or a seriously ill child with obvious signs of peritonism, radiographic examination should cease after the plain radiograph; and urgent surgery is indicated. In all other children with bilious vomiting and incomplete bowel obstruction, further investigation—usually in the form of an upper GI contrast study—is required. This examination is best performed with barium (single-contrast study).

The intestines in malrotation are malpositioned and the purpose of the upper GI study is to locate the position of the DJF. Meticulous radiological technique is required, and care must be taken not to overfill the stomach with contrast medium, as this can obscure the position of the DJF directly or secondarily by duodenal 'flooding' following rapid emptying of the stomach. The operator should aim to carefully define the position of the DJF on the first pass of contrast medium through the duodenum.

On a supine radiograph, the normal DJF lies to the left of the left-sided vertebral pedicles at the height of the duodenal bulb (Fig. 3-7A). When malrotation is present, the DJF is usually displaced inferiorly and to the right side (Fig. 3-7B). It is important to remember that the DJF can be displaced temporarily by a distended colon or stomach, an enlarged spleen, an indwelling naso-enteric tube or manual palpation.

The 'corkscrew' pattern of the duodenum and jejunum spiralling around the mesenteric vessels is pathognomonic for midgut volvulus on the upper GI study, the calibre of the bowel decreasing distal to the point of partial obstruction (Fig. 3-8). If there is an abrupt cut-off to the flow of contrast in the third part of the duodenum, volvulus cannot be excluded with certainty and these infants too must proceed directly to surgery.

Malfixation of the intestines invariably accompanies malrotation in an attempt to fix the gut in place. Peritoneal (Ladd's) bands stretch from the (sometimes high-lying) caecum and right colon, across the duodenum to the right upper quadrant and retroperitoneum. The Ladd's bands themselves can cause duodenal obstruction.

Ultrasound may demonstrate the dilated, fluid-filled stomach and proximal duodenum when obstruction is present. The relationship of the superior mesenteric vein (SMV) to the superior mesenteric artery (SMA) is abnormal in about two-thirds of patients with malrotation, when the vein lies ventral or to the left of the artery, a finding that is neither sensitive nor specific for malrotation. Ultrasound has also been proposed to confirm the (normal) retromesenteric position of the third part of the duodenum, and has been advocated as a screening tool in neonatal populations.[29] A volvulus may be demonstrated with ultrasound as the 'whirlpool sign'; colour Doppler studies show the SMV spiralling clockwise around the SMA.

Management

The standard operation for small bowel malrotation and volvulus is Ladd's procedure, whereby the bowel is exposed, untwisted and inspected. Any Ladd's bands are

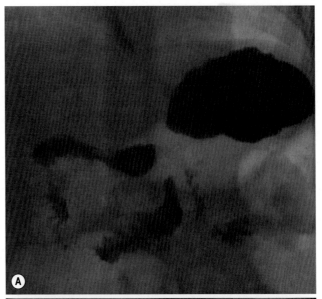

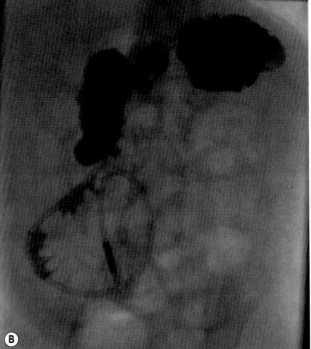

FIGURE 3-7 ■ Demonstration of (A) a normally sited duodeno-jejunal flexure and (B) a duodenojejunal flexure that is low lying and to the right of the expected position—as shown by the most distal curl of the feeding tube.

divided, and the base of the mesentery is widened. Finally, the bowel is returned to the abdomen, with the duodenum and jejunum to the right side, and the colon to the left; and a prophylactic appendicectomy is often performed.

In those patients with small bowel malrotation diagnosed incidentally on an upper GI contrast study performed for another indication, management is less certain. Many paediatric surgeons will opt to perform an elective Ladd's procedure.

It is important that radiologists understand that a Ladd's procedure does not result in a normal anatomical

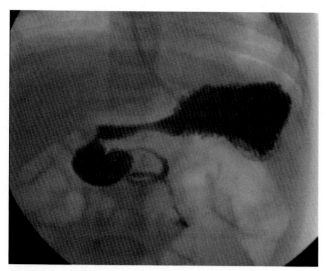

FIGURE 3-8 ■ **Small bowel malrotation and volvulus.** Upper GI contrast study demonstrates the classical 'corkscrew' pattern of the duodenum and jejunum spiralling around the mesenteric vessels. Note the change in bowel calibre at the level of the duodenojejunal flexure.

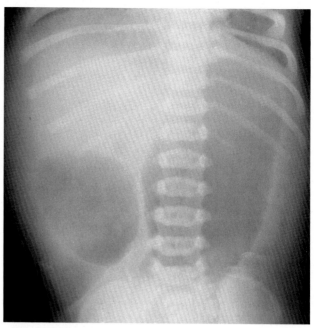

FIGURE 3-9 ■ **Duodenal atresia.** Supine radiograph shows the classical 'double bubble' appearance.

position of the bowel; the DJF will always be malpositioned in these patients and recurrent volvulus can occur if the mesenteric base is not sufficiently widened at the time of the first surgery.

Duodenal Atresia and Stenosis

Duodenal atresia (DA) is much more common than duodenal stenosis, and both are caused by failure of recanalisation of the duodenal lumen after the sixth week of fetal life. Duodenal obstruction may also be caused by webs or diaphragms. Extrinsic duodenal compression by an annular pancreas or preduodenal portal vein may contribute to the obstruction in some patients. Regardless of the cause, in 80% of cases, the level of the obstruction is just distal to the ampulla of Vater.

Associated anomalies are present in the majority of patients with DA or stenosis. Down's syndrome is present in 30% of patients and congenital heart disease in 20%. Malrotation is present in 20–30% of patients and can only be diagnosed prior to surgery if the duodenal obstruction is partial. Components of the VACTERL association may also be present, with OA coexisting in up to 10% of infants.

DA may be diagnosed antenatally when the dilated stomach and duodenal cap are seen. Fetal growth retardation, maternal polyhydramnios and consequent prematurity are common. Infants otherwise present early in the postnatal period with bilious vomiting and upper abdominal distension. Non-bilious vomiting occurs in those infants with a preampullary obstruction.

Radiographs show a gas-filled 'double bubble' of the stomach and duodenal cap (Fig. 3-9). If the obstruction is partial or in the rare cases of a bifid common bile duct straddling the atretic segment, then distal gas will be present.

In an upper GI study, duodenal stenosis is seen as a narrowed area in the second part of the duodenum, A duodenal web may be seen as a thin, filling defect extending across the duodenal lumen. Ultrasound can also be used to make the diagnosis, the examination made easier if the infant is first given clear fluids orally.

The treatment of both complete and incomplete duodenal obstruction is surgical.

Small Bowel Atresia and Stenosis

Jejunal and ileal atresias have a common aetiology and are thought to be due to an intrauterine vascular accident. The vascular insult may be a primary or secondary event (for example due to antenatal volvulus or intussusception). Jejunoileal atresias have an increased incidence in patients with gastroschisis and meconium ileus.

The 'apple peel' syndrome is thought to follow intrauterine occlusion of the distal SMA. There is a proximal jejunal atresia, with agenesis of the mesentery and absence of the mid-small bowel. The distal ileum spirals around its narrow vascular pedicle, an appearance which gives the syndrome its name. A malrotated microcolon is also usually present. A second, more complex type of intestinal atresia is the syndrome of multiple intestinal atresias with intraluminal calcifications.[30]

The majority of infants with a small bowel atresia present with bilious vomiting in the immediate postnatal period. With more distal atresias, abdominal distension and failure to pass meconium are more commonly recognised clinical features.

On the plain radiograph, there are dilated loops of small bowel down to the level of the atresia. The loop of bowel immediately proximal to the atresia may be disproportionately dilated and have a bulbous contour. A meconium peritonitis with calcification of the peritoneum will be present if an intrauterine perforation has occurred.

Management is surgical, with bowel resection and primary anastomosis if possible. In infants with multiple atresias, the surgeon aims to preserve as much of the bowel length as is feasible.

Abdominal Distension

Abdominal distension in the neonate may be due to mechanical or functional bowel obstruction, an abdominal mass lesion (Table 3-1), ascites or a pneumoperitoneum. A supine abdominal radiograph will show the distribution and calibre of the bowel loops, intra-abdominal calcifications (Table 3-2), the presence of pneumatosis or portal venous gas, any soft-tissue masses and a pneumoperitoneum.

Ultrasound will identify free fluid or the presence of a mass lesion, and is able to confirm the origin of the latter. The majority of neonatal abdominal masses are benign and arise in relation to the GU tract or are of hepatobiliary in origin.

TABLE 3-1   Causes of a Neonatal Intra-abdominal Mass Lesion

- Complicated meconium ileus
- Dilated bowel proximal to an obstruction
- Mesenteric or duplication cyst
- Abscess
- GU causes
  - Hydronephrosis
  - Renal cystic disease
  - Mesoblastic nephroma
  - Wilms' tumour
  - Adrenal haemorrhage
  - Neuroblastoma
  - Retroperitoneal teratoma
  - Ovarian cyst
  - Hydrometrocolpos
- Haemangioendothelioma
- Hepatoblastoma
- Choledochal, hepatic or splenic cysts

TABLE 3-2   Causes of Intra-abdominal Calcifications

- Complicated meconium ileus
- Intraluminal calcifications
  - Low obstruction
  - Anorectal malformations with a fistula to the urinary tract
- Adrenal
  - Haemorrhage
  - Neuroblastoma
  - Wolman's disease
- Hepatobiliary
  - Haemangioendothelioma
  - Hepatoblastoma
  - TORCH infections
- Duplication and mesenteric cysts
- Nephrocalcinosis
- Intravascular thrombus
- Teratomas

Necrotising Enterocolitis (NEC)

NEC is the term used to describe the (often severe) enterocolitis that primarily affects premature infants. The precise aetiology of the condition remains unknown, but a complex interaction of immaturity of the gut mucosa and immune response, impaired gut motility, colonisation of the bowel by pathogenic bacteria and intestinal ischaemia/hypoxia are all in part responsible.[31] There is an inverse relationship between birth weight and gestational age and the development of NEC. The condition is also seen in term infants, particularly those with intrauterine growth retardation, peripartum asphyxia, cyanotic congenital heart disease and gastroschisis.

NEC usually presents in the second week of life, following the commencement of enteral feeds. Initially superficial, the inflammatory process in NEC can extend to become transmural. Diffuse or discrete involvement of the bowel can occur, with the most commonly affected sites being the terminal ileum and colon. The clinical symptoms and signs are non-specific to begin with and include feeding intolerance, lethargy, hypoglycaemia, temperature instability, bradycardia, oxygen desaturation, increased gastric aspirates and gastric distension. Disease progression leads to vomiting, diarrhoea (often with the passage of blood or mucus in the stool) and eventually to shock.

The initial radiographic features of NEC are non-specific. One of the earliest findings is diffuse gaseous distension of both small and large bowel representative of an ileus. Serial radiographs will demonstrate fixed dilatation of one or more bowel loops, and thickening (oedema) and loss of distinction of the bowel walls as the disease progresses.

A more specific sign of NEC on the plain radiograph is intramural gas (pneumatosis intestinalis). Not all infants with pneumatosis will have NEC (Table 3-3). More extensive pneumatosis correlates with an increased severity of NEC. Portal venous gas is seen as branching

---

TABLE 3-3   Causes of Pneumatosis Intestinalis in the Neonate and the Older Child

- NEC
- Bowel ischaemia, inflammation and obstruction
- Cyanotic congenital heart disease
- Hirschsprung's disease
- Gastroschisis
- Anorectal atresia
- Inflammatory bowel disease
- Lymphoma
- Leukaemia
- CMV and rotavirus gastroenteritis
- Colonoscopy
- Caustic ingestion
- Short bowel syndrome
- Congenital immune deficiency states
- *Clostridium* infection
- Chronic granulomatous disease of childhood
- Chronic steroid use
- Post hepatic, renal or bone marrow transplant
- Collagen vascular disease
- Graft-versus-host disease
- AIDS

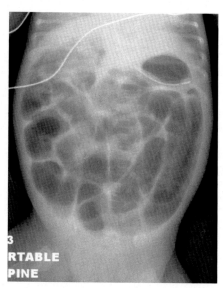

FIGURE 3-10 ■ **Necrotising enterocolitis.** Supine radiograph demonstrates multiple dilated loops of bowel and extensive pneumatosis.

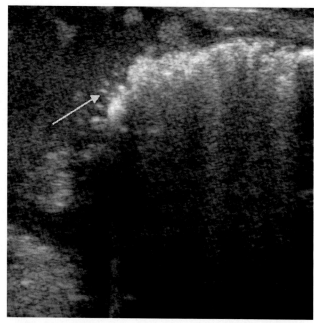

FIGURE 3-11 ■ **The use of ultrasound in the diagnosis of necrotising enterocolitis.** Echogenic dots representing intramural gas bubbles of pneumatosis intestinalis (arrow) in the oedematous bowel wall. (Image reproduced from Imaging in Medicine, August 2011;3(4): 393–410. With the permission of Future Medicine Ltd.)

linear lucencies over the liver that radiate from the region of the porta hepatis to the periphery of both lobes. It develops in around 30% of cases and is usually associated with severe NEC, although its presence does not necessarily imply a fatal outcome (Fig. 3-10).[32]

One-third of children with NEC will perforate, most commonly in the ileocaecal region. The supine, cross-table lateral view is useful to detect small amounts of free intraperitoneal air, as there is no need to reposition the infant when the image is taken. Air collects anteriorly, where it is seen as inverted triangles of air. Alternatively, a lateral decubitus radiograph may be used.

Ultrasound can detect signs of NEC before there are plain radiographic abnormalities.[32,33] Thickening of the bowel wall (≥ 2.7 mm), pneumatosis (seen either as echogenic 'dots' or dense echogenic lines within the bowel wall) (Fig. 3-11) and portal venous gas can all be observed. Colour Doppler will show both hyperaemic bowel wall, and the lack of bowel perfusion that accompanies ischaemia and necrosis. Free fluid will be seen clearly; debris within it may represent bowel content or pus, and has been shown to correlate with gangrene or perforation.[34]

Perforation in infants with NEC is not an absolute indication for surgical intervention. Peritoneal drains are used as a temporising measure in these critically ill infants, delaying the need for surgery and allowing time for systemic recovery. Surgery will be required in 20–40% of infants. Necrotic bowel is resected and as much bowel as possible is preserved.

A late complication of NEC is stricture formation, which occurs in up to a third of patients. Contrast studies (with water-soluble contrast media) are indicated to assess the calibre of the gut downstream prior to re-anastomosis of defunctioned bowel.

The overall mortality rate from NEC is approximately 30%, with this figure being even higher in very low birth weight infants.

Colon Atresia

Colon atresia is rare when compared with other intestinal atresias, and colonic stenosis is rarer still. Atresia has long been thought to be due to an in utero vascular accident;[35] however, Baglaj and colleagues have suggested compression of the bowel wall against the closing umbilical ring as an underlying cause.[6]

The affected infant presents after several feeds with abdominal distension, failure to pass meconium and vomiting.

The abdominal radiograph will show the features of a low intestinal obstruction, with the loop immediately proximal to the atretic segment being massively dilated. If multiple atresias are present, then the bowel will be distended only to the level of the most proximal atresia. A contrast enema usually demonstrates a distal microcolon, with obstruction to the retrograde flow of contrast at the point of the atresia.

The management of colon atresia is surgical.

Intra-abdominal Lymphangioma

Intra-abdominal lymphangiomas may be found in the mesentery, omentum or retroperitoneum, which explains the various names that are used to describe them (mesenteric and omental cysts being two of these). The most common location is in the ileal mesentery. These lesions are increasingly being diagnosed by antenatal imaging, meaning asymptomatic infants come for follow-up imaging early in the postnatal period.

Ultrasound will show a thin-walled, multiloculated cystic lesion that may be adherent to adjacent solid organs and bowel. There is no layering of the cyst wall, which helps to differentiate from an enteric duplication cyst. If the fluid within the cyst is chylous, infected or haemorrhagic, then it will be echogenic (see the section 'Mesenteric Cysts').

Megacystis-Microcolon-Intestinal Hypoperistalsis (Berdon's) Syndrome

This syndrome is a rare and severe form of functional intestinal obstruction. The aetiology of the condition remains obscure. The affected infants present with abdominal distension, bilious vomiting and delayed passage of meconium. Antenatal ultrasound shows a massively dilated bladder. Postnatally, an abdominal radiograph will show dilated small bowel with a large soft-tissue mass arising out of the pelvis. The megabladder and the degree of renal upper tract dilatation can be assessed by ultrasound. An upper GI contrast study will confirm malrotation and a short bowel. A contrast enema shows a non-obstructed microcolon. Treatment of this condition is largely unsuccessful—the mortality rate approaches 80%.

Delayed Passage of Meconium

All term infants should pass meconium in the first 24–48 h of life. Delayed or failed passage of the first stool is reported in premature infants, but may also be due to an underlying congenital bowel obstruction (Table 3-4), which will lead to progressive abdominal distension. The more common problems encountered include Hirschsprung's disease, functional immaturity of the colon, meconium plug syndrome, meconium ileus and peritonitis, and distal atresias.

In all cases, a supine abdominal radiograph will show the features of a low intestinal obstruction; there will be multiple, dilated loops of bowel down to the level of the obstruction. Differentiation between small and large bowel to determine the precise level of the obstruction is virtually impossible in the neonate, given that both may be of similar calibre and that the haustra are poorly developed.

Hirschsprung's Disease

Hirschsprung's disease is a neurocristopathy that presents as functional low bowel obstruction. It occurs due to the failure of caudal migration of neuroblasts in the developing bowel during the fifth through twelfth weeks of gestation. Histology reveals an absence of parasympathetic intrinsic ganglion cells in both Auerbach's and Meissner's plexuses in the bowel wall, which is associated with an increase in the number of acetylcholinesterase-positive nerve fibres in the aganglionic portions of the gut. The distal large bowel from the point of neuronal arrest to the anus is aganglionic. In about 75% of cases, the aganglionic segment extends only to the rectosigmoid region (short segment disease). Long segment disease involves a portion of the colon proximal to the sigmoid. Variants of Hirschsprung's disease include total colonic aganglionosis (TCA), which may involve the distal ileum also, and total intestinal Hirschsprung's disease. Ultrashort segment disease is rare and involves only the anus at the level of the internal sphincter. The existence of 'skip lesions' in Hirschsprung's disease is uncommon.[36]

A definitive diagnosis of Hirschsprung's disease is made by a suction or full-thickness rectal biopsy. Current treatment involves resection of the aganglionic bowel segment with a 'pull though' procedure, and anastomosis of the normally innervated gut close to the anal margin. The management of total intestinal Hirschsprung's disease is notoriously difficult and, at the present time, these patients are supported with parenteral nutrition.

Approximately 10% of children with Hirschsprung's disease have Down's syndrome. Other associations with Hirschsprung's disease include ileal, colonic and anorectal atresias, cleft palate, polydactyly, craniofacial anomalies, cardiac septal defects, multiple endocrine neoplasia types 2A and 2B and other neurocristopathies.[37]

Ninety per cent present in the neonatal period, with delayed passage of meconium, abdominal distension and vomiting. Stooling may follow a digital rectal examination or the insertion of a rectal thermometer, before the symptoms recur. Children with longer segment disease and TCA often present later, as their symptoms can paradoxically be milder and their diagnosis missed clinically.[38]

Severe bloody diarrhoea, sepsis and shock are associated with Hirschsprung's enterocolitis, which occurs in up to 30% of patients in both the pre- and postoperative periods. Enterocolitis is the leading cause of death in Hirschsprung's disease and has an increased frequency in long segment disease and those in whom the diagnosis was delayed.

Other postoperative complications of Hirschsprung's disease include anastomotic leaks, fistulae, abscesses and stenoses. Up to 10% of patients will eventually require a permanent colostomy.[37]

The abdominal radiograph will typically show a low bowel obstruction. A contrast enema should be performed. No pre-procedure bowel preparation is given, and there should be an interval of at least 48 hours since the last enema or rectal examination. The catheter tip is placed just inside the rectum. It is important that the catheter balloon is *not* inflated. A catheter balloon can obscure the diagnostic features or, worse, perforate the stiff, aganglionic bowel. The most important film is a lateral (or oblique) view of the rectum during slow filling (Fig. 3-12). In short segment disease the rectum will be

---

TABLE 3-4 Delayed Passage of Meconium

- Ileal atresia
- Meconium ileus
- Functional immaturity of the colon
- Colon atresia
- Anorectal malformations
- Hirschsprung's disease
- Megacystis–microcolon–intestinal hypoperistalsis syndrome
- Extrinsic compression of the distal bowel by a mass lesion
  - Mesenteric cyst
  - Enteric duplication cyst
- Paralytic ileus, sepsis, drugs and metabolic upset

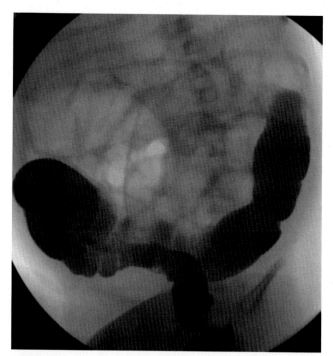

FIGURE 3-12 ■ **Rectosigmoid Hirschsprung's disease.** Supine oblique view, contrast enema. The cone-shaped transition zone and abnormal rectosigmoid ratio are demonstrated.

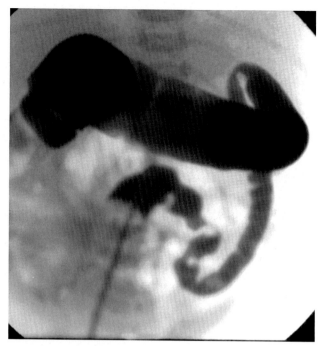

FIGURE 3-13 ■ **Small left colon syndrome.** Contrast enema shows a microcolon distal to the splenic flexure. The transition point is abrupt.

narrow and there will be a cone-shaped transition zone to the more proximal, dilated, ganglionated bowel. Irregular contractions may be seen in the denervated rectum. A useful calculation is the rectosigmoid ratio; the rectum should always be the most distensible portion of the bowel and have a diameter greater than that of the sigmoid colon (recto: sigmoid ratio > 1). In short segment disease, this ratio is reversed. The radiological features of Hirschsprung's disease may be absent in the neonate as it takes time for the ganglionated bowel to dilate.

Whereas coexistent enterocolitis, mucosal oedema, ulceration and spasm are not infrequently seen, an enema would obviously be absolutely contraindicated in the infant with fulminant colitis. Giant stercoral ulcers may also be seen in older children with a delayed presentation. Overall, the contrast enema has a reported sensitivity of 70% and a specificity of 83%;[39] however, the negative predictive value of a normal contrast enema in patients older than 1 month of age is 98%.[40]

In TCA the contrast enema may be entirely normal. Positive findings include shortening of a normal-calibre colon, with rounding of the contours of the hepatic and splenic flexures.

Functional Immaturity of the Colon and Meconium Plug Syndrome

Immature left colon (*syn.* small left colon) and meconium plug syndrome are relatively common causes of neonatal bowel obstruction. There is overlap in both the clinical features and radiology of the two conditions, and the terms are often used interchangeably in the literature. The former refers to a transient functional obstruction of the colon, which occurs as a result of immaturity of the myenteric plexus. It is common in the infants of diabetic mothers and in those whose mothers have a history of substance abuse. Meconium plug syndrome is a temporary colonic obstruction caused by plugs of meconium. It is associated with both cystic fibrosis and Hirschsprung's disease, both of which should either be confirmed or refuted if a diagnosis of meconium plug syndrome is made.[41] The infants of women who have received magnesium sulphate therapy and premature infants also have an increased incidence of meconium plug syndrome.[42]

In both conditions, the affected infants present with symptoms and signs of bowel obstruction. There is delayed passage of meconium. The plain radiograph shows distension of both small and large bowel loops to the level of the inspissated meconium plugs.

In small left colon syndrome, the contrast enema typically shows a microcolon distal to the splenic flexure, at which point there is an abrupt transition to a mildly dilated proximal colon (Fig. 3-13). The main differential diagnosis is long segment Hirschsprung's disease, and biopsy may be required.

In meconium plug syndrome, the lodged meconium plugs are the cause of the obstruction. The plugs lodge in the region of the splenic flexure, proximal to which there is colonic dilatation. There is no microcolon. The (water-soluble) contrast enema is therapeutic, and once the meconium plugs are passed, the infant recovers.

Meconium Ileus

Meconium ileus is a form of distal intestinal obstruction caused by inspissated pellets of meconium in the terminal ileum. Around 80–90% of infants with meconium ileus have cystic fibrosis and meconium ileus is the

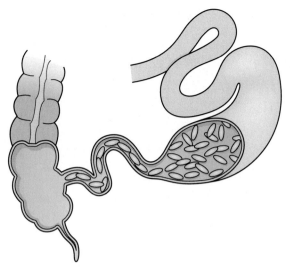

FIGURE 3-14 ■ **Diagrammatic representation of meconium ileus.** Pellets of desiccated meconium obstruct the terminal ileum, with the more proximal small bowel dilating. The unused colon is extremely narrow in calibre (a microcolon).

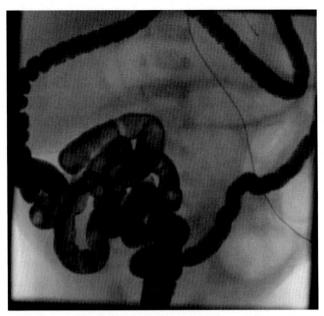

FIGURE 3-15 ■ **Meconium ileus.** Contrast enema demonstrates the empty microcolon. Contrast medium refluxes into the narrow terminal ileum, where pellets of meconium are outlined.

presenting feature of cystic fibrosis in 10–20% of affected patients. Children with the ΔF508 mutation have an increased incidence of meconium ileus, and those who are homozygous for this mutation have a higher incidence still.[43]

Over half of the affected infants have uncomplicated (or simple) meconium ileus. In utero these babies produce meconium that is thick and tenacious, and which fills and distends the small bowel loops. The meconium desiccates in the distal ileum and becomes impacted, causing a high-grade obstruction (Fig. 3-14). Failure of meconium to pass into the colon results in a functional microcolon, whereas more proximally the small bowel loops are dilated and filled with greenish-black meconium of a toothpaste-like consistency.

Meconium ileus is described as complicated when intrauterine volvulus, intestinal atresias, bowel necrosis, perforation or meconium peritonitis supervene. The presenting clinical symptoms and signs of non-complicated meconium ileus are those of a low bowel obstruction. The plain abdominal radiograph will show dilatation of small bowel loops, which are of varying calibre. Often, there is a 'soap bubble' appearance visible (classically in the right iliac fossa), which is caused by the admixture of meconium with gas.

The contrast enema in meconium ileus demonstrates a virtually empty microcolon. Reflux of contrast medium into the terminal ileum will show that it, too, is small in calibre and numerous pellets of meconium are outlined (Fig. 3-15). More proximal reflux of contrast medium will show the dilated mid-ileal loops. The contrast enema in uncomplicated meconium ileus may be therapeutic as well as diagnostic. Traditionally, 'neat' Gastrografin was the contrast medium of choice, but its hypertonicity led to fluid-balance problems. These days, Gastrografin is diluted to half-strength with saline or water, or another water-soluble contrast medium is substituted. If the infant's clinical condition remains stable, the enema can be repeated as necessary until the obstruction is relieved.

Volvulus of a heavy, meconium-laden loop of bowel occurs in about 50% of patients, and can lead to intestinal stenoses, atresias, necrosis and perforation. Perforation of bowel in utero leads to chemical (sterile) meconium peritonitis. The extruded bowel contents cause an intense inflammatory reaction, with fibrosis and calcification to follow. A meconium pseudocyst is formed when there is vascular compromise in association with an intrauterine volvulus; the ischaemic bowel loops become adherent and necrotic, and a fibrous wall develops around them. The presence of complicated meconium ileus may be suggested by the plain radiographic findings: intra-abdominal or scrotal calcifications, bowel wall calcification, prominent air–fluid levels and soft-tissue masses.

The management of meconium peritonitis is surgical.

Distal Ileal Atresia

Ileal atresia is thought to be due to a prenatal vascular insult. If the atresia is in the distal ileum, then the infant will present with abdominal distension and delayed passage of meconium. The plain radiograph will show a low obstruction with multiple dilated loops of bowel. The contrast enema will outline a microcolon and the contrast medium cannot be refluxed into the dilated small bowel. The condition is managed surgically.

Anorectal and Cloacal Malformations

Anorectal malformations (ARMs) are a not uncommon congenital abnormality of the hindgut. Their precise aetiology is unknown, but the condition results from maldevelopment of the cloacal structure early in the first trimester. The resulting cloacal membrane is too short and the distal cloaca absent, and it is these structures that are necessary for the formation of the lower rectum and anus.[44,45] The abnormality consists of anorectal atresia, with or without a fistulous connection between the atretic anorectum and the GU tract.

Associated congenital anomalies are common. The VACTERL sequence occurs in around 45% of patients, with around 80% of this group having GU tract abnormalities. Musculoskeletal abnormalities are seen in just under half of these VACTERL patients. Cloacal exstrophy and the OEIS complex (omphalocele, exstrophy, imperforate anus and sacral anomalies) are found in up to 5% of patients. Between 2 and 8% of patients have Down's syndrome, with the vast majority of these patients having imperforate anus without fistulae.[46] Currarino's triad is the association between an anorectal malformation, bony sacral anomalies and a presacral mass lesion.

In the past, ARMs were described as either high or low lesions, depending upon where the rectum ended relative to the levator ani muscles. These terms are gradually being replaced by a classification based upon the type of fistula that is present, as this gives information regarding the localisation of the atretic anorectum and has an important bearing upon surgical planning.[46,47] In male patients, the fistula may be to the prostatic or bulbar urethra or bladder neck. In females the fistula may be to the vaginal vestibule, with true posterior vaginal wall fistulae being extremely rare. Perineal fistulae may be present in infants of either sex, as may imperforate anus and rectal atresia or stenosis, the latter groups being without fistulae.

The diagnosis should be made clinically during the baby check immediately following delivery, and if a perineal or anal abnormality is detected, then immediate referral to the local paediatric surgery team is merited.

Should the paediatric surgical team not be able to distinguish between the type of ARM present after a period of 24 h, then the traditional cross-table lateral radiograph, with the infant in the prone position and the buttocks elevated may still have a role. A radiopaque marker is placed over the anal dimple and the distance between the pouch of rectal gas and the marker is measured. A distance of < 1.0 cm implies a more distal atresia. False interpretation of the film is obtained when the film is taken on the first day of life, when there has been insufficient time for gas to reach the rectum or if the infant had not been held prone for sufficient time to allow the gas to reach the tip of the rectal pouch. If the infant is crying or straining, the rectal pouch descends through the levator sling, which will also lead to errors in interpretation. Plain radiographs are useful if they demonstrate intravesical air (implying a rectovesical or rectourethral fistula in a boy). Transperineal ultrasound is also used to measure the distance of the rectal pouch from the perineum but interpretation suffers from similar problems to the radiograph.

Infants who have a perineal fistula usually undergo a posterior sagittal anoplasty within the first 24–48 h of life. All other children with ARMs will have a defunctioning colostomy performed, with the aim of surgery being to separate the GI and GU tracts and stop faecal contamination of the latter. Definitive surgery is postponed until a later stage, when the infant has grown and all other imaging investigations are complete.

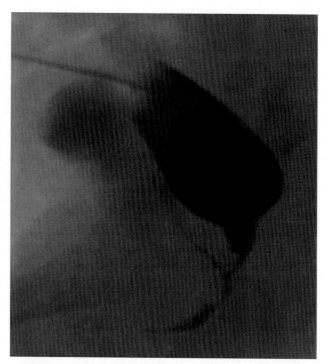

FIGURE 3-16 ■ **Rectourethral fistula.** Augmented pressure colostogram in a male infant with a high anorectal malformation. Contrast medium is seen passing through the fistula to the posterior urethra, with retrograde flow outlining the bladder.

In terms of defining the precise anatomy of the fistulous tract, the most useful investigation remains the augmented pressure colostogram. A Foley catheter is inserted into the distal segment of the colon and its balloon gently inflated so that it seals the stoma. With the patient in the lateral position, water-soluble contrast medium is hand-injected under mild pressure to distend the distal colon and define the fistulous tract. Interpretation of the images is made easier if there is a bladder catheter in situ, through which some contrast medium has been instilled; this gives anatomical markers for the bladder neck and the course of the urethra (Fig. 3-16).

The cloacal malformation occurs only in female patients. Examination of the perineum reveals a single opening into which the urethra, vagina and rectum drain. Defining the anatomy of these lesions is difficult, but ultrasound, pelvic MRI examinations and contrast studies of the cloaca all play a role. As these girls are all managed with an initial colostomy, then combined fluoroscopic studies of an augmented pressure colostogram, micturating cystourethrogram and 'cloacogram', with images obtained in both the lateral and anteroposterior positions are possible.

Ancillary radiological investigations in infants with ARMs include ultrasound of the GU tract, an echocardiogram along with radiographs of the chest and spine. A tethered spinal cord is seen in almost 50% of patients with ARMs, irrespective of the degree of lesion complexity.[48,49] Ultrasound of the spine is an excellent screening technique in the first few months of life. MRI of the spine and pelvis is extremely helpful to assess not only the spine but also the pelvic organs and pelvic floor muscles.

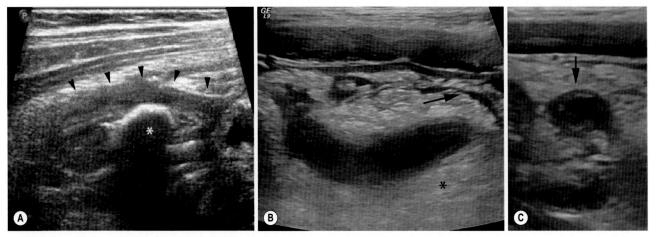

FIGURE 3-17 ■ **Sonographic findings in acute appendicitis.** (A) A longitudinal image showing a thickened appendix (arrowheads) with an appendicolith, casting an acoustic shadow (asterisk). (B, C) Sonographic appearance of a necrotic appendix with surrounding hyperechoic, inflamed mesenteric fat (asterisk) and some free fluid (arrow) suggestive of perforation. The axial view clearly shows a thickened appendix (arrow) with only two remaining layers of the appendix wall due to necrosis.

THE INFANT AND OLDER CHILD

Abdominal Pain

Abdominal pain can have numerous causes, and functional abdominal pain is not uncommon in childhood. However, important entities that may require treatment must be ruled out. One of the challenges in childhood is to accurately define the type, intensity and frequency of pain because children and adolescents have poor ability to recall episodes of abdominal pain, and also to localise and characterise the pain. Therefore the role of radiology is even more important in helping to establish the diagnosis.

The imaging approach will be tailored by the clinical information and the age-specific entities that may cause abdominal pain in childhood. In the majority of cases ultrasound is the primary technique of choice in both chronic and acute abdominal pain. Because of little body fat, children are ideally suited for ultrasound and superb images of excellent quality can be produced. Sonography is therefore a potentially powerful diagnostic tool in children; it is fast, cheap and does not expose the child to radiation. Magnetic resonance imaging (MRI) may be a complementary tool if ultrasound is unable to give sufficient diagnostic information.

The availability of MRI is sometimes limited and, occasionally, abdominal CT imaging may be necessary, especially in acute abdominal pain. However, a restrictive attitude towards the use of CT is important because of the radiation exposure. Plain abdominal radiography after the neonatal period should be reserved for the queries of intestinal obstruction and free intraperitoneal gas (with perforation).

Acute Appendicitis

Appendicitis is the most common cause for acute surgery in childhood. Thirty to 40% of children do not present with the typical findings of appendicitis.[50] Therefore

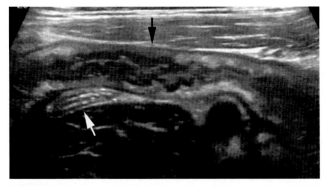

FIGURE 3-18 ■ Sonographic findings in a 12-year-old girl with suspected appendicitis showing a thickened terminal ileum (black arrow) with reduced peristalsis and a normal appendix (white arrow).

imaging is often necessary to confirm or suggest the diagnosis. Use of imaging has reduced the false-positive appendectomy rates from 20–30% to 4–8%.[51] Ultrasound should be the primary imaging technique and performing a comprehensive ultrasound examination will make CT examination redundant in most cases.[52,53] The ultrasound should be performed with a high-frequency linear transducer using a graded compression technique. The primary criteria of acute appendicitis are typically a tubular, blind-ending, non-compressible structure with maximal outer diameter over 6 mm. Other findings include wall hyperaemia or hypoperfusion (depending on the degree of inflammation/necrosis), surrounding hyperechoic mesenteric fat and the presence of an appendicolith (Fig. 3-17).[54]

CT is rarely necessary but may be an important diagnostic tool in difficult cases where ultrasound is unable to clarify and the clinical situation enforce acute surgery. Sonographical mimics of acute appendicitis may be acute salpingitis in teenage girls or terminal ileitis (see below) (Fig. 3-18).

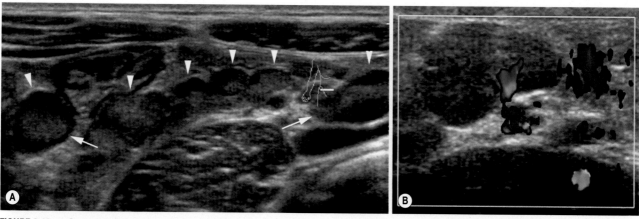

FIGURE 3-19 ■ **Sonographic appearances of mesenteric lymphadenitis.** (A) Multiple, unremarkable mesenteric lymph nodes (arrowheads) with preserved hyperechoic fatty hilum (arrows). (B) Normal hilar flow is seen on Doppler examination.

Mesenteric Lymphadenitis

Mesenteric lymphadenitis is a common cause of abdominal pain in childhood and may present as subacute or acute abdomen. The symptoms are caused by swelling of mesenteric lymph nodes as a reaction to a trivial, often asymptomatic viral infection. On ultrasound, multiple enlarged lymph nodes are seen in the root of the mesentery. The hyperechoic, fatty hilus is preserved and there is normal Doppler signal within the lymph nodes (Fig. 3-19). Mesenteric lymphadenitis is a diagnosis of exclusion and should be established and based on ultrasound findings in the absence of any other plausible explanations for the abdominal pain.[55]

Inflammatory Bowel Disease

The diagnosis of inflammatory bowel disease (IBD) encompasses Crohn's disease, ulcerative colitis and unclassified IBD. IBD is thought to develop as a result of dysregulation of the immune response to gut flora in a genetically susceptible host. The most common symptoms of inflammatory bowel disease are chronic diarrhoea, fever and weight loss but it may also present as acute or subacute abdominal pain. The gold standard for diagnosing IBD is ileocolonoscopy with biopsy. Imaging plays a role in establishing the extent of the disease, to assess possible complications and to select candidates for potential surgery.

Ultrasonography (US). In children ultrasound is the first imaging tool of choice, especially if the diagnosis is unknown. A comprehensive ultrasound to look for bowel wall thickening (BWT) has a strong negative predictive value for IBD. The sensitivity and specificity for BWT on US depends on the threshold used. A small bowel wall thickness greater than 1.5–3 mm and a colonic wall thickness over 2–3 mm is considered to be pathological. Colour Doppler US may reveal hyperaemia of the inflamed bowel and this finding may enhance the diagnosis (Fig. 3-20). Other signs of IBD on US include lack of bowel stratification, altered echogenicity of the bowel wall, hyperechoic mesenteric fat and enlarged lymph nodes. One should always look for complications of the disease, e.g. abscesses and fistula; however, the sensitivity for these features on US is low. US is a quick, radiation-free and easily available technique, but is highly operator dependent and the findings are not necessarily reproducible. The technique also has limited value in obese children and in the presence of gaseous distension of bowel.

Conventional Barium Studies. Conventional barium studies have largely been replaced by other imaging techniques such as MRI and US and play a very limited role in imaging of IBD in children because the techniques are stressful, give a high radiation dose to the patient and are unable to demonstrate extraluminal disease. Small bowel follow through (SBFT) may still play a role in the assessment of bowel obstruction but ultra-low-dose MDCT and capsule endoscopy have replaced SBFT for this indication. Barium enteroclysis should only be performed when the child is unable to undergo an MRI (Fig. 3-21).

Magnetic Resonance Imaging (MRI). The preferred technique for small bowel assessment on MRI is MR enterography. A comprehensive MRI has a high specificity and a sensitivity for bowel inflammation and includes no ionising radiation.[56] This technique is normally well tolerated by children from 6–7 years and older. Sufficient bowel distension is important for a proper assessment of the bowel wall. MR enteroclysis may be an alternative if the child is unable to drink the relatively large amount of fluid required to distend the small bowel. A low-residue diet should be given three days prior to the examination with nil per mouth from 24 h before the imaging.

MRI can estimate the length and localisation of the affected bowel and detect both intra- and extraluminal disease. However, if there is a clinical suspicion of a perianal fistula and/or abscess, dedicated pelvic MR fistulography may be required for detection and delineation of the fistula. A dynamic MRI sequence should be included to find possible bowel strictures, as this may change the treatment approach from medical to surgical. Table 3-5 shows the standard MRI sequences recommended for imaging in IBD. Motion artefacts due to lack of patient cooperation or bowel peristalsis may distort the

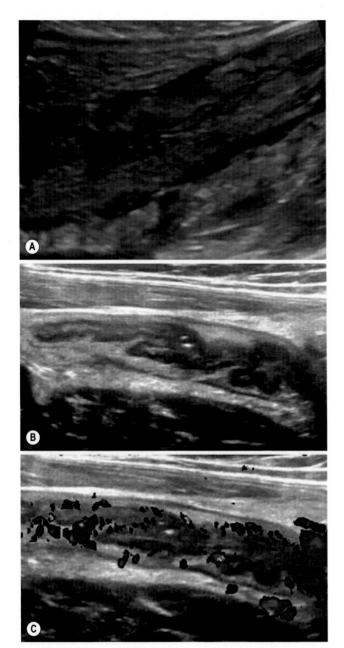

FIGURE 3-20 ■ Terminal ileitis. Ultrasound shows marked thickening of the terminal ileum and increased echogenicity of the bowel wall (A). A slightly thickened distal ileum with reduced peristalsis (B). Colour Doppler examination revealed hyperaemic bowel wall in the inflamed bowel segment (C).

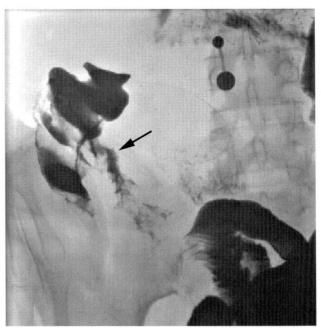

FIGURE 3-21 ■ Barium follow through (BFT) in terminal ileitis. BFT shows a narrowed and irregular bowel lumen in terminal ileitis (arrow).

TABLE 3-5 **MRI Sequences for Imaging of Inflammatory Bowel Disease**

- Hydrographic images: T2-weighted gradient echo (balanced steady-state free precession), in the axial and coronal planes. Alternatively, an ultrafast spin-echo sequence: half-Fourier single-shot turbo spin echo, in the axial and coronal planes
- Dynamic images: cine heavily T2-weighted gradient echo (balanced steady-state free precession) free breathing sequence
- Diffusion-weighted images in the axial plane, b-value >800
- Contrast series: T1W fat-suppressed images in the axial and coronal planes, pre- and post-contrast administration

---

TABLE 3-6 **MRI Signs of Inflammatory Bowel Disease**

*Bowel Loop Appearance
- Fixed
- Dilated
- Pseudo-sacculation appearance
- Strictures

*Bowel Wall
- Thickness
- Focal lesions (ulceration, pseudo-polyps, mural abscess)
- Enhancement pattern after gadolinium injection (mucosal alone, layered, global, serosal hypervascularity)
- Restricted diffusion
- Extramural signs: fibro-fatty proliferation, distended and enhancing mesenteric vessels fistula, abscess, enlarged lymph nodes

---

images. Controversies exist regarding MRI's ability to determine disease activity, both due to lack of a gold standard and because acute and chronic disease may coexist in the same bowel loop.[57] The development of new imaging techniques such as diffusion-weighted imaging (DWI) have shown to increase the sensitivity and specificity for both intraluminal and extraluminal disease in IBD (Fig. 3-22).[58] MRI signs of IBD are listed in Table 3-6.

Computed Tomography (CT). CT enteroclysis and CT enterography have become widely used techniques

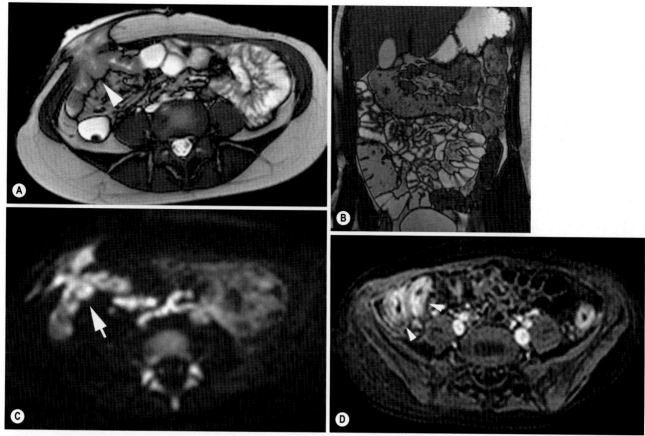

FIGURE 3-22 ■ **Inflammatory bowel disease.** MRI of Crohn's disease. (A) Axial hydrographic sequence showing thickening of the small bowel adjacent to the ileostomy (arrowhead). (B) Diffusion-weighted image of the same bowel segment with high signal suggestive of restricted diffusion. (C) Imaging in IBD should include hydrographic cine images to assess bowel peristalsis. (D) Contrast-enhanced T1W image showing contrast enhancement of thickened bowel loops.

for small bowel investigation in adults. These techniques should be avoided in children due to the high radiation dose. CT should be reserved for investigations of acute complications where US is deemed insufficient, for drainage of complex abscesses, or when the abscess is inaccessible for US-guided drainage.

Intussusception

Intussusception is a common surgical emergency in infants and young children. It is caused by telescoping of a segment of bowel (intussusceptum) into a more distal segment (intussuscipiens). The majority of children are under 1 year of age, with a peak incidence between 5 and 9 months of age; however, it may occur up to school age. Ileocolic intussusceptions are the most common type. Ileoileocolic, ileoileal and colocolic are much less common. Most (over 90%) have no lead point and are due to lymphoid hypertrophy, usually following a viral infection.

Secondary lead points (which include nasojejunal tubes, Meckel's diverticulum, intestinal polyp, duplication cyst and lymphoma) occur in 5–10% of patients. In very young infants or children over 6–7 years of age, intussusception is more likely to be caused by a secondary lead point. The clinical presentation of intussusception varies. The classical clinical signs of colicky abdominal pain, bloody stools and a palpable abdominal mass are present in less than 50% of the children. Intussusception must be treated as a surgical emergency. The clinical situation may deteriorate rapidly, particularly in infants, and may become life-threatening with hypovolaemia and shock. Prolonged symptom duration will reduce the likelihood of successful reduction.[59] Intussusception is diagnosed with ultrasound, with a sensitivity and specificity of 100% in several reported studies, even when performed by inexperienced radiologists, if properly trained.[60,61] The characteristic appearance of intussusception makes its diagnosis or exclusion very easy.

The intussusceptum is usually found just deep to the anterior abdominal wall, most often on the right side of the midline. Sonography must be performed with a high-frequency linear array transducer. The intussusception forms a mass of 3–5 cm in diameter, with a 'target appearance' in the transverse plane and a 'sandwich appearance' in the longitudinal plane. The characteristic 'crescent in doughnut' sign, a hyperechoic semilunar structure caused by the mesenteric fat pulled into the intussusceptum, facilitates the differentiation from mimickers of intussusception, like bowel wall thickening, stools and the psoas muscle (Fig. 3-23). Lymph nodes and fluid may be seen between within the intussuceptum and in some studies

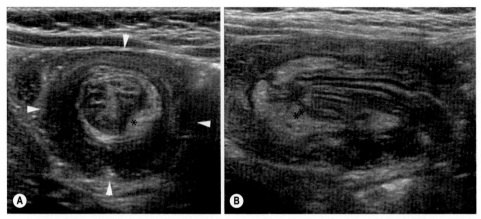

FIGURE 3-23 ■ **Intussusception is easily appreciated on ultrasound.** (A) The axial view shows the 'doughnut'—or 'target sign' (arrowheads)—caused by the multiple layers of bowel and the pathognomonic hyperechoic semilunar appearance of the mesenteric fat within the intussusceptum (asterisk). (B) The longitudinal view reveals the typical 'sandwich' appearance caused by the multiple layers of bowel wall and mesenteric fat (asterisk).

have been found to be associated with decreased hydrostatic reduction rate. Bowel necrosis is difficult to assess by ultrasonography, even with power Doppler examination of the bowel wall. Free intraperitoneal fluid is commonly seen in patients with intussusception and is therefore an unreliable indirect sign of bowel ischaemia. Ultrasonography should not only be performed to establish the diagnosis but also to look for secondary lead points and other intra-abdominal pathology unrelated to the intussusception. However, no sonographic features, including the presence of a secondary lead point, should preclude an attempt at reduction. In a well-hydrated, haemodynamically stable child the only contraindications for hydrostatic or pneumatic reduction are the presence of free intraperitoneal air or frank clinical signs of peritonitis.

The role of plain radiography in the diagnosis of intussusception is controversial. The 'classic' radiographic features of intussusception include a soft-tissue mass contrasting an air-filled bowel loop, the so-called 'meniscus sign' (Fig. 3-24). There may be dilated, gas-filled bowel loops proximal to the intussusceptum, and absence of gas within the caecum may suggest an ileocaecal intussusception. However, the caecum may be difficult to localise in a child, and the sigmoid is located on the left side of the abdomen in almost 50% of children and may be indistinguishable from the caecum on a plain radiograph. Abdominal radiographs should therefore not be routinely used in intussusception. The presence of free intraperitoneal gas is extremely rare in children with intussusception, and may be assessed by a quick fluoroscopic 'frame grab' performed before the fluoroscopically guided reduction.[61]

Image-guided reduction can be performed using a pneumatic technique or by contrast enema, under fluoroscopy or ultrasound guidance. Most centres in the UK use pneumatic reduction under fluoroscopy guidance, but the choice of technique varies across Europe and should be based on experience and expertise of the radiologist who performs the reduction (Fig. 3-25).[62] The use of sedation is also controversial. Animal studies have suggested that the use of sedation may lead to

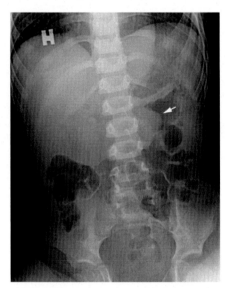

FIGURE 3-24 ■ **Intussusception.** An abdominal radiograph in a child with intussusception may show a soft-tissue mass contrasting an air-filled bowel loop, the so-called 'meniscus sign' (arrow); however, the diagnosis is made by ultrasound and the role of radiography in intussusception is controversial.

increased perforation rates; however, a prospective clinical study found an increased success rate and no difference in complications when using deep sedation with pneumatic reduction of intussusception in children.[63] Regardless of the technique used, one should aim at (and expect) a successful reduction rate over 80%.

Constipation

Constipation is probably the most common gastrointestinal problem in infants and children. Childhood functional constipation has an estimated prevalence of 3% in the Western world. The symptoms are typically infrequent painful defecation, faecal incontinence and abdominal pain.[64] This can lead to encopresis or faecal soiling, and occasionally can cause acute, severe abdominal pain.

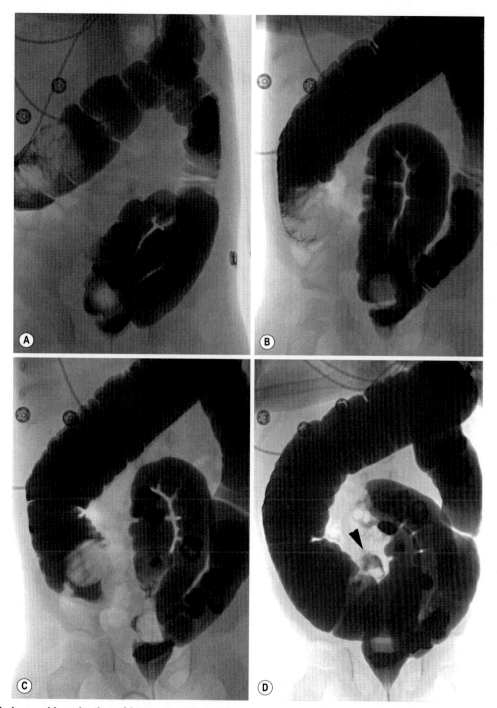

FIGURE 3-25 ■ **Hydrographic reduction of intussusception.** (A) Contrast defect in the proximal colon transversum due to the intussusceptum. (B) Further reduction of the intussusception into the colon ascendens. (C) Small contrast defect in the caecum. Normally the last part of the reduction is the most difficult due to oedema of the ileocaecal valve. (D) Contrast filling of the terminal ileum (arrowhead) as a sign of successful reduction. Proper filling of proximal small bowel loops is advised to ensure complete reduction.

Less than 5% of children with constipation have an underlying disease. The diagnosis of constipation is essentially clinically and radiological investigations play a very limited role in the work-up of constipation, and should not routinely be performed in children with functional constipation.[65] The plain abdominal radiograph will demonstrate the degree of faecal loading and dilatation of the large bowel; however, the presence of faecal loading on the plain radiograph does not necessarily indicate constipation, and several studies show that plain radiographs have a low sensitivity and specificity for diagnosing constipation.

Radiological investigations should only be performed in a carefully selected group of patients where an underlying cause is suspected. US should be the first imaging tool in chronic abdominal pain when radiological work-up is indicated. US gives a good overview of the bowel and intra-abdominal organs and can help differentiate a faecal mass from a pathological mass. Other imaging techniques described for the evaluation of constipation include the measurement of colonic transit time using radiopaque markers, fluoroscopy and MRI defecography. These are only indicated in highly selected cases.[66]

Intestinal Motility Disorders

'Intestinal motility disorder' is a term used to describe a variety of abnormalities that have, in common, reduced motility of the bowel and no organic occlusion of the bowel lumen. They can be divided into acute and chronic disorders.

Acute Dysmotility. Acute dysmotility includes paralytic ileus in which there is temporary cessation of peristalsis in the gut. This simulates intestinal obstruction, as there is failure of propagation of intestinal contents. Acute gastroenteritis can simulate small bowel obstruction by causing a local paralytic ileus, with dilatation of the affected segment of bowel and multiple fluid levels on an erect plain radiograph of the abdomen.

Chronic Motility Disorders. Chronic motility disorders include primary abnormalities of the bowel—Hirschsprung's disease (aganglionosis), hypoganglionosis which is rare and mimics Hirschsprung's disease, and neuronal intestinal dysplasia, which is a defect of autonomic neurogenesis characterised by an absent or rudimentary sympathetic ganglion innervation of the gut or by hyperplasia of cholinergic nerve fibres and hyperplasia of neuronal bodies in intramural nerve plexuses.

Chronic Intestinal Pseudo-obstruction. Chronic intestinal pseudo-obstruction (CIP) is rare and represents a spectrum of diseases that have in common clinical manifestations consisting of recurrent symptoms mimicking bowel obstruction over weeks or years. The age of presentation varies from the newborn to adulthood. The condition is due to a visceral neuropathy or myopathy, which can be familial or non-familial, resulting in a lack of coordinated intestinal motility. Megacystis–microcolon–intestinal hypoperistalsis syndrome is the most severe form of CIP and is usually fatal in the first year of life. Plain radiographs of the bowel will show loops of bowel with pronounced dilatation (Fig. 3-26). The diagnosis is made by intestinal manometry and biopsy. A contrast medium enema can exclude mechanical obstruction in children with acute symptoms.[67]

Henoch-Schönlein Purpura

Henoch-Schönlein purpura (HSP) is an acute, small vessel vasculitis that occurs almost exclusively in childhood. The manifestations are purpuric skin lesions (without thrombocytopenia), gastrointestinal manifestations, arthritis or nephritis. In most cases the changes of HSP are completely reversible and healing takes place in 3–4 weeks.[68]

Abdominal pain is a common symptom, and the GI involvement is caused by oedema, bleeding, ulceration and intussusception of the intestine. Ultrasound is the

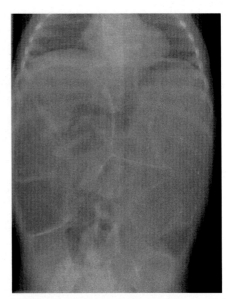

FIGURE 3-26 ■ Chronic intestinal obstruction. Multiple, hugely dilated bowel loops throughout the abdomen in a child with chronic intestinal pseudo-obstruction. (Small, dense pellets from intestinal transit time examination are seen within the bowel loops on the left side of the abdomen.)

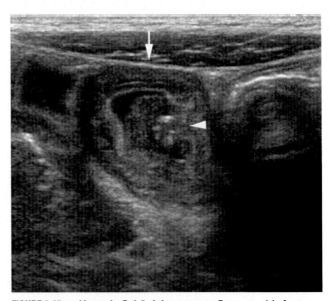

FIGURE 3-27 ■ Henoch–Schönlein purpura. Sonographic features of bowel wall thickening (arrow) due to intramural haemorrhage (arrowhead) in a child with Henoch-Schönlein purpura.

imaging technique of choice in HSP and will detect most surgical cases.[69] The sonographic features of HSP are uni- or multifocal thickening of the bowel wall accompanied by reduced peristalsis with normal or slightly dilated bowel loops between the thickened segments (Fig. 3-27).[70] Some patients have a small amount of intraperitoneal free fluid. Intussusception is easily seen on US, with a sensitivity of up to 100%.[61] Intussusceptions in HSP are most often ileoileal, hence not amenable to pneumatic or hydrostatic reduction. However, small bowel intussusception often reduces spontaneously. Ileo-coloc intussusception may also occur and should be treated as idiopathic intussusception (see above). Radiographs may show signs of thickened bowel wall (Fig. 3-28) but are less sensitive to these changes than US.

Abdominal Distension

Enteric Duplication Cysts

Enteric duplication cysts are uncommon congenital anomalies and are due to abnormal canalisation of the GI tract. They can occur anywhere along the length of the gut but are most frequent in the ileum where they lie along the mesenteric border and share a common muscle wall blood supply. They have a mucosal lining and 43% contain ectopic gastric mucosa. The majority of duplication cysts do not communicate with the GI tract. Duplication cysts may be diagnosed antenatally. If small and non-obstructing, they may not cause any symptoms.

Clinically they usually present in the first year of life with vomiting or abdominal pain. Infection or haemorrhage into the cyst can cause it to enlarge and suddenly cause pain. A duplication cyst may act as a lead point of intussusception. An abdominal radiograph is useful to assess bowel obstruction or signs of bowel obstruction and may show displacement of bowel loops or even a soft-tissue mass; however, the cyst itself is normally not seen on plain radiographs (Fig. 3-29). US will demonstrate the cyst, which is usually spherical in shape and less often tubular. The cyst is typically anechoic but may have echogenic contents if there has been a bleeding into the cyst. The classical feature of an intestinal duplication cyst is the presence of bowel wall lining the cyst with an inner echogenic mucosal layer and an outer hypoechoic muscular layer (Fig. 3-30).[71] This 'double layer sign' on

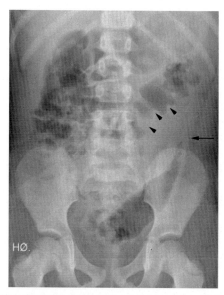

FIGURE 3-28 ■ Radiographic features of bowel wall thickening. 'Thumbprint' appearances of the transverse colon (arrowheads) and narrowing of the lumen (arrow).

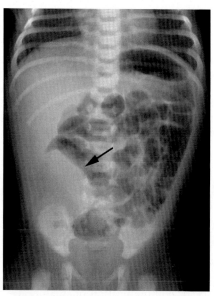

FIGURE 3-29 ■ Intestinal duplication cyst. The initial radiograph in a child with an intestinal duplication cyst showed a round soft-tissue mass on the right side of the abdomen (arrow) and slightly dilated bowel loops. The child presented with abdominal distension and increased regurgitation.

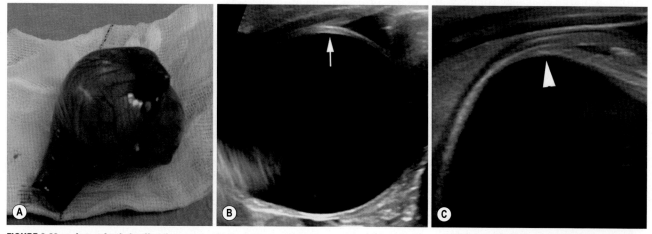

FIGURE 3-30 ■ Intestinal duplication cyst. (A) Pathological specimen of a resected duplication cyst. (B) Sonographic features of the duplication cyst showing an anechoic cyst with a 'double layer' sign of the cyst wall. (C) Magnified image of the cyst wall revealing multiple layers in keeping with an intestinal duplication cyst.

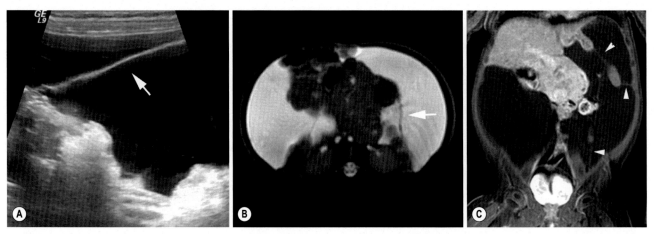

FIGURE 3-31 ■ Imaging characteristics of mesenteric lymphangioma. (A) Ultrasound of the abdomen shows a large, septated fluid-filled structure with debris. (B) T2W MRI shows a large, septated cystic mass, displacing the bowel cranially and towards the mid-abdomen. (C) T1W fat-saturated MRI after administration of intravenous contrast shows subtle enhancement of the intracystic septae.

US is characteristic for intestinal duplication cysts (Figs. 3-4 and 3-30B). However, the sonographic appearance of other intra-abdominal cysts may mimic the double layer sign. Therefore, thorough examination with a high-frequency transducer to identify the split hypoechoic muscularis propria layer (or all five layers of the cyst wall) increases the specificity in making the sonographic diagnosis of a true duplication cyst (Fig. 3-31C).[72] ^{99m}Tc-pertechnetate is taken up by ectopic gastric mucosa and is helpful in diagnosing duplication cysts presenting with gastrointestinal bleeding.[73]

Mesenteric Cysts

Mesenteric cysts (intra-abdominal lymphangioma) have been discussed in 'The Neonate' section. Pathologically there is lack of communication of small bowel or retroperitoneal lymphatic tissue with the main lymphatic vessels, resulting in formation of a cystic mass. They most often present in childhood and children are more likely to present acutely with pain, abdominal distension, fever or anorexia due to haemorrhage into the cyst, infection, or torsion. Large cysts may compress the ureters or lead to bowel obstruction.[74]

Plain abdominal radiographs show a soft-tissue mass, which displaces adjacent bowel loops. Occasionally the cyst wall is calcified. US examination demonstrates a thin-walled, uni- or multilocular cystic mass that may be adherent to the solid organs and bowel. The cyst wall consists of a single layer, which contrasts with the double-layered wall seen with enteric duplication cysts. If the intracystic fluid is chylous, infected, or haemorrhagic, then echogenic debris will be present. MRI or CT can more precisely define the anatomical margins of the cyst, but again, MRI is the preferred imaging method due to radiation protection. MRI can also characterise the cyst content, which will vary according to the cyst content.

Occasionally, large mesenteric lymphangiomas may be misinterpreted as septated ascites; however, the thin septae contain small vessels and may enhance following

the administration of intravenous contrast material. Imaging with US, MRI or CT is sensitive to this diagnosis (Fig. 3-31).[75]

Non-bilious Vomiting

Vomiting is not a disease but a symptom that can be caused by numerous conditions, both gastrointestinal and extragastrointestinal (Table 3-7). Vomiting is the forceful ejection of gastric contents from the stomach up the oesophagus, and through the mouth, and is never physiological but the underlying condition may be harmless.

Gastro-oesophageal reflux is the backflow of undigested food from the stomach and up the oesophagus and is common in infants and children and may be normal up to 18 months of age. GOR can occur in healthy children without causing any symptoms. However, GOR may mimic or trigger vomiting. Radiological investigations should be performed when there are warning signals requiring investigation in infants with either GOR or vomiting, to rule out underlying causes that need treatment (Table 3-8).

Gastro-oesophageal Reflux Disease

GORD is present when the reflux of gastric contents causes troublesome symptoms and/or complications. Diagnosing GORD may be difficult, particularly in infants and young children. There is no agreed perfect method for detecting GORD but the diagnosis is usually made on the basis of questionnaires, 24 h pH monitoring and impedance measurements. Both ultrasound and fluoroscopy with contrast medium may show the presence of GOR, but radiological investigations play no role in establishing the diagnosis of GORD.

Barium contrast study of the upper gastrointestinal tract is useful to confirm or rule out anatomical abnormalities of the upper gastrointestinal tract in the presence of GORD, such as malrotation with intermittent volvulus or hiatus hernia (Fig. 3-32).[76]

TABLE 3-7   Causes of Vomiting in Children

*Obstructive Gastrointestinal Causes
- Pyloric stenosis
- Malrotation with intermittent volvulous
- Intestinal duplication cyst
- Antral or duodenal web
- Severe constipation
- Foreign body
- Incarcerated hernia

*Non-obstructive Gastrointestinal Causes
- Gastroenteritis
- Achalasia
- Gastroparesis
- Peptic ulcer
- Eosinophilic oesophagitis or gastritis
- Food allergy
- Inflammatory bowel disease
- Appendicitis or pancreatitis

*Neurological Disorders
- Increased intracranial pressure
- Childhood migraine

*Infections
- All infections in childhood may cause vomiting, particularly in the younger child

*Metabolic and Endocrine Disorders
*Renal
- Obstructive nephropathy
- Renal failure

*Cardiac
- Heart failure
- Vascular rings

*Others
- Munchausen syndrome by proxy
- Child neglect or abuse
- Self-induced vomiting
- Cyclic vomiting syndrome

TABLE 3-8   Warning Signals Requiring Investigation in Children with Regurgitation or Vomiting

- Bilious vomiting
- Gastrointestinal bleeding
- Consistently forceful vomiting
- Onset of vomiting after 6 months of life
- Failure to thrive
- Diarrhoea
- Severe constipation
- Fever
- Lethargy
- Hepatosplenomegaly
- Bulging fontanelle
- Macro-or microcephaly
- Seizures
- Abdominal tenderness or distension
- Documented or suspected genetic or metabolic disorder

Organoaxial Torsion and Gastric Volvulus

Sometimes, particularly in younger children, **organoaxial** torsion of the stomach may be the cause of forceful regurgitation or vomiting. The ligaments anchoring the

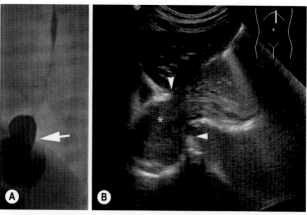

FIGURE 3-32 ■ **Hiatus hernia can be diagnosed on ultrasound or an upper gastrointestinal contrast study.** (A) Fluoroscopic image of a sliding hiatus hernia (arrow). (B) Sonographic appearance of the hiatus hernia with widening of the oesophageal hiatus (arrowheads) through which the stomach slides to protrude into the thoracic cavity (asterisk).

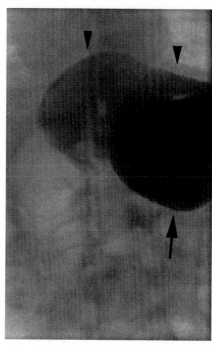

FIGURE 3-33 ■ **Organoaxial torsion of the stomach.** Fluoroscopic contrast study showing organoaxial torsion of the stomach. The greater curvature is in an inverse position (arrowheads) and the antrum of the stomach is flipped caudally (arrow).

stomach are dynamic to allow expansion. Absence of one or more ligaments and ligamentous laxity increase the risk of gastric volvulus. In **organoaxial** torsion, the stomach flips upward along its long axis and the gastrooesophageal junction and pylorus maintain their normal position. There is no risk of ischaemia; however, there may be full or partial obstruction of the gastric outlet. Gastric distension or gas-filled colon may predispose to this condition. A fluoroscopic barium study will reveal a distended stomach where the greater curvature is positioned superior to and to the right of the lesser curvature (Fig. 3-33). The condition is normal in infancy

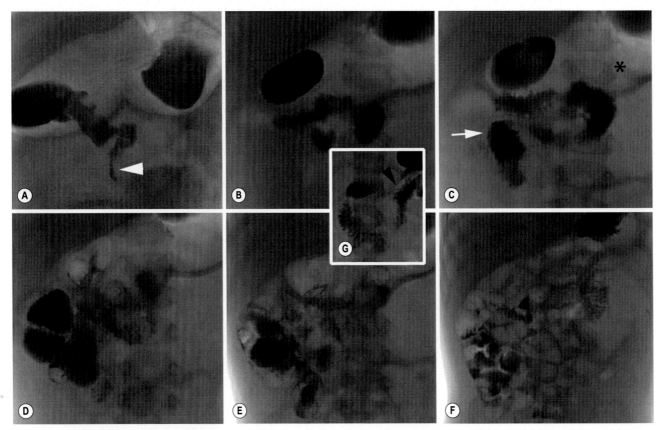

FIGURE 3-34 ■ **(A–G) Malrotation without volvulus.** An upper gastrointestinal contrast study performed in an 18-month-old girl with intermittent abdominal pain and failure to thrive. The initial, lateral image shows contrast passing to the D2, which turns caudally (arrowhead). Normally the DJF should be placed to the left of the spine, at the level of the duodenal bulb (asterisk). In this patient the duodenum did not have the normal U-shape and the DJF was located low, on the right side of the abdomen. Delayed images show the entire small intestine on the right side of the abdomen. The small image shows a normal, U-shaped duodenum with a normal DJF (arrowhead).

and can be seen as an incidental finding. In symptomatic older children gastropexy may be required.

Mesenteroaxial volulus is a rare entity where the stomach twists transversely around its mesenteric axis, causing close approximation of the gastro-oesophageal junction and pylorus. This is always a surgical emergency, causing gastric obstruction with high risk of ischaemia. The child presents acutely with vomiting and abdominal pain and distension.[77]

Malrotation with Chronic Intestinal Obstruction or Intermittent Volvulus

Malrotation with midgut volvulus is described in detail under 'The Neonate' section. It is, however, important to emphasise that even though symptomatic malrotation most frequently presents in the neonatal period with midgut volvulus, it may also occur in the older child with either acute or chronic symptoms.[78] The chronic presentation is a diagnostic challenge. The most common symptoms are crampy abdominal pain, failure to thrive, recurrent vomiting and signs of malabsorbtion. The symptoms may be non-specific and diagnostic delay is common. Pathophysiology of these chronic symptoms may relate to intestinal obstruction from Ladd's bands or from venous and lymphatic congestion in intermittent

volvulus.[79] Surgical treatment is recommended in all patients, even when asymptomatic due to the lifelong risk of complications.[80] The diagnosis can normally be made from an upper gastrointestinal barium examination (Fig. 3-34) but is occasionally seen on cross-sectional imaging investigations for chronic abdominal complaints.

Hypertrophic Pyloric Stenosis

Hypertrophic pyloric stenosis (HPS) is the commonest surgical cause of vomiting in infants. It typically presents with projectile vomiting 2–8 weeks after birth. It is caused by hypertrophy of the pyloric muscle and mucosa with an elongated, narrow pyloric canal that fails to relax, which leads to gastric outlet obstruction. Boys are more frequently affected than girls, and there is a five-fold increased risk with a first-degree relative with this condition. The classic clinical presentation is a dehydrated, cachectic child with a palpable 'olive'-shaped mass in the upper abdomen. However, there has been a change in the epidemiology over the last decades and children are admitted to hospital before they get severe symptoms and so the 'olive' mass is seen in less than 30% of the patients.[81] Ultrasound is the first technique of choice when there is clinical suspicion of HPS, and has replaced barium studies in diagnosing this condition, with a

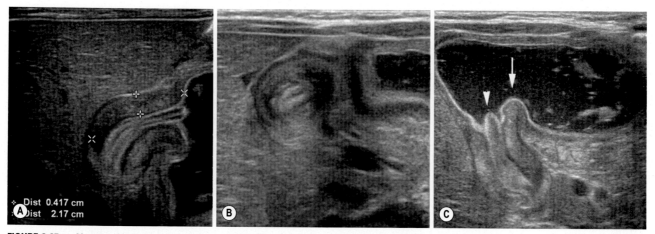

FIGURE 3-35 ■ Hypertrophic pyloric stenosis (HPS). Sonographic appearances diagnostic of HPS with an elongated and thickened pyloric muscle (A, B). A longitudinal image of the pyloric muscle shows the hypertropic mucosa (arrowhead) and the hypertropic muscle (arrow) protruding into the fluid-filled stomach (C).

reported sensitivity and specificity of up to 98 and 100%, respectively.[82] US allows assessment of the pyloric morphology and pyloric movement. The morphological features include a hypoechoic, thickened pyloric muscle, measuring more than 3 mm in transverse diameter and an elongated pyloric canal greater than 12 mm in length (Figs. 3-35A and B). The obstructed pyloric canal is lined with hypertrophic, hyperechoic mucosa. The hypertrophic muscle typically bulges into the antrum of a fluid-filled stomach, creating the so-called 'shoulder sign', and the double-layered hypertrophic mucosa protrudes into the stomach, creating the so-called 'nipple sign' (Fig. 3-35C). The sonographic appearance of the hypertrophied pylorus resembles that of the uterine cervix and is sometimes referred to as the 'cervix sign' (Fig. 3-35C). Abnormal, exaggerated peristaltic waves due to the stomach trying to force its contents past the narrowed pyloric outlet is also seen on real-time US. The treatment is surgical pyloromyotomy most often performed laparoscopically.[83]

Omphalomesenteric (Vitelline) Duct Remnants

The omphalomesenteric (vitelline) duct is a normal fetal structure that connects the midgut to the extraembryonic yolk sac. The omphalomesenteric duct usually involutes in the mid first trimester. Its persistence can give rise to a variety of congenital malformations. The majority of symptomatic omphalomesenteric ducts occur in boys and 60% of patients present before the age of 10. The clinical presentation depends on the exact underlying malformation.

Meckel's diverticulum is the most common end result of the spectrum of omphalomesenteric duct anomalies. Other presentations include umbilicoileal fistula, umbilical sinus and umbilical cyst. There may also be a fibrous cord running from the ileum to the umbilicus. Small bowel obstruction from this cord is the most common cause of ileus in otherwise healthy children and adolescents. Rarely, the entire duct remains patent. The symptoms present in the neonatal period with discharge of faeces from the umbilicus, or the ileum can prolapse onto the anterior abdominal wall.

Meckel's Diverticulum

The most common type of omphalomesenteric duct remnant is the Meckel's diverticulum, which arises on the antimesenteric border of the ileum. This contrasts with the enteric duplication cysts that are located on the mesenteric border of the small bowel. The diverticulum is present in 2–4% of the population. The size of Meckel's diverticula varies, with those greater than 5 cm in length being considered 'giant'. Most are located within 60 cm of the ileocaecal junction. All the layers of the intestine are contained within their walls and frequently contain islands of gastric and/or pancreatic mucosa. The most common presentations are melaena caused by hemorrhage from peptic ulceration, and ileus due to intussusception or volvulus around a Meckel's diverticulum. Meckel's diverticula may also become entrapped within an inguinal hernia, which has become known as Littre's hernia. Patients may present with abdominal pain, and occasionally peritonitis caused by diverticulitis or perforation. The diagnosis of Meckel's diverticulum is difficult to establish preoperatively and the investigations should be tailored by the clinical presentation. The Meckel's diverticula that haemorrhage contain ectopic gastric mucosa in 95% of cases and ^{99m}Tc-pertechnetate scintigraphy can be diagnostic. Plain radiographs can diagnose the presence of ileus and occasionally a soft-tissue mass may be seen (Fig. 3-36); however, the diagnosis is most often made intraoperatively. Occationally, enteroliths may be seen as peripheral calcifications with radiolucent centres. This is the most specific feature for Meckel's diverticulum on plain radiographs. An ultrasound is often performed if the clinical situation allows for further investigation. The diverticulum itself may not be identified on US; however, abscess formation and signs of inflammation with hyperechoic mesenteric fat may be seen in acute diverticulitis. Intussusception caused by a Meckels's diverticulum will also be identified with US. CT is occasionally performed in the evaluation of intestinal obstruction or peritonitis; however, the diverticulum itself is most often difficult to identify. Conventional barium studies may be useful in patients with chronic, persistent symptoms and negative cross-sectional or nuclear imaging. The characteristic feature of a Meckel's diverticulum is a saccular, blind-ending pouch on the antimesenteric border of the ileum with a triradiate fold pattern converging with the ileum. Neoplasms arising in Meckel's diverticula are very rare and do not occur in childhood.[84]

Gastrointestinal Malignancies

Primary gastrointestinal tumours are rare in childhood. Colorectal cancer or gastrointestinal stromal tumours (GIST) may occasionally be seen in children but are most often part of a syndrome. Lymphomas account for 10–15% of all childhood cancers. Extranodal involvement is frequently seen in non-Hodgkin's lymphoma (NHL) and more frequently seen in children compared to adults. The gastrointestinal tract is the most common

site of manifestation. The distal ileum, caecum, appendix and ascending colon are most commonly affected and the involvement may be multifocal (Fig. 3-37). There is marked bowel wall thickening with stenosis or dilatation of the affected segment. The lymphomatous infiltrate is hypoechoic on ultrasound and shows soft-tissue attenuation with sparse contrast enhancement on CT or MRI, and diffusion-weighted sequences show restricted diffusion (Fig. 3-38). In contrast to inflammatory causes of bowel wall thickening, loss of stratification appears early in lymphomatous involvement of the bowel wall. Mesenteric and retroperitoneal lymph node involvement may be seen in both Hodgkin's lymphoma (HL) and NHL. Ascites is commonly seen. The spleen is frequently involved in both HL and NHL. Liver involvement rarely occurs without splenic involvement and is most commonly seen in NHL. The imaging findings in diffuse lymphomatous involvement of the liver and spleen are non-specific. On both MRI and US the parenchyma may be normal or show a hazy, salt-and-pepper appearance. There may or may not be hepatosplenomegaly.[85]

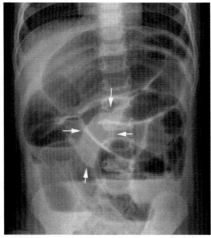

FIGURE 3-36 ■ **Meckel's diverticulum.** Abdominal radiograph of a 2-year-old boy with acute abdominal pain and clinical signs of peritonitis. The image shows dilated bowel loops and gas–fluid levels suggestive of mechanical ileus. Meckel's diverticulum can be seen as a saccular soft-tissue shadow in the mid-abdomen (arrows).

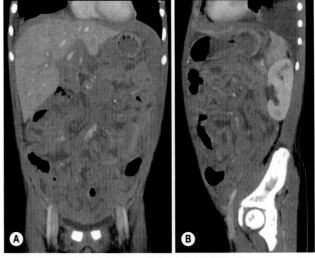

FIGURE 3-37 ■ **Small bowel lymphoma (A, B).** A coronal and sagittal reformatted contrast-enhanced abdominal CT examination of a 12-year-old boy with non-Hodgkin's lymphoma, presenting with abdominal pain, showing multifocal thickening of the intestinal wall and ascites. Pleural effusion is also present.

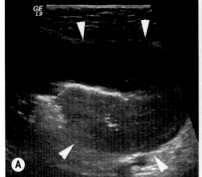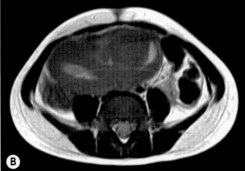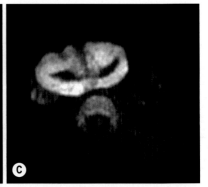

FIGURE 3-38 ■ **Focal lymphomatous involvement of the small bowel.** (A) Ultrasound revealed a very thick, hypoechoic bowel wall with loss of normal stratification (arrowheads). MRI of the same patient showed a slightly dilated loop of bowel with marked bowel wall thickening, which returned an intermediate signal on a T2W image (B) and a high signal on a diffusion-weighted image in keeping with restricted diffusion (C).

THE IMMUNOCOMPROMISED CHILD

Various abdominal complications can be encountered in young cancer patients following chemotherapy. They often present with diffuse abdominal complaints but may also be asymptomatic. The most common abdominal complications of chemotherapy in childhood are listed in Table 3-9. Some of the entities are rare, and some are specific for children undergoing chemotherapy. It is therefore important to recognise the signs of these complications to improve patient's outcome.

Gallstones, sludge or crystals may be seen as an incidental finding and may be related to the specific drug used or to prolonged illness. The findings may disappear spontaneously. Cholelcystitis may occur as a complication of cholelithiasis; however, acalculous cholecystitis is more commonly seen. The gall bladder is best evaluated with US using the high-frequency linear transducer. Gallstones are freely moving, hyperechoic objects with posterior shadowing within the gall bladder (Fig. 3-39). Sludge is seen as a hyperechoic, liquid material and

crystals or sludge balls may resemble gallstones but without posterior shadowing. Acalculous cholecystitis is diagnosed by the presence of a clinically painful gall bladder, and US showing wall oedema with or without overdistension of the gall bladder.

Liver steatosis is a common finding, particularly in children undergoing treatment for acute lymphatic leukaemia. The steatosis may be focal or diffuse. It is important to differentiate liver fatty infiltration from diffuse leukaemic liver infiltration. Focal liver steatosis will follow a typical distribution with hyperechogenic areas on US, due to fat deposition around the main branches of porta hepatis. Steatosis is easily diagnosed on MRI, where there will be loss of signal on the opposed-phase images relative to the in-phase images on proton shift sequences.[86]

Liver fibrosis and siderosis may also occur as a consequence of treatment for childhood malignancies. In both liver fibrosis and siderosis the liver will be hyperechoic relative to the kidney. Siderosis is caused by heamosiderine deposition within the liver, which, due to the ferromagnetic effect of haemosiderin, will return low signal on both T1 and T2 sequences.

Veno-occlusive disease is a rare entity but a severe complication related to chemotherapy with indirect, non-specific findings on imaging. It affects the small hepatic vessels and sinusoids, leading to high resistance within the liver and, importantly, thrombi within the large vessels are not seen. On imaging there may be hepatomegaly, periportal oedema, reversed portal venous flow, high RI within the hepatic artery and ascites. The diagnosis is made by biopsy.

Typhilitis is an opportunistic infection of the bowel caused by the patient's own intestinal flora. It typically occurs in a neutropenic patient and most often affects the terminal ileum and caecum, but may be seen in any part of the bowel. It presents as bowel wall thickening, with or without dilatation of the proximal bowel. Ultrasound is the technique of choice to diagnose and follow up patients with typhilitis but CT may be used in an acute

TABLE 3-9	Abdominal Complications of Chemotherapy in Childhood

***Gall bladder**
• Sludge or sludge balls
• Stones
• Acalculous cholecystitis

***Liver**
• Steatosis
• Siderosis
• Veno-occlusive disease

***Typhilitis**
***Pancreatitis**
***Fungal Oesophagitis**

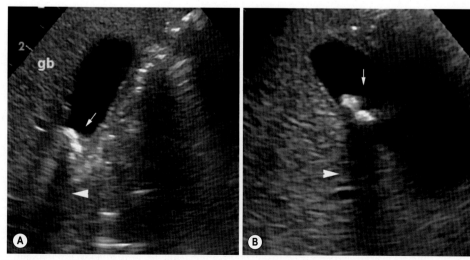

FIGURE 3-39 ■ **Gallstones.** Abdominal ultrasound of a 1-year-old child on chemotherapy for leukaemia, (A) in the supine position and (B) in the decubitus position, revealed two hyperechoic, mobile, round structures (arrows) with posterior shadowing (arrowheads) in keeping with gallstones.

setting to rule out other entities like pneumatosis intestinalis and bowel perforation.[87]

Gastrointestinal Manifestations of Acquired Immune Deficiency Syndrome

Opportunistic infections account for most of the GI tract manifestations of acquired immune deficiency syndrome (AIDS) in children.

Primary lymphoma and Kaposi's sarcoma occur in the adult GI tract but are relatively rare in human immunodeficiency virus (HIV)-infected children. The most common symptoms include acute or chronic diarrhoea, failure to thrive, oesophagitis due to *Candida* invasion, and, less often, cytomegalovirus (CMV) or herpes simplex virus. Imaging is usually not required.[88] Abdominal lymphadenopathy is common in paediatric AIDS and can be idiopathic (where no causative agent is found). Infection, Kaposi's sarcoma and lymphoma also cause lymph node enlargement. Lympadenopathy is the most common finding in intra-abdominal manifestations of tuberculosis in children. US is useful in the evaluation of abdominal lymphadenopathy.[89] Cross-sectional imaging may be required to evaluate the extent of the abdominal disease and potential solid organ involvement.

ABDOMINAL MANIFESTATIONS OF CYSTIC FIBROSIS

The gastrointestinal manifestations of cystic fibrosis (CF) are primarily caused by the abnormal viscous luminal secretions within hollow viscera, and the excretory ducts of solid organs. Abdominal complications of cystic fibrosis can present at any age from neonates to adolescence. The first manifestation of CF may be meconium ileus, which presents in the neonatal period (see 'The Neonate' section). An equivalent to meconium ileus, appearing later in life, is the distal intestinal obstruction syndrome (DIOS). Plain radiographs will reveal faecal impaction in

the distal small ileum and right colon with various degrees of proximal small bowel dilatation (Fig. 3-40). Intussusception occurs in 1% of all patients with CF and may manifest as recurrent abdominal pain. Intussusception is diagnosed with US (see above) and is most often ileocolic. Symptomatic small bowel intussusception that necessitates surgery occurs more frequently in children with cystic fibrosis[90] (Fig. 3-41). Fibrosing colonopathy is related to the use of pancreatic enzyme replacement therapy and is also seen more frequently in children with DIOS. A fluoroscopic barium enema study will reveal multiple colonic strictures and irregularities of the colonic mucosa. Enlargement of the appendix is seen in most

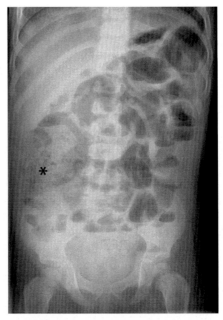

FIGURE 3-40 ■ Distal intestinal obstruction syndrome (DIOS) in a 2-year-old child with cystic fibrosis, presenting with abdominal pain. The plain abdominal radiograph shows faecal impaction (asterisk) in the distal small bowel and proximal colon with dilated small bowel proximal to the obstruction.

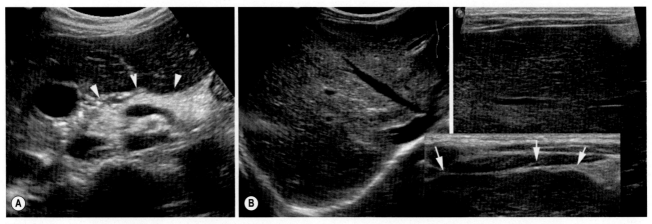

FIGURE 3-41 ■ Sonographic findings in cystic fibrosis. (A) A hyperechoic, small pancreas (arrowheads) is a frequent finding in patients with cystic fibrosis and pancreatic insufficiency. Sonographic findings in cystic fibrosis liver disease include increased echogenicity due to fatty infiltration (B). Careful examination with a high-frequency linear transduser may reveal coarse echogenicity (B) and nodular surface of the liver (small image, arrows) as early signs of cirrhossis.

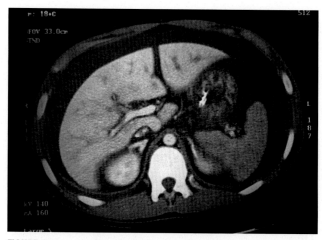

FIGURE 3-42 ■ **Hypoperfusion complex.** Axial CT showing peri-portal low attenuation, small IVC, diminished and patchy enhancement of the spleen, intense enhancement of the adrenal glands and kidneys and a haemoperitoneum.

asymptomatic patients with CF. This is caused by intra-luminal mucus stagnation. US will show an increased diameter of the appendix but without thickening of the appendiceal wall and there is absence of periappendiceal inflammation. Appendicitis occurs less frequently in patients with CF. The symptoms are often misinterpreted as DIOS or masked due to the use of antibiotics. The diagnostic delay leads to increased risk of complications.[91] Exocrine pancreatic insufficiency is seen in up to 95% of children with CF at 1 year of age. The most common findings are fatty replacement or fibrosis; hence the imaging findings vary from a large, lobulated pancreas with fatty infiltration to a small fibrotic panceas. Pancreatic cysts are also a frequent finding as a result of obstructed exocrine ducts. Pancreatic cystosis, where the pancreas is completely replaced by cysts, may be seen. Hepatobiliary involvement is also common in CF and ranges from asymptomatic gallstones to biliary cirrhosis. Hepatosteatosis is the most common abnormality of the liver parenchyma.[92]

ABDOMINAL TRAUMA

Blunt abdominal trauma accounts for 80% of traumatic injuries in childhood. Computed tomography is the imaging method of choice in the evaluation of abdominal and pelvic injury after blunt trauma in haemodynamically stable children. CT classification systems for grading intra-abdominal injuries apply to children as well as adults; however, children are more often treated conservatively. Ultrasound may play a role in follow-up of abdominal trauma, and the application of intravenous ultrasound contrast enhances the sensitivity and specificity of organ injuries and ongoing haemmorhage. Plain radiographs have low sensitivity in detecting intra-abdominal injuries, but may reveal free intraperitoneal gas; however, when bowel perforation is suspected, CT is the technique of choice.

Multi-phase CT should be avoided in children due to the high radiation burden. The morphological

characteristics of the paediatric abdomen, abdominal wall and rib cage may lead to different injuries following blunt trauma than normally seen in adults.

The liver is the most commonly affected viscus in blunt trauma in children, followed by splenic injuries. The kidneys are often affected and injuries to the vessels or collecting system typically result from deceleration, because the kidneys in children have greater laxity than in adults.

Bowel injuries and pancreatic injuries are rare in children but can be seen due to compression of the rib cage against the spine. Another mechanism for pancreatic and bowel injury in children is the direct impact from a bicycle handlebar to the abdomen. Associated rib fractures may not always be seen due to the high elasticity of the growing skeleton. Lap-belt ecchymoses represent an important high-risk marker for injury, particularly to the lumbar spine, bowel and bladder.[93] Young children have a relatively high centre of gravity, which produces shearing forces by the seat belt.

The **hypoperfusion complex** or shock bowel is due to poorly compensated hypovolaemic shock, which results in dilated, fluid-filled loops of bowel, and is a more frequent finding in children than adults. On CT there is intense contrast enhancement of the bowel wall mucosa and thickening of the bowel wall. The major abdominal blood vessels and kidneys also show intense enhancement, and the calibre of the aorta and inferior vena cava are reduced. Enhancement of the spleen and pancreas is decreased due to splanchnic vasoconstriction (Fig. 3-42).[94] Always be aware of the possibility of non-accidental injury (NAI) in children with abdominal trauma. NAI is described in Chapter 6, 'Paediatric Musculoskeletal Trauma: The Radiology of Non-accidental and Accidental Injury'.

LIVER

Imaging Techniques

US

Grey-scale US allows detailed assessment of the liver parenchyma provided that every section is imaged systematically[95,96] and a high-frequency linear probe is used. The linear probe is particularly helpful for evaluation of the liver surface (e.g. undulations seen in cirrhosis), small parenchymal focal lesions (e.g. small fungal foci (Fig. 3-43), small or diffuse metastases) and diffuse parenchymal processes (e.g. congenital hepatic fibrosis (Fig. 3-44). A curved or vector probe is helpful for assessing the deeper liver in older children. Lower-frequency probes may be necessary if there is dense hepatic fibrosis.

Colour Doppler is mandatory and is used to assess the hepatic and portal veins and the hepatic artery, the presence of collateral vessels (e.g. cavernoma following extrahepatic portal vein occlusion or recanalisation of fetal veins in portal vein hypertension) and varices. Pulsed-wave Doppler is routinely used to evaluate flow in the portal vein. When traces are difficult to obtain in the moving child, colour Doppler will at least establish

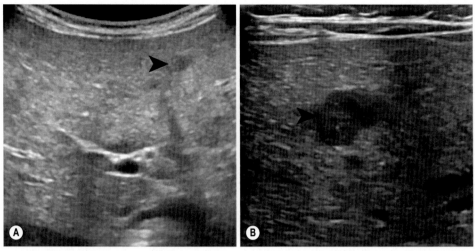

FIGURE 3-43 ■ US in a neutropenic child with spiking temperature. (A) The focal fungal lesion (arrowhead) in the liver is easily missed with a low-frequency (5–2 MHz) curvilinear transducer. (B) The lesion (arrowhead) is more conspicuous with a high-frequency (9.5 MHz) linear transducer.

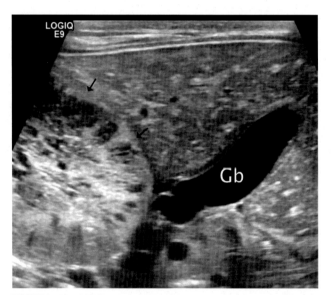

FIGURE 3-44 ■ US in an infant with congenital hepatic fibrosis shows lace-like hyperechoic bands throughout the liver. There is associated polycystic kidney disease. Arrows, enlarged polycystic right kidney; Gb, gall bladder.

the flow direction. Twinkling (artefact) seen on colour Doppler is useful to detect calcifications, gallstones and bile duct hamartomas. The sensitivity increases when the focal zone is set deep to the abnormality and with higher colour write priority.[95] Microbubble-based intravenous US contrast media are thought to increase the diagnostic accuracy of US, but are currently only used off-label.[96]

MRI

Provided adequate preparation, MRI allows high-resolution (submillimetre, isotropic) high-contrast imaging of the liver. Respiratory gating is used whenever possible. Useful pulse sequences include short tau inversion recovery (STIR) fast spin-ech, volumetric T2-weighted spin-echo with variable refocusing pulse

flip-angle (CUBE, SPACE, VISTA), in-phase and opposed-phase spoiled gradient-echo, diffusion-weighted imaging and T1-weighted gradient-echo before and after intravenous administration of contrast medium (possibly with several post-contrast acquisitions, as in adults to detect, for example, centripetal enhancement in infantile haemangioma and rapid washout in neoplasms).

Non-contrast-enhanced angiographic techniques include selective inversion followed by balanced steady-state free-precession acquisition (NATIVE, TRANCE, FBI). This technique depends on inflow of fresh spins, and may therefore require several acquisitions with varying placement of the inversion volume. The technique is promising for portal venography.

Hepatocyte-specific contrast agents are promising for detection of small lesions and lesion characterisation, and for functional assessment of biliary drainage, but are currently restricted to off-label use (Fig. 3-45).[97,98]

CT

CT should be restricted in children (1) due to its generally poor soft-tissue contrast, (2) because paucity of body-fat in young children hampers identification of tissue planes and (3) for radiation protection. If used, protocols need to be in place to minimise the radiation dose. No pre-contrast run and only one post-contrast run is indicated—with very few exceptions.

Angiography

Angiography is very rarely indicated for diagnosis and, as such, is only performed in specialist centres.

Imaging Anatomy

The neonatal liver is hypoechoic to the kidneys. This reverses during infancy. The umbilical vein and the ductus venosus are patent in the premature and early newborn (< 48 h), and in two-thirds up to 1 week of age.

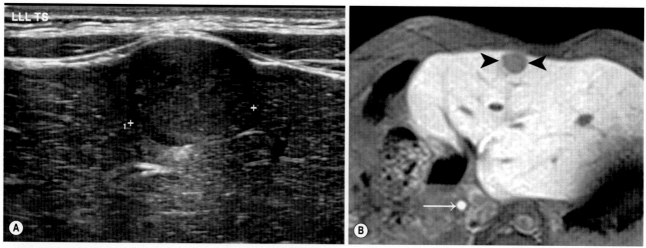

FIGURE 3-45 ■ **Imaging in a 3-year-old with Beckwith–Wiedemann syndrome and previously resected hepatoblastoma.** (A) During off-treatment surveillance, a 15-mm subcapsular nodule (between markers) is seen with high-frequency US in the left lobe of the liver. (B) Axial spoiled gradient-echo MRI 20 min following intravenous injection of gadoxetic acid (a hepatocyte-specific contrast agent) demonstrates normal enhancement of surrounding liver, but no enhancement in the nodule (arrowheads). Recurrent hepatoblastoma was therefore suspected, and confirmed histopathologically. Note contrast material in the common bile duct (arrow).

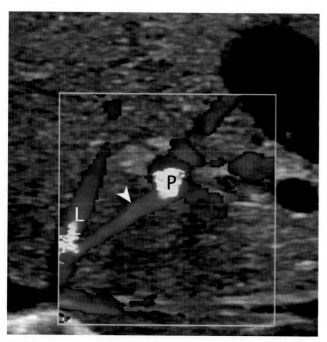

FIGURE 3-46 ■ Duplex Doppler sonography in a neonate demonstrates a patent ductus venosus (arrowhead) between the portal vein (P) and the left hepatic vein (L) just distal to the inferior vena cava. Anatomical variation is common in this fetal umbilicosystemic shunt.

TABLE 3-10	Suggested Upper Limit of Normal Sonographic Measurement of Liver Size in Children[83]	

Age (months)	Suggested Upper Limit for the Longitudinal Dimension (mm) of the Right Lobe of the Liver in the Midclavicular Sagittal Plane
1–3	90
4–6	95
7–9	100
12–30	105
36–59	115
60–83	125
84–107	130
108–131	135
132–179	140
180–200	145

The limits are based on an ethnically homogeneous material. Considerable intra- and inter-observer variation need to be accounted for.

Patency beyond 2–3 weeks is abnormal. The ductus venosus is seen as a vascular channel between the left portal branch and the left hepatic vein/inferior vena cava (Fig. 3-46). There is considerable variation in the size of normal livers, and measurements are difficult to standardise. Uncritical application of reference measurements is therefore not advised; however, Table 3-10 gives an idea of the upper limit of normal. Portal vein sonographic diameter after 1–3 h of fasting in the supine position was found to range in mm (age group): 3–5 (at birth), 4–8 (1 year), 6–8 (5 years), 6–9 (10 years), 7–11 (15 years).[99] Similar findings were done in a more recent cohort, supine, after at least 2-h fasting, where the 5–95 centiles in mm (age group) were 3.0–6.4 (0–12 months), 4.3–8.3 (1–5 years) and 5.0–10.8 (5–10 years).[100]

Liver Involvement in Congenital Malformation and Infections, Syndromes and Systemic Conditions

Right cardiac isomerisms are associated with two right lobes of the liver, left isomerisms with midline liver and preduodenal portal vein and with biliary and splenic abnormalities (see the sections 'Biliary System' and 'Spleen').[101] Congenital infections (*Toxoplasma*, rubella,

CMV, herpes virus and other) may involve the liver: hepatosplenomegaly, focal calcifications. One differential diagnosis is Aicardi–Goutières syndrome. Periportal hyperechogenicity is non-specific and commonly seen in response to systemic inflammation, and abdominal inflammation in particular.

Non-obstructive Jaundice

Non-obstructive jaundice may be caused by increased production of bilirubin, insufficient conjugation, transport, excretion and/or drainage. All these factors may contribute to physiological jaundice in the neonate with an immature liver. Only prolonged jaundice (beyond 2 weeks) without a clear cause (neonatal hepatitis, haemolytic conditions, sepsis, etc.) requires imaging investigation in the neonate. (Idiopathic) neonatal hepatitis is an increasingly obsolete terms for non-obstructive causes of jaundice,[102] and it follows that the sonographic manifestations are highly variable, e.g. with hyperechoic liver parenchyma and poor visualisation of peripheral portal branches.[103] Severe hepatitis with poor biliary excretion may lead to a small gall bladder and may therefore be confused with biliary atresia (see the section 'Biliary System').

In childhood, the differential is wide and includes metabolic disease (e.g. glycogen storage disorders, Wilson's disease, tyrosinaemia, alpha-1-antitrypsin deficiency) and cystic fibrosis.

The role of imaging is limited in hepatitis: findings are non-specific. However, follow-up to detect and quantify secondary fibrosis (see the section 'Chronic Liver Disease') may be useful.

Infection

Imaging has a more well-defined role in focal infection for detection, image-guided drainage and assessment of treatment response. Estimated globally, liver abscesses in children are most frequently pyogenic (80%; most commonly caused by *Staphylococcus aureus*) and amoebal (most frequently *Entamoeba histolytica*). Fungal causes (often multifocal and involving the spleen) are most likely in the immunocompromised child.[104] US with a high-frequency linear probe is mandatory in febrile neutropaenia since the clinical and laboratory diagnosis is more difficult due to the poor immune response (Fig. 3-43). Repeat US is indicated if the cause remains occult.

In chronic granulomatous disease, the child is susceptible to catalase-positive infections (*Staphylococcus aureus*, fungi and other) and responds with formation of granulomata rather than typical abscesses. It follows that imaging findings are heterogeneous on a spectrum from multilocular to homogeneous, solid (enhancing) lesions, solitary or multifocal, of highly variable size. Calcification is a common sequela post-resolution of acute infection.[105]

Parasitic infections (e.g. *Echinococcus* sp.) are endemic in many parts of the world, and imaging findings are similar to those in adults. Tuberculous infections of the liver are rare.

Chronic Liver Disease

Cirrhosis

Hepatic cirrhosis is advanced fibrosis with anatomical distortion that causes hepatocyte dysfunction. In children, cirrhosis, due to increased intrahepatic vascular resistance, is the leading cause of portal hypertension. As in adults, cirrhosis predisposes for hepatocellular carcinoma. The most common cause of cirrhosis in children is cholestasis, which may be due to biliary anomalies (biliary atresia, persistent intrahepatic cholestasis), cystic fibrosis or long-term total parenteral nutrition.[106–108] Other causes of cirrhosis are necrosis (neonatal, viral and autoimmune hepatitis) and constitutional metabolic disease (e.g. Wilson's disease, alpha-1 antitrypsin deficiency, tyrosinaemia). Non-alcoholic fatty liver disease as a cause of cirrhosis is on the increase in developed countries.[109,110]

Cirrhosis is suggested by typical appearances of a hyperechoic, nodular parenchyma and an undulating surface, atrophy of the right lobe, hypertrophy of the caudate and left lobes, widening of the fissures and of the gall bladder fossa. Doppler investigation of the portal vein is an important part of the investigation (see 'Portal Vein' section).

Imaging is important in surveillance for malignant transformation to hepatocellular carcinoma. US is the primary imaging technique, but is limited to detecting growth of individual nodules, which may be challenging.

MRI has higher, albeit not perfect, accuracy. Regenerative nodules are similar to normal liver on T1- and T2-weighted sequences, opposed-phase sequences and following contrast administration. The steatotic nodule may disclose itself by a high fat concentration, i.e. relatively higher signal intensity on T1- and T2-weighted images, low in opposed phase.

The siderotic nodule has relatively low signal intensity on all sequences due to iron deposition. The hallmark of dysplastic nodules and hepatocellular carcinoma are high signal intensity of T2-weighted images, marked enhancement in the arterial phase following intravenous administration of contrast medium, and rapid washout.[111]

Hepatocyte-specific MRI contrast agents are not licensed for use in children, but there is mounting evidence for their contribution to increasing the diagnostic accuracy for focal lesions, including in cirrhosis (Fig. 3-45).[97,98]

Fibrosis

Non-invasive grading of fibrosis remains difficult. Quantification has been explored by observation of the propagation of mechanical waves (shear-wave velocity) in tissues and subsequent estimation of tissue stiffness (elastography). The feasibility in children has been shown with stand-alone devices and integrated with grey-scale US.[112] Although elastography distinguishes normal and fibrotic liver, there is significant overlap among the intermediate stages of fibrosis.[113] Elastography by MRI has been described in children (using a reduced drive power in children younger than 1 year).[114] However, there are still no normal references for children, so accurate data are not available.

All techniques require standardisation, since several factors other than fibrosis influence liver stiffness, e.g. degree of hydration, postprandial portal flow.

Non-alcoholic Fatty Liver Disease (NAFLD)

In the developed world NAFLD is now one of the most frequent indications for referral for chronic liver disease in children and young people and evidence suggests it is associated with progressive liver disease and cirrhosis.[115] The course from simple steatosis to non-alcoholic steatohepatitis (NASH), possibly via fibrosis to cirrhosis, is poorly understood. Grading of hepatic steatosis is accurate using signal loss in opposed-phase MRI as a severity measurement.[116] The method is also feasible in children, and the range for hepatic fat fraction in obese children without NAFLD was up to 4.7% in one study.[117]

Fibropolycystic Liver Disease

Fibropolycystic liver disease is a spectrum of overlapping phenotypes caused by ductal plate developmental abnormalities. There is variable association with polycystic kidney disease. Secondary cirrhosis is rare. More common complications include portal hypertension, cholangitis and mass effect. Manifestation generally progresses from the peripheral to the central liver. Entities include the following.

Congenital hepatic fibrosis manifests as periportal fibrosis, biliary dysplasia and autosomal recessive polycystic kidney disease (Fig. 3-44). Both the hepatic and renal involvement are variable.[111] US may show mild dilatation of hilar bile ducts. Hepatopetal collateral veins without extrahepatic portal vein occlusion is seen in one-third of affected children.[118] There may be hepatic artery widening and regenerative nodules.

Autosomal dominant polycystic disease was considered 'adult-type' polycystic disease but is now recognised in children, who are often asymptomatic. The liver is usually enlarged and diffusely involved with heterogeneous cysts. Complications are rare in children, but may include infection and rupture of cysts, bleeding and mass effect. Secondary portal hypertension is rare.

Choledochal malformations (see the section 'Biliary System') overlap with fibropolycystic liver disease, in particular in Caroli's syndrome (type 5 choledochal malformation) where there is congenital hepatic fibrosis.

In **hepatoportal sclerosis** US may show a hyperechoic zone (representing fibrosis) surrounding the portal veins with a hypoechoic zone separating it from normal-appearing liver.[119] This entity may have alternative presentation with hepatic nodules.[111]

Biliary hamartomas are uniform cystic lesions < 15 mm in diameter with thin rim enhancement.[120] These may be seen on US and MRI, and are sometimes incidental findings. The entity has not been comprehensively described in children.

Suprahepatic Chronic Liver Disease

Venous stasis is the common denominator for this group, which includes congestive heart failure. Specific entities include the following.

Veno-occlusive disease is associated with antineoplastic therapy and myeloablation. There are no recognised specific imaging findings. However, the severity is correlated with degree of splenomegaly, ascites and flow in the paraumbilical vein and with signs of portal hypertension.[121]

Budd–Chiari syndrome is hepatic venous obstruction due to thrombosis of hepatic veins or of the inferior vena cava. It may be constitutional (primary, associated with myeloproliferative disease) or secondary (hepatic neoplasms and infections). Thrombus is demonstrated on US and Doppler in the acute phase, whereas obliterated veins, reversed flow and collaterals are seen in chronic phase.[111] On CT and MRI there may be heterogeneous arborating enhancement in portal venous phase following contrast medium administration.

Portal Vein

Portosystemic Shunts

Congenital extrahepatic portosystemic shunts, total (type 1) and partial (type 2), are rare.[122] Shunting is to the inferior vena cava, renal vein, iliac veins or azygos system. Establishing the type is important for surgery: total shunts should not be ligated as they represent the sole mesenteric venous return. Several associated congenital anomalies are recognised (e.g. cardiac, gastrointestinal, genitourinary, vascular).[123] Other congenital abnormalities include hypoplasia and atresia, absence of a portal branch and intrahepatic developmental connections between portal and hepatic veins.

Portosystemic shunts are clinically important to recognise since untreated they may cause pulmonary hypertension, hepatopulmonary syndrome and hepatic encephalopathy. US with Doppler is the first technique of choice, with CT or MRI angiography, and catheter portovenography reserved for special cases and for preoperative planning.

Extrahepatic Portal Vein Occlusion

Acquired extrahepatic portal vein occlusion is more common and is, after cirrhosis, the second most common cause of portal hypertension in children. Known causes are umbilical venous catheter, abdominal infection, inflammation, trauma, surgery and neoplasms (hepatoblastoma and hepatocellular carcinoma). The liver is often functionally normal (depending on aetiology), but may be small. The primary finding is cavernous transformation at the porta hepatis and associated signs of portal hypertension.

Portal Hypertension

Slow portal venous flow (< 15–18 mm/s) and loss of respiratory pulsatility suggests portal hypertension, but these findings are unreliable in extrahepatic portal vein occlusion if there is a rich collateral network.[124] US, MRI and CT may all demonstrate varicose veins and aneurysmal dilatations. There is hepatofugal flow with engorged veins in the lesser omentum, at the spleen and gastro-oesophageal junction, recanalised or non-obliterated umbilical vein and/or ductus venosus (Fig. 3-46), and splenomegaly. There is low or absent portovenous flow and high hepatic artery flow.[111] Thickening of the lesser omentum (sagittal sonogram at the level of the coeliac origin) to more that 1.7 times the diameter of the aorta may be seen but it is a non-specific sign.[125]

Portal Venous Gas

US is the most sensitive technique for detecting portal venous gas, seen as hyperechoic dots flowing with the portal blood. When visible on radiographs (or CT) it may be easier to recognise its arborating pattern to within a few centimetres of the hepatic capsule. This is different from biliary gas, which usually collects centrally.[126] The gas may originate from bowel lumen (obstruction), bowel wall (ischaemia or pneumatosis), intra-abdominal abscesses or from gas-forming organisms in the portal venous system itself.

Necrotising enterocolitis is the most common cause in neonates, the gas bubbling from the pneumatotic bowel wall into mesenteric veins. Portal venous gas seen on radiographs is associated with a higher frequency of operative intervention, but not with mortality from necrotising enterocolitis.[127]

Portal venous gas beyond the early stage following liver transplant in children may suggest developing intestinal lymphoproliferative disease.[128]

Preduodenal Portal Vein

There are many case reports of a preduodenal portal vein as an incidental finding or as a cause of duodenal obstruction. It seems associated with other developmental abnormalities, such as the heterotaxia syndromes.

Mass Lesions

Primary liver tumours are rare in children. Before 3 years of age the most common entities are vascular neoplasms, hepatoblastoma, teratoma, rhabdoid tumour and mesenchymal hamartoma; however, primary liver tumours are very rarely malignant in the first few months of life. After 3 years of age the diagnostic distribution becomes increasingly similar to that in adults. Hepatocellular carcinoma occurs, and is associated with cirrhosis. Only lesions that are specific to children are described here.

Imaging Features

Ossification may be seen in teratomas and hepatocellular carcinomas. Fatty content is almost pathognomonic of teratomas. A solid mass with cyst-like low attenuation on CT and/or high signal intensity on T2-weighted MRI suggests undifferentiated sarcoma.[129] Calcification is not a useful discriminator as it is seen in hepatoblastoma, hepatocellular carcinoma, rapidly involuting congenital haemangiona, teratoma and infection.[130]

Hepatoblastoma (Fig. 3-47)

Hepatoblastoma is very uncommon in the first few months of life and after 3 years of age. Known associations include Beckwith–Wiedemann syndrome and biliary atresia. The diagnosis is suggested when there is thrombocytosis and raised serum alpha-fetoprotein (AFP) for age (raised AFP is also associated with the rarer yolk sac tumour). Final diagnosis (tissue) and staging need to be performed in a specialist environment. Staging is based on the number of adjoining liver sections free from tumour, venous encasement/invasion, rupture and metastases.[131] Metastases are most commonly to the lungs, so chest CT is part of the staging procedure.

Vascular Neoplasms

Infantile haemangioma of the liver is similar to those in other locations (e.g. skin) and is associated with multiple skin haemangiomas.[132] Lesions have low vascular resistance and therefore high flow velocities on pulsed-wave

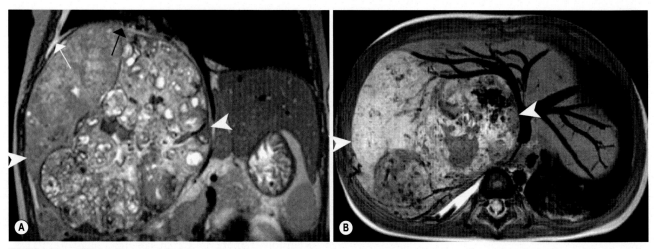

FIGURE 3-47 ■ **MRI in a 2-year-old with a hepatoblastoma shows a large, heterogeneous mass (arrowheads) in the right lobe of the liver.** (A) Coronal reconstruction of volumetric T2-weighted spin-echo. Note the infiltration of the right hemidiaphragm (black arrow) and the secondary pleural fluid (white arrow). (B) Thick-slab minimum intensity projection in the axial plane of the same sequence demonstrates the relation between tumour and the hepatic veins, the basis for local staging in hepatoblastoma.

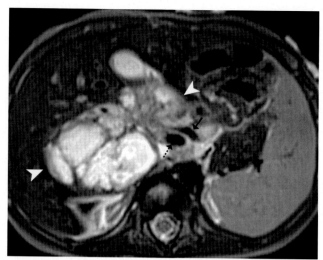

FIGURE 3-48 ■ **MRI in a 2-month-old with a partly exophytic liver mass.** T2-weighted MRI shows the heterogeneous lesion (arrowheads) with large hyperintense components corresponding to cystic spaces. Tumour encases the inferior vena cava (dashed arrow) and the portal vein (arrow). Mesenchymal hamartoma was established following biopsy. Along with infantile haemangioma and hepatoblastoma, this is one of the top differential diagnoses for a solitary liver tumour in a child younger than 3 years.

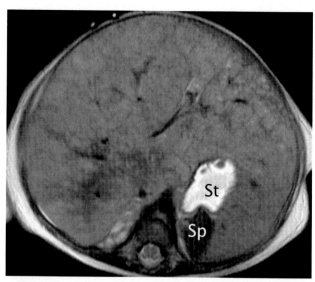

FIGURE 3-49 ■ Axial T2-weighted MRI in an infant with metastatic neuroblastoma shows diffuse infiltration of the liver, which has enlarged to hug the spleen (Sp) and stomach (St).

Doppler,[133] and even arteriovenous shunting. The flow dynamics explain the association with high-output heart failure. On repeated MRI after gadolinium administration there is typically centripetal enhancement. All techniques should demonstrate a non-infiltrating lesion without perilesional oedema.[134]

Congenital haemangiomas are similar on imaging to infantile haemangiomas but may specifically demonstrate vascular aneurysms and thrombosis.[134] The subgroup of rapidly involuting congenital haemangioma (RICH) may present thick, irregular rim enhancement on CT and MRI.[135] These usually involute completely by 14 months of age, as opposed to non-involution congenital haemangioma (NICH).

Mesenchymal Hamartoma (Fig. 3-48)

The majority of children with mesenchymal hamartoma present clinically before the age of 2 years with a palpable mass. Imaging demonstrates variable a mixed cystic/solid mass, which may be very large. Solid may be seen in the youngest. Multifocal variants are known.

Liver Metastases and Other Multifocal Lesions

Liver metastases in children are most frequently from neuroblastoma (Fig. 3-49), lymphoproliferative disease, nephroblastoma and sarcomas. Differentials for multifocal liver lesions include multifocal vascular neoplasm, infection, regenerating nodules, focal nodular hyperplasia, angiomyolipoma, fibropolycystic disease and peliosis hepatis.

Trauma

CT has higher sensitivity than US for liver lacerations.[136] The liver is the most commonly injured organ (particularly the right lobe) in paediatric abdominal trauma due to the soft rib cage. Liver injury accounts for about half of deaths caused by abdominal trauma in children.[137] In children, particularly in the youngest, non-accidental (inflicted) injury needs to be remembered as a possible differential diagnosis. There are no pathognomonic signs. However, the left lobe of the liver is thought most commonly injured due to compression against the spine during a direct impact.[138] (See also the section 'Trauma' under 'Spleen'.)

Transplant

It is important to detect signs of infarction, rejection, post-transplantation lymphoproliferative disorder (PTLD), and vascular and biliary complications.[139] PTLD is frequent in childhood recipients at 9–14%.[140] Apart from typical findings of lymphoproliferation, gas in the portal vein has been suggested a sign of PTLD following liver transplantation.[128] Biliary complications are common (around one-quarter of liver transplantations), and usually present in the first 3 months after transplantation as leakage, stenosis, gallstones, sludge, biloma or infection.

Arterial stenosis or thrombosis occurs in about one-fifth of children. At colour Doppler there is high flow velocity and turbulence across a stenosis, and parvus tardus distally. Portal vein complications are seen in fewer than one-tenth. Significant narrowing may be defined as a reduction of the lumen to less than 50%, but one needs to account for possible differences in vascular calibres due to size mismatch between donor and recipient.

BILIARY SYSTEM

Imaging Techniques

US is the first technique of choice for investigating the biliary system. It may even depict the intrapancreatic portion and the ampulla of Vater. However, for complete biliary anatomy, MR cholangiopancreatography (MRCP) is indicated. Rather than thick-slab multi-direction techniques, volumetric heavily T2-weighted spin-echo images are preferred as they have exquisite resolution and allow multiplanar post-processing. Functional MRI of biliary drainage with a hepatocyte-specific contrast agent has been shown feasible and is promising, e.g. in diagnosis of biliary atresia; however, it is not yet licensed for clinical use in children.[97]

Specific radioisotope imaging in children is performed when there is suspicion of biliary atresia (see 'Jaundice' section), and derivatives of Tc-labelled iminodiacetic acid (IDA) are used. These are actively taken up and excreted by hepatocytes. Infants younger than 2 months with biliary atresia typically have prompt hepatic extraction, no visualisation of a gall bladder, prolonged hepatic tracer retention and no intestinal excretion of tracer.

Imaging Anatomy

The suggested upper limit of normal for the common bile duct diameter is about 2 mm in infants, 4 mm in children and 7 mm in adolescents; the gall bladder length should be at least 1.5 cm in neonates.[141,142]

Jaundice

Jaundice may be caused by increased haemoglobin breakdown (e.g. haemolytic disorders), poor liver function (e.g. immature liver, hepatitis) and/or poor excretion or drainage (e.g. atresia, obstruction). Jaundice is therefore physiological in the newborn due to increased breakdown and an immature liver. However, jaundice beyond 2 weeks is suspicious for liver disease.[143] Of infants with surgical jaundice, about 80% have biliary atresia, and most of the remaining have inspissated bile syndrome or choledochal malformation.[144] Important differential diagnostic imaging findings are summarised in Table 3-11.

Biliary Atresia (Fig. 3-50)

Biliary atresia has an incidence of 1 in 8000–18,000 live births (more common in East and South-East Asia) and is the most common cause of childhood liver transplant.[102] There may be atresia of the common bile duct (type I), common hepatic duct (type II) or intrahepatic ducts (type III), rarely of the cystic duct. A subgroup has an associated cyst at the porta hepatis and may be sonographically similar to choledochal malformation.[145] Importantly, atresia does not cause biliary dilatation or sludge as opposed to choledochal malformations. The main differential diagnoses in a jaundiced infant without biliary dilatation or sludge are neonatal hepatitis and persistent intrahepatic cholestasis. Associated abnormalities (in about one-fifth) include congenital heart disease, preduodenal portal vein, polysplenia, situs inversus and absent

TABLE 3-11   Important, but not Comprehensive, Imaging Differential Diagnosis in Infantile Jaundice

Imaging Finding	Biliary Dilatation	Normal Gall Bladder	Hyperechoic Structure at the Porta Hepatis (Triangular Cord)	Biliary Drainage on Radioisotope Scan
Neonatal hepatitis	No	Yes	No	May be detectable
Biliary atresia	No	Rarely	Usually	None
Choledochal malformation	Variable	Usually	No	Usually seen

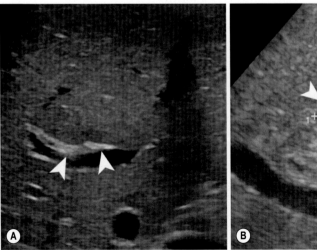
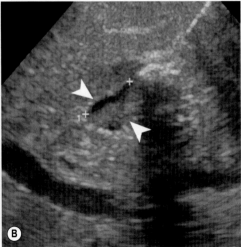

FIGURE 3-50 ■ **Typical US findings of biliary atresia in an infant with persistent jaundice.** (A) The fibrous atretic plate (arrowheads) is present at the porta hepatis (triangular cord sign). Note that there is no biliary dilatation. (B) A small (about 10 mm) gall bladder (arrowheads) with abnormal wall.

vena cava. The natural history is of progressive fibrosis, cirrhosis and portal hypertension. However, if portoenterostomy (Kasai's procedure) is performed before 8 weeks of age, about half reach adolescence without needing transplant.[146]

The definitive diagnosis is by intraoperative cholangiography. Preoperative percutaneous transhepatic cholecystocholangiography combined with liver biopsy in cholestatic infants has a sensitivity of 100% and a specificity of 93% for diagnosing biliary atresia.[147]

The sonographic signs are (1) absent or abnormal (<1.5 cm fasting and/or no normal wall) gall bladder, (2) a hyperechoic structure ('triangular cord') that represents a fibrous remnant of the extrahepatic bile ducts at the porta hepatis and (3) a wide hepatic artery (diameter > 2 mm at the porta hepatis).[148–153]

In infants up to 3 months of age with conjugated hyperbilirubinaemia, a negative triangular cord sign and normal gall bladder morphology on US has a high negative predictive value (> 90%) for excluding extrahepatic biliary atresia.[154]

Radioisotope studies have high sensitivity but a false-positive rate above 20%. The poor specificity is mostly due to poor biliary excretion/drainage in other conditions, e.g. metabolic disease, infection, persistent intrahepatic cholestasis, total parenteral nutrition and neonatal hepatitis.[155]

Choledochal Malformation (Choledochal Cyst (Fig. 3-51))

Choledochal malformations comprise a spectrum of conditions with overlapping expressions in which there is abnormal widening of the biliary tract without acute obstruction. About 80% manifest clinically during childhood. Malignant transformation in children is not documented.[156] The incidence is 1 : 100,000–200,000, but as high as 1 : 1000 in Japan.[157,158]

In infants younger than 3 months with extrahepatic biliary dilatation and conjugated hyperbilirubinaemia, bile duct diameter < 3 mm suggests a non-surgical cause, whereas diameter > 4 mm suggests choledochal malformation. The intermediate cases are often associated with inspissated bile syndrome.[159]

Most commonly there is spherical or fusiform dilatation of the extrahapatic ducts (type 1).[156] A common pancreaticobiliary channel may be seen sonographically[160] and with MRCP, and flux of pancreatic excretions via this into the common bile duct is thought to be a pathogenetic factor. The clinically most important differential diagnosis for a cyst at the porta hepatis is cystic biliary atresia.[145] Other differential diagnoses include duodenal duplication cyst and lymphangioma.

Other variants demonstrate a cystic diverticulum from the common bile duct (type 2), cholodochocele into the duodenum (type 3) or a combination of intra- and extrahepatic dilatation (type 4). Choledochal malformations may be part of the fibropolycystic spectrum (see 'Liver' section). Indeed, Caroli's disease is an association between intrahepatic segmental duct dilatations (type 5 choledochal malformation), (congenital) hepatic fibrosis and cystic kidney disease. Intrahepatic focal biliary dilatation can be recognised by the central dot sign, which represents the encased adjoining portal vein branch. Differential diagnoses to intrahepatic choledochal malformation include sclerosing cholangitis (see later) and recurrent pyogenic cholangitis.[161]

There may be complications like cholangitis (due to stagnant bile), biliary obstruction (calculi), cirrhosis (secondary to obstruction) and cholangiocarcinoma in adults.[162] Surgical treatment is usually hepatoenterostomy.

Inspissated Bile

In infants and young children, obstruction (partial or total) by stagnant-formed bile may be associated with

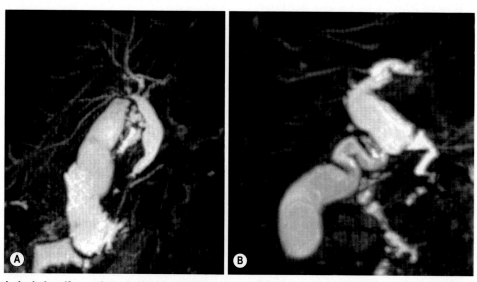

FIGURE 3-51 ■ **Choledochal malformations depicted with thick-slab maximum intensity projections of volumetric heavily T2-weighted fast spin-echo images.** (A) Fusiform widening of the extrahepatic bile ducts (type 1). (B) Widening of the common hepatic duct and central intrahepatic bile ducts (type 4).

prematurity, haemolysis, functional intestinal obstruction (e.g. Hirschsprung's disease), cystic fibrosis and total parenteral nutrition. It is usually idiopathic in infants (inspissated bile syndrome). US demonstrates the (slightly) echogenic bile with no acoustic shadowing, and the secondary biliary dilatation (mainly extrahepatic). There may be increased periportal echogenicity if long-standing. Choledochal malformation is the main differential diagnosis in infants.

Persistent Intrahepatic Cholestasis

This is a spectrum of inherited disorders that need to be considered in infantile jaundice. It includes Alagille syndrome: paucity of intrahepatic bile ducts associated with butterfly vertebrae, congenital heart disease, ocular and/or facial anomalies. There is no documented role for imaging in these conditions; however, this may change with the introduction of hepatocyte-specific contrast agents.[97]

Other causes of biliary obstruction include external compression by cystic (e.g. duplication cysts) or solid (e.g. enlarged lymph nodes) masses. Biliary neoplasms are rare in children (see 'Neoplasia' section).

Sludge and Gallstones

The prevalence of gallstones increases with age; they are rare in children unless there is an underlying cause, such as haemolytic disorders, obesity, cystic fibrosis, small bowel disease, choledochal malformation or total parenteral nutrition. There may not be a developmental continuum from sludge to stone formation.[163]

Spontaneous Perforation of the Bile Ducts

This is a very rare condition. The clinical presentation is increasing ascites, irritability and variable mild jaundice in a young infant. The hepatobiliary radioisotope image demonstrates extrabiliary pooling, and US or MRI may verify coinciding loculated fluid and possibly underlying causes, such as choledochal malformation, gallstone and biliary stenosis.[164]

Cholangitis

Cholangitis in children prompts a search for predisposing conditions. These include anatomical abnormalities (choledochal malformation), congenital hepatic fibrosis, biliary obstruction (gallstone, inspissated bile), congenital immunodeficiency and complications following surgery and transplantation.

Sclerosing Cholangitis

The pathology and imaging findings are similar to those in adults: a beaded appearance of alternating strictures and dilatation of intra- and extrahepatic bile ducts. Primary sclerosing cholangitis is associated with ulcerative colitis in up to 80% (may be metachronous). Conversely, inflammatory bowel disease is found in around

half of children with sclerosing cholangitis.[165] Secondary sclerosing cholangitis may be seen in Langerhans cell histiocytosis. Clinical presentation is usually after 2 years of age, but a neonatal form is well known. The differential diagnoses include primary biliary cirrhosis, autoimmune hepatitis, biliary atresia and graft-versus-host disease.

Sclerosing cholangitis leads to progressive cholestasis and cirrhosis. The risk a person with primary sclerosing cholangitis has for developing cholangiocarcinoma is estimated at 0.6–1.5% per year.[166]

Neoplasia

Biliary neoplasms are rare in children. Biliary rhabdomyosarcoma is suspected when there is a mass at the porta hepatis and associated proximal biliary dilatation. It rarely invades the portal vein. Cystic variants are known. Cholangiocarcinoma is an important differential diagnosis in children with sclerosing cholangitis. It is unlikely to arise in childhood from choledochal malformation.

PANCREAS

Imaging Techniques

US usually allows complete depiction of the pancreas in children. The pancreatic tail is seen through a splenic acoustic window. Islet cell neoplasm and other small lesions, however, are not commonly visible, and may also not be seen on MRI. Complete imaging in suspected cases therefore involves radioisotope studies. The pancreatic ducts may be difficult to visualise on MRCP unless the exocrine pancreas is stimulated using intravenous secretin; however, care should be taken in case of recent pancreatitis, which may be exacerbated by secretin.

Imaging Anatomy

Pancreatic size is variable, volumetric references unavailable, and sonographic measurements have unknown reliability. The pancreas may appear large relative to the size of the child. Suggested anteroposterior dimensions on US are (infants–teenagers, cm) 1–2 (head and tail) and 0.6–1.1 (body) with standard deviations of around 0.4 cm.[167] Suggested normal pancreatic duct diameters are 1.1 mm in toddlers to 2.1 mm in late teens, with standard deviations of about 0.2 mm.[168]

Congenital Abnormalities and Associations

Pancreas Divisum (Fig. 3-52)

This is a common, and often uncomplicated, variant. The embryonal ventral and dorsal anlagen have separate ducts that normally connect. This failing, two separate ducts persist. Since the smaller dorsal anlage develops into the larger part (body, tail, part of the head), its duct (of Santorini) may provide inadequate draining capacity through the minor papilla, which may predispose to recurrent acute pancreatitis. However, such an association is disputed (in adults).[169]

Annular Pancreas (Fig. 3-53)

Annular pancreas, i.e. pancreatic tissue encasing the second part of the duodenum, results from erroneous migration of the anlagen. It may result in duodenal obstruction and is a differential diagnosis for the double bubble sign. Associated anomalies are common in children (71%) and differ from those in adults, the most common being trisomy 21, intestinal and cardiac anomalies that often require surgery.[170]

Other

Agenesis of the dorsal anlage is suggested by a short rounded pancreatic head and absence of the body and tail. It is associated with insulin-dependent diabetes mellitus, possibly through a gene mutation.[171] Ectopic pancreatic tissue may exist and is most frequently located in the wall of the stomach, duodenum or jejunum.

Systemic Disorders

Cystic Fibrosis

High-viscosity secretions cause distal obstruction and inevitable destruction of the pancreas in children with cystic fibrosis. The main imaging findings are atrophy and/or fat replacement (Fig. 3-54); however, fibrous tissue and calcifications may be seen.[107] Pancreatitis is a less common complication, occurring in just over 1% of patients with cystic fibrosis.[172]

Other

Diffuse enlargement of the pancreas may be seen in children with Beckwith–Wiedemann syndrome, which also predisposes to pancreatoblastoma, albeit seen very rarely. Both autosomal dominant polycystic kidney disease and von Hippel–Lindau disease may manifest with pancreatic cyst(s).

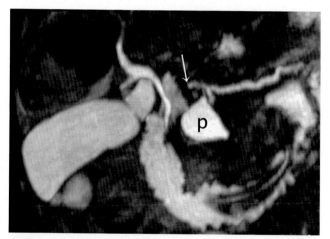

FIGURE 3-52 ■ **Thick-slab heavily T2-weighted fast spin-echo in a child following acute pancreatitis.** A pseudocyst (p) is seen. The pancreatic duct from the tail, body and proximal head appears to drain exclusively through the duct of Santorini, which narrows abruptly near the minor papilla (arrow).

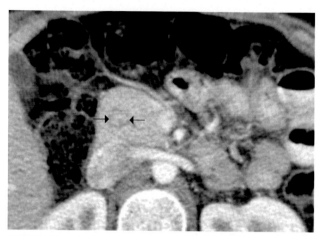

FIGURE 3-53 ■ **Contrast-enhanced CT in a toddler with symptoms of partial upper gastrointestinal obstruction demonstrates annular pancreas.** The second part of the duodenum (arrows) is completely encircled by pancreatic tissue.

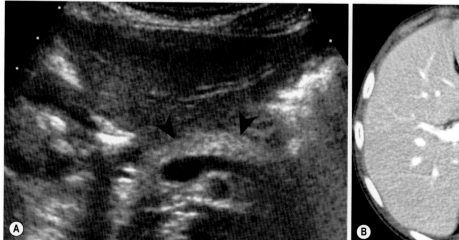
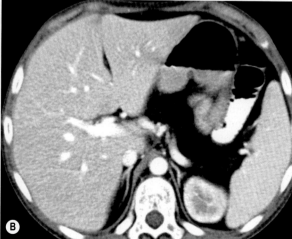

FIGURE 3-54 ■ **Fatty replacement of the pancreas in a child with cystic fibrosis.** (A) Sonogram demonstrates a small, hyperechoic pancreas (arrowheads). (B) Contrast-enhanced CT shows a fat-attenuated pancreas. Gradual destruction happens during childhood due to stagnant secretions, and may also manifest as fibrosis and calcification.

Pancreatitis

Underlying conditions differ in children. In acute pancreatitis they include congenital biliary abnormalities, viral infections, systemic disease (e.g. Henoch-Schönlein purpura and other vasculitides, metabolic and other hereditary disease) and pancreatic duct abnormalities; however, about one-third are idiopathic.[173] Apart from playing a role in the acute stage (as in adults), imaging in children is directed towards uncovering any underlying anatomical abnormality, for which MRI is used.

Conditions associated with chronic pancreatitis include cystic fibrosis, Shwachman–Diamond syndrome and other hereditary disorders.

Trauma

Children are more prone to pancreatic injury, which may manifest as laceration, transection and/or acute pancreatitis. As with any injury in childhood, non-accidental causes need to be considered, particularly in the youngest.

Congenital Hyperinsulinism

Congenital hyperinsulinism is caused by diffuse or focal inappropriate secretion of insulin. [16]F-fluoro-DOPA PET may differentiate the two—important for planning surgical options (partial or complete resection of the pancreas).[174] Co-registration of PET with MRCP images allows assessment of the relation between a focal lesion and the common bile duct.

Neoplasms

Pancreatoblastoma is rare, even in predisposed children with Beckwith–Wiedemann syndrome. Presentation is usually in infants or young children with a heterogeneous solid/cystic mass and variable enhancement.

Solid and papillary epithelial neoplasms (Frantz tumour) is most often seen in adolescent or young adult females. Imaging usually shows a large well-defined mass with cystic-haemorrhagic degeneration, calcifications and low-signal intensity (fibrous) rim on MRI (Fig. 3-55).

Islet cell tumours are associated with multiple endocrine neoplasia type 1 and with von Hippel–Lindau disease. Functioning entities in children are insulinoma (most common; Fig. 3-56), gastrinoma, VIPoma and glucagonoma. These are often small and undetectable on US, CT and MRI, so imaging in suspected cases need to include radioisotope studies.

SPLEEN

Imaging Techniques

US (high-frequency linear transducer) is best for detecting small parenchymal lesions, such as focal fungal infection. MRI is preferred for further investigation of larger (>1 cm) uncertain lesions.

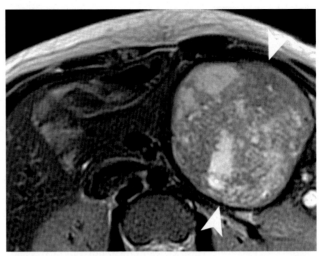

FIGURE 3-55 ■ Solid-cystic and papillary neoplasm (Frantz tumour; arrowheads) in an adolescent girl. Axial T2-weighted fast spin-echo MRI shows a heterogeneous hyperintense mass with a thick hypointense (fibrotic) rim.

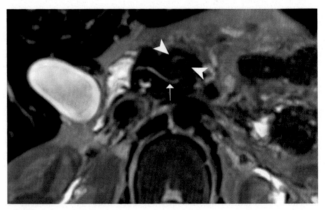

FIGURE 3-56 ■ MRI in a 9-year-old boy with pancreatic insulinoma. Axial T2-weighted MRI (grey scale) with overlay of diffusion-weighted (b, 1000) MRI (red tones) shows the insulinoma (arrowheads) because of its mildly restricted water diffusion. Note also how tumour deflects the main pancreatic duct (arrow) posteriorly.

Imaging Anatomy

Accessory spleens are common and of no interest. In the neonate the spleen is hypointense both on T1- and T2-weighted MRI. With increasing white pulp-to-red pulp ratio, its MRI contrast becomes similar to that in adults by 8 months of age. Table 3-12 suggests upper size limits. High-frequency US may demonstrate the spotted appearance of a reactive spleen (Fig. 3-57), which should not be mistaken for multifocal lesions.

Imaging Findings

Splenomegaly

Splenomegaly has a wide differential, as in adults. In children one also needs to consider mononucleosis, depositional disorders (Gaucher's disease, mucopolysacharidosis,

TABLE 3-12	Suggested Upper Limit of Normal Sonographic Measurement of the Spleen in Children[177]	
Age (months)	Suggested Upper Limit for the Sonographic Longitudinal Diameter (Coronal Orientation) of the Spleen (mm)	
1–3	70	
4–6	75	
7–9	80	
12–30	85	
36–59	95	
60–83	105	
84–107	105	
108–131	110	
132–155	115	
156–179	120	
180–200	120	

The limits are based on an ethnically homogeneous material. Considerable intra- and inter-observer variation need to be accounted for.

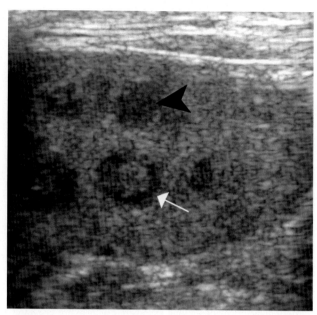

FIGURE 3-58 ■ US with a high-frequency linear transducer in a child with acute lymphoblastic leukaemia and febrile neutropenia shows several hypoechoic (arrowhead) and target lesions (arrow) suggestive of fungal infection.

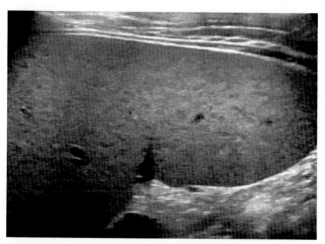

FIGURE 3-57 ■ US in a 10-year-old with falciparum malaria shows an enlarged spleen with a spotted appearance, which is commonly seen in reactive states and should not be mistaken for focal lesions.

Niemann–Pick disease), Langerhans cell histiocytosis and other conditions.

Wandering Spleen

Wandering spleen is associated with prune-belly syndrome, surgery and gastric volvulus, and predisposes to splenic torsion and infarction.

Focal Lesions

Most focal lesions (solitary or multifocal) in the spleen are infectious: abscesses and fungal infection (Fig. 3-58). Granulomata and hydatid cysts often contain calcification. (See also 'Neoplasia' section.)

Lateralisation Disorders (Fig. 3-59)

Both asplenia and polysplenia are associated with congenital heart disease.[101] Asplenia is more commonly associated with immunodeficiency and polysplenia with azygos continuation of IVC, preduodenal portal vein, bilateral left-sidedness of the lungs and biliary atresia. On US the spleen should be located near the greater curvature of the stomach, regardless of its situs. Radioisotope studies can be used to confirm asplenia.

Infarction

Splenic infarction may occur in disorders with massive sequestration (sickle-cell anaemia), deposition (storage disorders) or infiltration (leukaemia).

Trauma

Trauma epidemiology and mechanisms are different in children than in adults, but imaging is similar. The focused abdominal sonography for trauma (FAST) technique has low (50%) negative predictive value for abdominal injury in haemodynamically stable children post trauma, as compared with CT.[175]

More comprehensive, but still fast (median imaging time 5 min), US, performed by sonographers, in non-selected children post trauma, soon after arrival in an emergency department was reported as highly accurate, but less sensitive, in a prospective study, for any abdominal traumatic injury compared with a combination of CT, peritoneal lavage and laparotomy, with a negative predictive value of 91% for haemoperitoneum.[176]

Non-accidental injury is always an important differential, particularly in the younger age groups.[177] In children with abdominal injury following abuse, the frequency of injury to the spleen has been reported to come third, after small bowel and liver.[138]

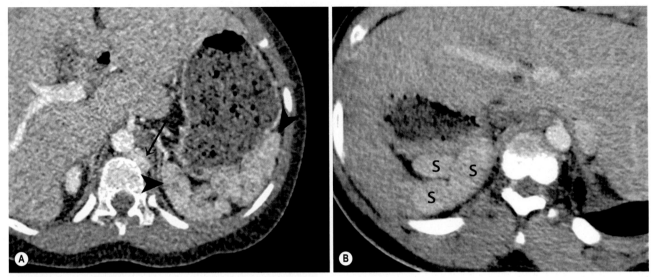

FIGURE 3-59 ■ Polysplenia on CT. (A) Multiple spleens (between arrowheads) in this child are associated with minor congenital heart disease and azygos (arrow) continuation of interrupted IVC. (B) Visceral situs inversus, multiple spleens (s) which in this child with primary ciliary dyskinesia was associated with major congenital heart disease and bronchial isomerism (Kartagener's syndrome).

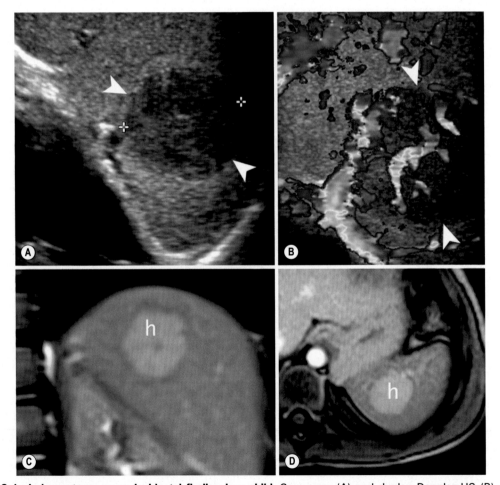

FIGURE 3-60 ■ Splenic hamartoma as an incidental finding in a child. Sonogram (A) and duplex Doppler US (B) demonstrate a vascularised well-demarcated, hypoechoic lesion (arrowheads). (C) Coronal T2-weighted MRI shows the lesion (h) as an almost geometrical figure (hexagon) with a fine hypointense perimeter and centre (resembling focal nodular hyperplasia of the liver). (D) There is homogeneous enhancement of the lesion (h) 3 min after intravenous administration of gadoteric acid.

Neoplasia

Most splenic neoplasms are benign. Cystic lesions are usually epidermoid/dermoid cysts, lymphangioma or splenic (epithelial) cysts. Solid lesions include haemangioma and hamartoma (Fig. 3-60). Malignant tumours are most commonly lymphoproliferative disease. Metastases and primary splenic angiosarcoma are rare.

REFERENCES

1. Sadler TW, Feldkamp ML. The embryology of body wall closure: relevance to gastroschisis and other ventral body wall defects. Am J Med Genet Part C (Semin Med Genet) 2008;148C:180–5.
2. Sadler TW. The embryologic origin of ventral body wall defects. Semin Pediatr Surg 2010;19:209–14.
3. Christison-Lagay ER, Kelleher CM, Langer JC. Neonatal abdominal wall defects. Semin Fetal Neonatal Med 2011;16:164–72.
4. Loane M, Dolk H, Bradbury I, et al. Increasing prevalence of gastroschisis in Europe 1980-2002: a phenomenon restricted to younger mothers? Paediatr Perinat Epidemiol 2007;21:363–9.
5. Suver D, Lee SL, Shekherdimian S, et al. Left-sided gastroschisis: higher incidence of extraintestinal congenital anomalies. Am J Surg 2008;195:663–6.
6. Baglaj M, Carachi R, MacCormack B. Colonic atresia: a clinico-pathological insight into its etiology. Eur J Pediatr Surg 2010;20(2):102–5.
7. Howell KK. Understanding gastroschisis: an abdominal wall defect. Neonatal Netw 1998;17(8):17–25.
8. Mortellaro VE, St. Peter SD, Fike FB, et al. Review of the evidence on the closure of abdominal wall defects. Pediatr Surg Int 2011;27:391–7.
9. Phillips TM. Spectrum of cloacal exstrophy. Semin Pediatr Surg 2011;20:113–18.
10. Sawaya D, Goldstein S, Seetharamaiah R, et al. Gastrointestinal ramifications of the cloacal exstrophy complex: a 44-year experience. J Pediatr Surg 2010;45:171–6.
11. Stec AA. Embryology and bony and pelvic floor anatomy in the bladder exstrophy-epispadias complex. Semin Pediatr Surg 2011;20:66–70.
12. Newman B, Bender TM. Esophageal atresia/tracheoesophageal fistula and associated congenital esophageal stenosis. Pediatr Radiol 1997;27(6):530–4.
13. Salomon LJ, Sonigo P, Ou P, et al. Real-time fetal magnetic resonance imaging for the dynamic visualization of the pouch in esophageal atresia. Ultrasound Obstet Gynecol 2009;34:471–4.
14. Holland AJA, Fitzgerald DA. Oesophageal atresia and tracheo-oesophageal fistula: current management strategies and complications. Paediatr Respir Rev 2010;11:100–7.
15. Luo C-C, Lin J-N, Wang C-R. Evaluation of oesophageal atresia without fistula by three-dimensional computed tomography. Eur J Pediatr Surg 2002;161:578–80.
16. Wen Y, Peng Y, Zhai R-Y. Application of MPVR and TL-VR with 64-row MDCT in neonates with congenital EA and distal TEF. World J Gastroenterol 2011;17(12):1649–54.
17. Soye JA, Yarr J, Dick AC, et al. Multidetector row computed tomography three-dimensional volume reformatted 'transparency' images to define an upper pouch fistula in oesophageal atresia. Pediatr Radiol 2005;35(6):624–6.
18. Zhao R, Li K, Shen C, et al. The outcome of conservative treatment for anastomotic leakage after surgical repair of esophageal atresia. J Pediatr Surg 2011;46:2274–8.
19. Rintala RJ, Sistonen S, Pakarinen MP. Outcome of esophageal atresia beyond childhood. Semin Pediatr Surg 2009;18:50–6.
20. Briganti V, Oriolo L, Mangia G, et al. Tracheomalacia in esophageal atresia. Usefulness of preoperative imaging evaluation for tailored surgical correction. J Pediatr Surg 2006;41:1624–8.
21. Gatzinsky V, Jönsson L, Ekerljung L, et al. Long-term respiratory symptoms following oesophageal atresia. Acta Paediatr 2011;100:1222–5.
22. Natsuga K, Nishie W, Shinkuma S, et al. Plectin deficiency leads to both muscular dystrophy and pyloric atresia in epidermolysis bullosa simplex. Hum Mutat 2010;31(10):E1687–E1698.
23. Shah A, More B, Buick R. Pyloric duplication in a neonate: a rare entity. Pediatr Surg Int 2005;21:220–2.
24. Sutcliffe J, Munden M. Sonographic diagnosis of multiple gastric duplication cysts causing gastric outlet obstruction in a pediatric patient. J Ultrasound Med 2006;25:1223–6.
25. Terui K, Iwai J, Yamada S-I. Etiology of neonatal gastric perforation: a review of 20 years' experience. Pediatr Surg Int 2012;28:9–14.
26. Lin C-M, Lee H-C, Kao H-A, et al. Neonatal gastric perforation: report of 15 cases and review of the literature. Pediatr Neonatol 2008;49(3):65–70.
27. Metzger R, Metzger U, Fiegel HC, et al. Embryology of the midgut. Semin Pediatr Surg 2011;20:145–51.
28. Levin TL, Liebling MS, Ruzal-Shapiro C, et al. Midgut malfixation in patients with congenital diaphragmatic hernia: what is the risk of midgut volvulus? Pediatr Radiol 1995;25(4):259–61.
29. Yousefzadeh DK, Kang L, Tessicini L. Assessment of retromesenteric position of the third portion of the duodenum: an US feasibility study in 33 newborns. Pediatr Radiol 2010;40:1476–84.
30. Bilodeau A, Prasil P, Cloutier R, et al. Hereditary multiple intestinal atresia: thirty years later. J Pediatr Surg 2004;39:726–30.
31. Neu J, Walker WA. Necrotizing enterocolitis. N Engl J Med 2011;364:255–64.
32. Epelman M, Daneman A, Navarro OM, et al. Necrotizing enterocolitis: review of state-of-the-art imaging findings with pathologic correlation. Radiographics 2007;27:285–305.
33. Silva CT, Daneman A, Navarro OM, et al. Correlation of sonographic findings and outcome in necrotizing enterocolitis. Pediatr Radiol 2007;37:274–82.
34. McBride WJ, Roy S, Brudnicki A, et al. Correlation of complex ascites with intestinal gangrene and perforation in neonates with necrotizing enterocolitis. J Pediatr Surg 2010;45:887–9.
35. Winters WD, Weinberger E, Hatch EI. Atresia of the colon in neonates: radiographic findings. Am J Roentgenol 1992;159(6):1273–6.
36. Doi T, O'Donnell A-M, McDermott M, et al. Skip segment Hirschsprung's disease: a rare phenomenon. Pediatr Surg Int 2011;27:787–9.
37. Kenny SE, Tam PK, Garcia-Barcelo M. Hirschsprung's disease. Semin Pediatr Surg 2010;19:194–200.
38. Sarioglu A, Tanyel FC, Buyukpamukcu N, et al. Colonic volvulus: a rare presentation of Hirschsprung's disease. J Pediatr Surg 1997;32(1):117–18.
39. De Lorijn F, Kremer LCM, Reitsma JB, et al. Diagnostic tests in Hirschsprung's disease: a systematic review. J Pediatr Gastroenterol Nutr 2006;42(5):496–505.
40. Reid JR, Buonomo C, Moreira C, et al. The barium enema in constipation: comparison with rectal manometry and biopsy to exclude Hirschsprung's disease after the neonatal period. Pediatr Radiol 2000;30:681–4.
41. Burge D, Drewett M. Meconium plug obstruction. Pediatr Surg Int 2004;20:108–10.
42. Krasna IH, Rosenfeld D, Salerno P. Is it necrotizing enterocolitis, microcolon of prematurity, or delayed meconium plug? A dilemma in the tiny premature infant. J Pediatr Surg 1996;31(6):855–8.
43. Blackman SM, Deering-Brose R, McWilliams R, et al. Relative contribution of genetic and non-genetic modifiers to intestinal obstruction in cystic fibrosis. Gastroenterology 2006;131(4):1030–9.
44. Kluth D. Embryology of anorectal malformations. Semin Pediatr Surg 2010;19:201–8.
45. Kluth D, Fiegel HC, Metzger R. Embryology of the hindgut. Semin Pediatr Surg 2011;20:152–60.
46. Levitt MA, Peña A. Anorectal malformations. Orphanet J Rare Dis 2007;2:33.
47. Holschneider A, Hutson J, Peña A, et al. Preliminary report on the International Conference for the Development of Standards for the Treatment of Anorectal Malformations. J Pediatr Surg 2005;40:1521–6.
48. Uchida K, Inoue M, Matsubara T, et al. Evaluation and treatment for spinal cord tethering in patients with anorectal malformations. Eur J Pediatr Surg 2007;17(6):408–11.
49. Miyasaka M, Nosaka S, Kitano Y, et al. Utility of spinal MRI in children with anorectal malformation. Pediatr Radiol 2009;39:810–16.

50. Hennelly KE, Bachur R. Appendicitis update. Curr Opin Pediatr 2011;23(3):281–5.
51. Hernandez JA, Swischuk LE, Angel CA, et al. Imaging of acute appendicitis: US as the primary imaging modality. Pediatr Radiol 2005;35(4):392–5.
52. Holscher HC, Heij HA. Imaging of acute appendicitis in children: EU versus U.S. ... or US versus CT? A European perspective. Pediatr Radiol 2009;39(5):497–9.
53. Bachur RG, Hennelly K, Callahan MJ, Monuteaux MC. Advanced radiologic imaging for pediatric appendicitis, 2005-2009: trends and outcomes. J Pediatr 2012;160(6):1034–8.
54. Goldin AB, Khanna P, Thapa M, et al. Revised ultrasound criteria for appendicitis in children improve diagnostic accuracy. Pediatr Radiol 2011;41(8):993–9.
55. Toorenvliet B, Vellekoop A, Bakker R, et al. Clinical differentiation between acute appendicitis and acute mesenteric lymphadenitis in children. Eur J Pediatr Surg 2011;21(2):120–3.
56. Griffin N, Grant LA, Anderson S, et al. Small bowel MR enterography: problem solving in Crohn's disease. Insights Imaging 2012;3(3):251–63.
57. Alexopoulou E, Roma E, Loggitsi D, et al. Magnetic resonance imaging of the small bowel in children with idiopathic inflammatory bowel disease: evaluation of disease activity. Pediatr Radiol 2009;39(8):791–7.
58. Gorincour G, Aschero A, Desvignes C, et al. Chronic inflammatory diseases of the bowel: diagnosis and follow-up. Pediatr Radiol 2010;40(6):920–6.
59. Fike FB, Mortellaro VE, Holcomb GW 3rd, St Peter SD. Predictors of failed enema reduction in childhood intussusception. J Pediatr Surg 2012;47(5):925–7.
60. Riera A, Hsiao AL, Langhan ML, et al. Diagnosis of intussusception by physician novice sonographers in the emergency department. Ann Emerg Med 2012;60(3):264–8.
61. Daneman A, Navarro O. Intussusception. Part 1: a review of diagnostic approaches. Pediatr Radiol 2003;33(2):79–85.
62. Daneman A, Navarro O. Intussusception. Part 2: An update on the evolution of management. Pediatr Radiol 2004;34(2):97–108; quiz 87.
63. Ilivitzki A, Shtark LG, Arish K, Engel A. Deep sedation during pneumatic reduction of intussusception. Pediatr Radiol 2012;42(5):562–5.
64. Tabbers MM, Boluyt N, Berger MY, Benninga MA. Clinical practice: diagnosis and treatment of functional constipation. Eur J Pediatr 2011;170(8):955–63.
65. Bardisa-Ezcurra L, Ullman R, Gordon J. Diagnosis and management of idiopathic childhood constipation: summary of NICE guidance. BMJ 2010;340:c2585.
66. Constipation Guideline Committee of the North American Society for Pediatric Gastroenterology, Hepatology and Nutrition. Evaluation and treatment of constipation in infants and children: recommendations of the North American Society for Pediatric Gastroenterology, Hepatology and Nutrition. J Pediatr Gastroenterol Nutr 2006;43(3):e1–13.
67. De Giorgio R, Cogliandro RF, Barbara G, et al. Chronic intestinal pseudo-obstruction: clinical features, diagnosis, and therapy. Gastroenterol Clin North Am 2011;40(4):787–807.
68. Saulsbury FT. Henoch-Schönlein purpura. Curr Opin Rheumatol 2001;13(1):35–40.
69. Chang WL, Yang YH, Lin YT, Chiang BL. Gastrointestinal manifestations in Henoch-Schönlein purpura: a review of 261 patients. Acta Paediatr 2004;93(11):1427–31.
70. Ha HK, Lee SH, Rha SE, et al. Radiologic features of vasculitis involving the gastrointestinal tract. Radiographics 2000;20(3):779–94.
71. Hur J, Yoon CS, Kim MJ, Kim OH. Imaging features of gastrointestinal tract duplications in infants and children: from oesophagus to rectum. Pediatr Radiol 2007;37(7):691–9.
72. Cheng G, Soboleski D, Daneman A, et al. Sonographic pitfalls in the diagnosis of enteric duplication cysts. Am J Roentgenol 2005;184(2):521–5.
73. Tong SC, Pitman M, Anupindi SA. Best cases from the AFIP. Ileocecal enteric duplication cyst: radiologic-pathologic correlation. Radiographics 2002;22(5):1217–22.
74. Wootton-Gorges SL, Thomas KB, Harned RK, et al. Giant cystic abdominal masses in children. Pediatr Radiol 2005;35(12):1277–88.
75. Konen O, Rathaus V, Dlugy E, et al. Childhood abdominal cystic lymphangioma. Pediatr Radiol 2002;32(2):88–94.
76. Vandenplas Y, Rudolph CD, Di Lorenzo C, et al. Pediatric gastroesophageal reflux clinical practice guidelines: joint recommendations of the North American Society for Pediatric Gastroenterology, Hepatology, and Nutrition (NASPGHAN) and the European Society for Pediatric Gastroenterology, Hepatology, and Nutrition (ESPGHAN). J Pediatr Gastroenterol Nutr 2009;49(4):498–547.
77. Oh SK, Han BK, Levin TL, et al. Gastric volvulus in children: the twists and turns of an unusual entity. Pediatr Radiol 2008;38(3):297–304.
78. Spigland N, Brandt ML, Yazbeck S. Malrotation presenting beyond the neonatal period. J Pediatr Surg 1990;25(11):1139–42.
79. Wanjari AK, Deshmukh AJ, Tayde PS, Lonkar Y. Midgut malrotation with chronic abdominal pain. N Am J Med Sci 2012;4(4):196–8.
80. Prasil P, Flageole H, Shaw KS, et al. Should malrotation in children be treated differently according to age? J Pediatr Surg 2000;35(5):756–8.
81. Sommerfield T, Chalmers J, Youngson G, et al. The changing epidemiology of infantile hypertrophic pyloric stenosis in Scotland. Arch Dis Child 2008;93(12):1007–11.
82. Niedzielski J, Kobielski A, Sokal J, Krakos M. Accuracy of sonographic criteria in the decision for surgical treatment in infantile hypertrophic pyloric stenosis. Arch Med Sci 2011;7(3):508–11.
83. Costa Dias S, Swinson S, Torrao H, et al. Hypertrophic pyloric stenosis: tips and tricks for ultrasound diagnosis. Insights Imaging 2012;3(3):247–50.
84. Levy AD, Hobbs CM. From the archives of the AFIP. Meckel diverticulum: radiologic features with pathologic correlation. Radiographics 2004;24(2):565–87.
85. Toma P, Granata C, Rossi A, Garaventa A. Multimodality imaging of Hodgkin disease and non-Hodgkin lymphomas in children. Radiographics 2007;27(5):1335–54.
86. Joy D, Thava VR, Scott BB. Diagnosis of fatty liver disease: is biopsy necessary? Eur J Gastroenterol Hepatol 2003;15(5):539–43.
87. Khoury NJ, Kanj V, Abboud M, et al. Abdominal complications of chemotherapy in pediatric malignancies: imaging findings. Clin Imaging 2009;33(4):253–60.
88. Haller JO, Cohen HL. Gastrointestinal manifestations of AIDS in children. Am J Roentgenol 1994;162(2):387–93.
89. Andronikou S, Welman CJ, Kader E. The CT features of abdominal tuberculosis in children. Pediatr Radiol 2002;32(2):75–81.
90. Munden MM, Bruzzi JF, Coley BD, Munden RF. Sonography of pediatric small-bowel intussusception: differentiating surgical from nonsurgical cases. Am J Roentgenol 2007;188(1):275–9.
91. Smyth RL, Ashby D, O'Hea U, et al. Fibrosing colonopathy in cystic fibrosis: results of a case-control study. Lancet 1995;346(8985):1247–51.
92. King LJ, Scurr ED, Murugan N, et al. Hepatobiliary and pancreatic manifestations of cystic fibrosis: MR imaging appearances. Radiographics 2000;20(3):767–77.
93. Sivit CJ. Imaging children with abdominal trauma. Am J Roentgenol 2009;192(5):1179–89.
94. Strouse PJ, Close BJ, Marshall KW, Cywes R. CT of bowel and mesenteric trauma in children. Radiographics 1999;19(5):1237–50.
95. Kim HC, Yang DM, Jin W, et al. Color Doppler twinkling artifacts in various conditions during abdominal and pelvic sonography. J Ultrasound Med 2010;29:621–32.
96. Riccabona M. Application of a second generation ultrasound contrast agent in infants and children? A European questionnaire-based survey. Pediatr Radiol 2012;42(12):1471–80.
97. Tamrazi A, Vasanawala SS. Functional hepatobiliary MR imaging in children. Pediatr Radiol 2011;41:1250–8.
98. Meyers AB, Towbin AJ, Serai S, et al. Characterization of pediatric liver lesions with gadoxetate disodium. Pediatr Radiol 2011;41:1183–97.
99. Patriquin HB, Perreault G, Grignon A, et al. Normal portal venous diameter in children. Pediatr Radiol 1990;20:451–3.

100. Soyupak S, Gunesli A, Seydaoğlu G, et al. Portal venous diameter in children: Normal limits according to age, weight and height. Eur J Radiol 2010;75:245–7.

101. Applegate KE, Goske MJ, Pierce G, Murphy D. Situs revisited: Imaging of the heterotaxy syndrome. Radiographics 1999;19:837–52; discussion 853–4.

102. Balistreri WF, Grand R, Hoofnagle JH, et al. Biliary atresia: Current concepts and research directions. Summary of a symposium. Hepatology 1996;23:1682–92.

103. Gubernick JA, Rosenberg HK, Ilaslan H, Kessler A. US approach to jaundice in infants and children. Radiographics 2000;20: 173–95.

104. Mishra K, Basu S, Roychoudhury S, Kumar P. Liver abscess in children: An overview. World J Pediatr 2010;6:210–16.

105. Garcia-Eulate R, Hussain N, Heller T, et al. CT and MRI of hepatic abscess in patients with chronic granulomatous disease. Am J Roentgenol 2006;187:482–90.

106. Akata D, Akhan O. Liver manifestations of cystic fibrosis. Eur J Radiol 2007;61:11–17.

107. Chaudry G, Navarro OM, Levine DS, Oudjhane K. Abdominal manifestations of cystic fibrosis in children. Pediatr Radiol 2006;36:233–40.

108. Akata D, Akhan O, Ozcelik U, et al. Hepatobiliary manifestations of cystic fibrosis in children: Correlation of CT and US findings. Eur J Radiol 2002;41:26–33.

109. Alisi A, Manco M, Vania A, Nobili V. Pediatric nonalcoholic fatty liver disease in 2009. J Pediatr 2009;155:469–74.

110. Sundaram SS, Zeitler P, Nadeau K. The metabolic syndrome and nonalcoholic fatty liver disease in children. Curr Opin Pediatr 2009;21:529–35 DOI: 10.1097/MOP.0b013e32832cb16f.

111. Pariente D, Franchi-Abella S. Paediatric chronic liver diseases: How to investigate and follow up? Role of imaging in the diagnosis of fibrosis. Pediatr Radiol 2010;40:906–19.

112. Noruegas MJ, Matos H, Gonçalves I, et al. Acoustic radiation force impulse-imaging in the assessment of liver fibrosis in children. Pediatr Radiol 2012;42:201–4.

113. Nobili V, Monti L, Alisi A, et al. Transient elastography for assessment of fibrosis in paediatric liver disease. Pediatr Radiol 2011; 41:1232–8.

114. Binkovitz LA, El-Youssef M, Glaser KJ, et al. Pediatric MR elastography of hepatic fibrosis: Principles, technique and early clinical experience. Pediatr Radiol 2012;42:402–9.

115. Barshop NJ, Francis CS, Schwimmer JB, Lavine JE. Nonalcoholic fatty liver disease as a comorbidity of childhood obesity. Ped Health 2009;3:271–81.

116. Qayyum A, Nystrom M, Noworolski SM, et al. MRI steatosis grading: Development and initial validation of a color mapping system. Am J Roentgenol 2012;198:582–8.

117. Pacifico L, Martino MD, Catalano C, et al. T1-weighted dual-echo MRI for fat quantification in pediatric nonalcoholic fatty liver disease. World J Gastroenterol 2011;17:3012–19.

118. Besnard M, Pariente D, Hadchouel M, et al. Portal cavernoma in congenital hepatic fibrosis. Angiographic reports of 10 pediatric cases. Pediatr Radiol 1994;24:61–5.

119. Gürkaynak G, Yildirim B, Aksoy F, Temuçin G. Sonographic findings in noncirrhotic portal fibrosis. J Clin Ultrasound 1998;26: 309–13.

120. Semelka RC, Hussain SM, Marcos HB, Woosley JT. Biliary hamartomas: Solitary and multiple lesions shown on current MR techniques including gadolinium enhancement. J Magn Reson Imaging 1999;10:196–201.

121. Lassau N, Auperin A, Leclere J, et al. Prognostic value of doppler-ultrasonography in hepatic veno-occlusive disease. Transplantation 2002;74:60–6.

122. Murray CP, Yoo SJ, Babyn PS. Congenital extrahepatic portosystemic shunts. Pediatr Radiol 2003;33:614–20.

123. Alonso-Gamarra E, Parrón M, Pérez A, et al. Clinical and radiologic manifestations of congenital extrahepatic portosystemic shunts: A comprehensive review. Radiographics 2011;31: 707–22.

124. Goyal N, Jain N, Rachapalli V, et al. Non-invasive evaluation of liver cirrhosis using ultrasound. Clin Radiol 2009;64:1056–66.

125. Patriquin H, Tessier G, Grignon A, Boisvert J. Lesser omental thickness in normal children: Baseline for detection of portal hypertension. Am J Roentgenol 1985;145:693–6.

126. Hoddick W, Jeffrey RB, Federle MP. CT differentiation of portal venous air from biliary tract air. J Comput Assist Tomogr 1982;6: 633–4.

127. Sharma R, Tepas JJ, Hudak ML, et al. Portal venous gas and surgical outcome of neonatal necrotizing enterocolitis. J Pediatr Surg 2005;40:371–6.

128. Wallot MA, Klepper J, Clapuyt P, et al. Repeated detection of gas in the portal vein after liver transplantation: A sign of EBV-associated post-transplant lymphoproliferation? Pediatr Transplant 2002;6:332–6.

129. Buetow PC, Buck JL, Pantongrag-Brown L, et al. Undifferentiated (embryonal) sarcoma of the liver: Pathologic basis of imaging findings in 28 cases. Radiology 1997;203:779–83.

130. Roebuck D. Focal liver lesion in children. Pediatr Radiol 2008;38(Suppl 3):S518–522.

131. Roebuck DJ, Aronson D, Clapuyt P, et al. 2005 PRETEXT: A revised staging system for primary malignant liver tumours of childhood developed by the SIOPEL group. Pediatr Radiol 2007;37:123–32.

132. Metry DW, Hawrot A, Altman C, Frieden IJ. Association of solitary, segmental hemangiomas of the skin with visceral hemangiomatosis. Arch Dermatol 2004;140:591–6.

133. Dubois J, Patriquin HB, Garel L, et al. Soft-tissue hemangiomas in infants and children: Diagnosis using Doppler sonography. Am J Roentgenol 1998;171:247–52.

134. Dubois J, Alison M. Vascular anomalies: What a radiologist needs to know. Pediatr Radiol 2010;40:895–905.

135. Roebuck D, Sebire N, Lehmann E, Barnacle A. Rapidly involuting congenital haemangioma (RICH) of the liver. Pediatr Radiol 2012;42:308–14.

136. Emery KH, McAneney CM, Racadio JM, et al. Absent peritoneal fluid on screening trauma ultrasonography in children: A prospective comparison with computed tomography. J Pediatr Surg 2001;36:565–9.

137. Schmidt B, Schimpl G, Höllwarth ME. Blunt liver trauma in children. Pediatr Surg Int 2004;20:846–50.

138. Raissaki M, Veyrac C, Blondiaux E, Hadjigeorgi C. Abdominal imaging in child abuse. Pediatr Radiol 2011;41:4–16; quiz 137–8.

139. Babyn PS. Imaging of the transplant liver. Pediatr Radiol 2010;40:442–6.

140. Faye A, Vilmer E. Post-transplant lymphoproliferative disorder in children: Incidence, prognosis, and treatment options. Paediatr Drugs 2005;7:55–65.

141. Hernanz-Schulman M, Ambrosino MM, Freeman PC, Quinn CB. Common bile duct in children: Sonographic dimensions. Radiology 1995;195:193–5.

142. McGahan JP, Phillips HE, Cox KL. Sonography of the normal pediatric gallbladder and biliary tract. Radiology 1982;144:873–5.

143. Mieli-Vergani G, Howard ER, Portman B, Mowat AP. Late referral for biliary atresia—missed opportunities for effective surgery. Lancet 1989;1:421–3.

144. Davenport M, Betalli P, D'Antiga L, et al. The spectrum of surgical jaundice in infancy. J Pediatr Surg 2003;38:1471–9.

145. Caponcelli E, Knisely AS, Davenport M. Cystic biliary atresia: An etiologic and prognostic subgroup. J Pediatr Surg 2008;43: 1619–24.

146. Hartley JL, Davenport M, Kelly DA. Biliary atresia. Lancet 2009;374:1704–13.

147. Jensen MK, Biank VF, Moe DC, et al. HIDA, percutaneous transhepatic cholecysto-cholangiography and liver biopsy in infants with persistent jaundice: Can a combination of PTCC and liver biopsy reduce unnecessary laparotomy? Pediatr Radiol 2012;42: 32–9.

148. Tan Kendrick AP, Phua KB, Ooi BC, et al. Making the diagnosis of biliary atresia using the triangular cord sign and gallbladder length. Pediatr Radiol 2000;30:69–73.

149. Kanegawa K, Akasaka Y, Kitamura E, et al. Sonographic diagnosis of biliary atresia in pediatric patients using the 'triangular cord' sign versus gallbladder length and contraction. Am J Roentgenol 2003;181:1387–90.

150. Humphrey TM, Stringer MD. Biliary atresia: US diagnosis. Radiology 2007;244:845–51.

151. Choi SO, Park WH, Lee HJ, Woo SK. 'Triangular cord': A sonographic finding applicable in the diagnosis of biliary atresia. J Pediatr Surg 1996;31:363–6.

152. Aziz S, Wild Y, Rosenthal P, Goldstein RB. Pseudo gallbladder sign in biliary atresia—an imaging pitfall. Pediatr Radiol 2011;41:620–6; quiz 681–2.

153. Lee MS, Kim MJ, Lee MJ, et al. Biliary atresia: color doppler US findings in neonates and infants. Radiology 2009;252:282–9.

154. Mittal V, Saxena AK, Sodhi KS, et al. Role of abdominal sonography in the preoperative diagnosis of extrahepatic biliary atresia in infants younger than 90 days. Am J Roentgenol 2011;196:W438–45.

155. Howman-Giles R, Uren R, Bernard E, Dorney S. Hepatobiliary scintigraphy in infancy. J Nucl Med 1998;39:311–19.

156. Makin E, Davenport M. Understanding choledochal malformation. Arch Dis Child 2012;97:69–72.

157. Stringer MD, Dhawan A, Davenport M. Choledochal cysts: Lessons from a 20 year experience. Arch Dis Child 1995;73:528–31.

158. Miyano T, Yamataka A. Choledochal cysts. Curr Opin Pediatr 1997;9:283–8.

159. Fitzpatrick E, Jardine R, Farrant P, et al. Predictive value of bile duct dimensions measured by ultrasound in neonates presenting with cholestasis. J Pediatr Gastroenterol Nutr 2010;51:55–60.

160. Chapuy S, Gorincour G, Roquelaure B, et al. Sonographic diagnosis of a common pancreaticobiliary channel in children. Pediatr Radiol 2006;36:1300–5.

161. Brancatelli G, Federle MP, Vilgrain V, et al. Fibropolycystic liver disease: CT and MR imaging findings. Radiographics 2005;25:659–70.

162. Bloustein PA. Association of carcinoma with congenital cystic conditions of the liver and bile ducts. Am J Gastroenterol 1977;67:40–6.

163. Wesdorp I, Bosman D, de Graaff A, et al. Clinical presentations and predisposing factors of cholelithiasis and sludge in children. J Pediatr Gastroenterol Nutr 2000;31:411–17.

164. Lee MJ, Kim MJ, Yoon CS. MR cholangiopancreatography findings in children with spontaneous bile duct perforation. Pediatr Radiol 2010;40:687–92.

165. Wilschanski M, Chait P, Wade JA, et al. Primary sclerosing cholangitis in 32 children: Clinical, laboratory, and radiographic features, with survival analysis. Hepatology 1995;22:1415–22.

166. LaRusso NF, Shneider BL, Black D, et al. Primary sclerosing cholangitis: Summary of a workshop. Hepatology 2006;44:746–64.

167. Siegel MJ, Martin KW, Worthington JL. Normal and abnormal pancreas in children: US studies. Radiology 1987;165:15–18.

168. Chao HC, Lin SJ, Kong MS, Luo CC. Sonographic evaluation of the pancreatic duct in normal children and children with pancreatitis. J Ultrasound Med 2000;19:757–63.

169. Bertin C, Pelletier AL, Vullierme MP, et al. Pancreas divisum is not a cause of pancreatitis by itself but acts as a partner of genetic mutations. Am J Gastroenterol 2012;107:311–17.

170. Zyromski NJ, Sandoval JA, Pitt HA, et al. Annular pancreas: Dramatic differences between children and adults. J Am Coll Surg 2008;206:1019–25; discussion 1025–7.

171. Haldorsen IS, Vesterhus M, Raeder H, et al. Lack of pancreatic body and tail in HNF1B mutation carriers. Diabet Med 2008;25:782–7.

172. De Boeck K, Weren M, Proesmans M, Kerem E. Pancreatitis among patients with cystic fibrosis: Correlation with pancreatic status and genotype. Pediatrics 2005;115:e463–9.

173. Pezzilli R, Morselli-Labate AM, Castellano E, et al. Acute pancreatitis in children. An Italian multicentre study. Dig Liver Dis 2002;34:343–8.

174. Arnoux JB, Verkarre V, Saint-Martin C, et al. Congenital hyperinsulinism: Current trends in diagnosis and therapy. Orphanet J Rare Dis 2011;6:63.

175. Coley BD, Mutabagani KH, Martin LC, et al. Focused abdominal sonography for trauma (FAST) in children with blunt abdominal trauma. J Trauma 2000;48:902–6.

176. Richards JR, Knopf NA, Wang L, McGahan JP. Blunt abdominal trauma in children: Evaluation with emergency US. Radiology 2002;222:749–54.

177. Konuş OL, Ozdemir A, Akkaya A, et al. Normal liver, spleen, and kidney dimensions in neonates, infants, and children: Evaluation with sonography. Am J Roentgenol 1998;171:1693–8.

CHAPTER 4

IMAGING OF THE KIDNEYS, URINARY TRACT AND PELVIS IN CHILDREN

Owen Arthurs • Marina Easty • Michael Riccabona

OVERVIEW

In this chapter, we cover the important areas of renal, urinary tract and pelvic imaging in children, emphasising the importance of congenital abnormalities and the need for minimising radiation burden and optimising image quality.

Ultrasound (US) is the preferred method for imaging the paediatric population, due to the ease of availability, lack of ionising radiation, reproducibility and because it is usually well tolerated. Modern US is often the only modality required to make a diagnosis, with the high frequency probes and new technology producing exquisite anatomical details in children who are ideal subjects. Alternatively, US can be used to direct other imaging modalities, such as functional assessment of the urinary tract by ^{99m}Tc-MAG3 dynamic imaging.

Intravenous urography (IVU) is now rarely used. Fluoroscopic micturating cystourethrography (MCUG) is essential to exclude bladder outflow obstruction such as in posterior urethral valves and urethral pathology, and to assess for vesicoureteric reflux (VUR). Contrast-enhanced voiding urosonography (ce-VUS) with microbubble contrast is used in some European countries rather than a fluoroscopic examination for VUR assessment, avoiding the radiation burden from conventional MCUG. Direct isotope cystography using ^{99m}Tc-pertechnetate is a low-dose functional study used to assess VUR, particularly in girls, where urethral anatomy is usually normal. Older, continent and cooperative children may benefit from an indirect radionuclide cystogram, IRC, as part of their dynamic ^{99m}Tc-MAG3 renogram, as a non-invasive means of assessing for VUR.

Cross-sectional imaging—computed tomography (CT) and magnetic resonance imaging (MRI)—is crucial in tumour imaging, for disease staging and prognostication as well as for imaging complications. CT is used much less frequently in children than in adults for urolithiasis: indeed, only severe trauma imaging relies on CT in children. The role of MRI is increasing both for anatomical and functional diagnostic information, particularly in cooperative older children, and where nuclear medicine is not available.

Conventional angiography is reserved for specific clinical indications, and is invasive with a high radiation burden. CT and MR angiography (MRA), however, have emerged as replacements for angiography for many diagnostic purposes.

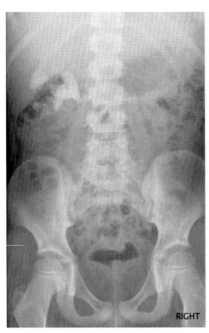

FIGURE 4-1 ■ Renal calculus. Plain abdominal radiograph of a large staghorn calculus in the right kidney.

Here we review the relative strengths and weaknesses of these techniques, illustrated using specific pathologies and recommend imaging algorithms.

IMAGING TECHNIQUES

Plain Radiography

Radiographs still have a role to play in babies with congenital renal anomalies, particularly in those cases associated with skeletal anomalies, such as vertebral segmentation anomalies and pubic diastasis (in bladder exstrophy). They may show renal tract calculi (Fig. 4-1) where the exposure should be coned to the kidneys, ureters and bladder (so-called 'KUB film').

Age-appropriate exposure settings and electronic filtering (in digital radiography equipment) are essential.

Ultrasound

Ultrasound is the most useful way of providing anatomical information about the intra-abdominal, pelvic and retroperitoneal structures. The ability to delineate and recognise normal and abnormal findings is directly related to the skill of the ultrasonographer and the equipment used, including high-frequency transducers, and familiarity examining children in a conducive environment, with knowledge of the spectrum of diseases in childhood being paramount. Several European guidelines regarding standard paediatric urinary tract US are available.[1]

Standard Technique

In the young child, ideally a full bladder is necessary, which usually requires at least 30–60 min of encouraged

---

Well-hydrated patient, full bladder, adequate equipment & transducer, training, etc.

↓

Urinary bladder: size (volume), shape, ostium, wall, bladder neck, include distal ureter & retrovesical space/ internal genitalia

Optional: CDS for urine inflow, perineal US, scrotal US ...

↓

Kidneys: lateral and/or dorsal, longitudinal and axial sections, parenchyma? Pelvicalyceal system?
Standardised measurements in 3 planes & volume calculation.
If dilated: + max. axial pelvis & calyxdiameter, narrowest parenchymal width + ureteropelvic junction

Optional: (a)CDS & duplex Doppler

↓

Post-void evaluation
Bladder: residual volume, bladder neck, shape & configuration
Kidneys: dilatation of pelvicalyceal system/ureter changed?

Optional: ce-VUS, 3DUS ...

Note: Cursory US of entire abdomen is recommended for first study, and in mismatch of findings and query

FIGURE 4-2 ■ US of the urinary tract. ESPR imaging recommendations for standard paediatric sonography of the urinary tract. US = ultrasound, CDS = colour Doppler sonography, ce-VUS = contrast-enhanced voiding urosonography, 3DUS = three-dimensional ultrasound. (Adapted from Riccabona M, Avni F E, Blickman J G, et al 2008 Imaging recommendations in paediatric uroradiology: minutes of the ESPR workgroup session on urinary tract infection, foetal hydronephrosis, urinary tract ultrasonography and voiding cystourethrography, Barcelona, Spain, June 2007. Pediatr Radiol 38(2).138–145.[1])

fluid intake to allow adequate hydration. Any US examination of the abdomen should begin by imaging the bladder, to fortuitously attempt to capture a full bladder (as the infant in nappies may void at any time). The distended bladder provides an acoustic window for the lower urinary tract, bladder neck and ureteric orifices (vesicoureteric junction), distal ureters, internal genitalia, retrovesical space, pelvic musculature and vessels (Fig. 4-2).[1]

It is customary to measure pre- and post-micturition bladder volumes, as incomplete voiding may be related to bladder dysfunctions and urinary tract infections, and the presence of pre- and/or post-micturition upper tract dilatation. Normal age-related changes in the kidney must be appreciated. The neonatal kidneys lack renal sinus fat over the first 6 months of life, and the medullary pyramids are typically large and hypoechoic relative to the cortex (the opposite to that found in older children and adults), which may be mistaken for pelvicalyceal dilatation or 'cysts' (Fig. 4-3). The normal neonatal renal cortex is also hyper- to iso-echoic relative to the adjacent normal liver, which again can often be reversed in adults. The neonatal renal pyramids may be echogenic, a transient physiological appearance in up to 5% of newborns, and should not be mistaken for nephrocalcinosis, although it can be seen in older infants with dehydration.[2] The

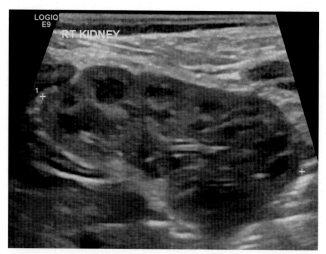

FIGURE 4-3 ■ **Normal neonatal kidney.** Oblique US image of a normal neonatal kidney. The medullary pyramids are hypo-echoic relative to the cortex (the opposite to that found in older children and adults), which may be mistaken for pelvicalyceal dilatation.

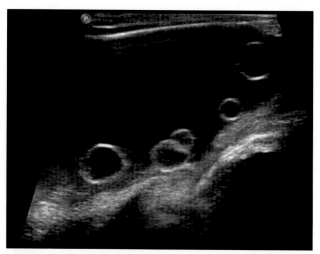

FIGURE 4-5 ■ **Ovarian cysts.** US of a neonatally physiologically large ovarian cyst with daughter cysts.

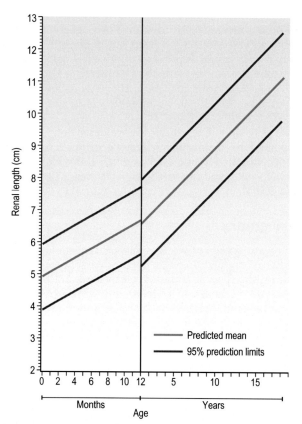

FIGURE 4-4 ■ **Renal growth chart.** Normal reference sizes and 95th centiles given by age of child.

average newborn kidney is approximately 4.5 cm in length, and measurements of bipolar renal lengths can be compared against age/height/weight indexed charts (Fig. 4-4). As the paediatric kidney is more spherical than the ellipsoid adult kidney, renal volumes may be a better assessment using the equation:

$$\text{Kidney Volume} = 0.523 \ (\pi/6) \times \text{length} \times \text{width} \times \text{depth}$$

Colour Doppler sonography (CDS) of the renal vessels is particularly important in assessing perfusion in a variety of conditions, including infection (segmental perfusion impairment), trauma (hilar vascular injury), biopsy (post-biopsy complications), renal failure, urolithiasis tumours, renal transplants and hypertension, and for the vascular anatomy in hydronephrosis (HN). High-frequency linear transducers yield better images in smaller children, especially in the prone position and should be performed for detailed analysis in all examinations.[1]

Normal Gonadal Imaging in Girls

Normal pelvic structures can be difficult to visualise in children: visualisation of the ovaries by US depends on their location, size and the age of the girl—they are more easily seen in the first few months of life. Ovarian volume is usually under 1 mL in the neonate, and 2–4 mL in the prepubertal child. Ovaries typically look heterogeneous due to the presence of follicles, and larger follicles can appear as small ovarian 'cysts' which are normal at all ages (Fig. 4-5). After puberty, ovarian volumes of 5–15 mL are normal, with normal primordial follicles <10 mm in diameter, and stimulated follicles 10–30 mm in diameter.

The normal uterus also changes dramatically with hormonal changes, and is the most useful guide to pubertal staging. The neonatal uterus is prominent due to circulating maternal oestrogens, typically measuring 2–4.5 cm in length, with thickened and clearly visible endometrial lining (Fig. 4-6A). By 1 year of age it becomes smaller, has changed to the prepubertal tubular appearances: the fundus and cervix are the same size and the endometrium is no longer visible (Fig. 4-6B). At puberty, the fundus starts to enlarge, becomes up to three times the size of the cervix, with a total uterine length of 5–7 cm and the typical adult pear-like shape. The endometrial appearances will clearly vary with the phase of the menstrual cycle.

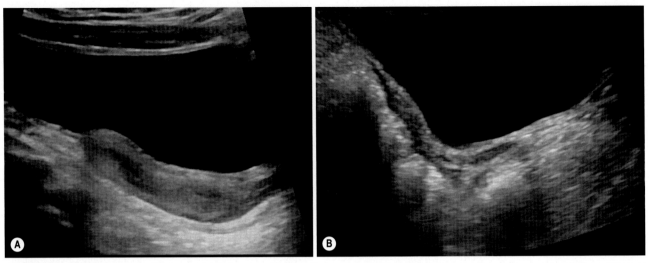

FIGURE 4-6 ■ Normal uterus. (A) Sagittal US image of normal neonatal uterus, which is prominent due to circulating maternal oestrogens with a clearly visible endometrial lining. (B) Sagittal US image of the infantile uterus which has a prepubertal tubular appearance: the fundus and cervix are the same size and the endometrium is no longer visible.

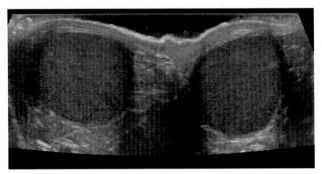

FIGURE 4-7 ■ Normal testes. Axial US image of normal prepubertal testes.

The vagina may be visualised by US if airfilled, (shown as a linear bright echo), or if fluid filled. On MRI the vagina is best seen on sagittal T2-weighted spin-echo MRI. As with the uterus, the appearance and the thickness of the vaginal epithelium and the signal from the vaginal wall change with the age and the phases of the menstrual cycle. Ultrasound genitography with saline filling of the vagina, or 3D US can be used for uterine anomalies, and perineal US for vagina and urethral pathology.[3,4]

Normal Gonadal Imaging in Boys

The prostate has an ellipsoid homogeneous appearance, but is difficult to see in newborns, as are the seminal vesicles. As the processus vaginalis remains open for some time after birth (and may never close completely), hydroceles are considered a normal physiological finding in the newborn. Cryptorchidism is discussed later in this chapter.

The normal testis changes in appearance during childhood. It has a homogeneous hypoechoic echotexture and is spherical/oval in shape during the neonatal period, measuring <10 mm in diameter (Fig. 4-7). The epididymis and mediastinum testis are usually not seen at this point, but are clearly identified by puberty. Testicular size in adolescence ranges from 3 to 5 cm in length and from 2 to 3 cm in depth and width (2–4 mL in total). Testicular flow, as measured by Doppler US, also changes with age. The testis in infants shows very low-velocity colour flow, which can be difficult to see despite optimised slow-flow settings, and even normal prepubertal testes may show not exhibit low-velocity flow on power Doppler US. Technically it may be difficult to identify abnormalities in a single testis given the wide range of normal values, and thus a side-by-side comparison can be most useful.

Cystography

There are several ways to visualise the bladder in the paediatric population. The method of choice depends both on the type of pathology suspected and the age of child. All methods, apart from the ^{99m}Tc-MAG3 IRC, require a bladder catheter, which becomes more unpleasant for both child (and the carer who observes) as the child gets older. The modern MCUG, using pulsed fluoroscopy, digital image amplifiers and last image hold, means that high-quality imaging is now available at an acceptably low radiation dose (Table 4-1).

The direct isotope cystogram is useful in the assessment of VUR in young babies (before toilet training), particularly in girls where there is no need to demonstrate the urethral anatomy, or for screening other family members when the index of suspicion for reflux is high.

Micturating (Voiding) Cystogram (MCUG/VCUG)

Indications. If the male baby is found (on US) to have significant bilateral hydronephrosis (HN), a dilated ureter, a pathological urethra or a thick-walled bladder,

TABLE 4-1   **Comparison of Relative Radiation Doses from Urological Examinations**

	DRL (MBq)	Effective Dose (mSv)	Equivalent CXR (0.02 MSv)	Equivalence to NBR (2.6 mSv/year)	Equivalence to a Return Transatlantic Flight (0.1 mSv)
AXR	N/A	0.7	35	3.3 months	7
MCUG in girls	N/A	0.9	45	4.2 months	9
MCUG in boys	N/A	1.5	75	6.9 months	15
DIC	20 MBq	0.3	15	1.4 months	3
DMSA	80 MBq	1.0	50	4.6 months	10
MAG3 renogram	100 MBq	0.7	35	3.3 months	7
MAG3 transplant	200 MBq	1	50	4.6 months	10
DTPA transplant	330 MBq	2	100	9.2 months	20
CT abdomen/pelvis	N/A	10	500	3.85 years	100

CXR = chest radiograph, AXR = abdominal radiograph, DIC = direct radio-isotope cystogram, N/A = not applicable or available. MBq = megabequerel. NBR = national background radiation dose (approximate for UK).

an MCUG is then performed.[5] MCUG is also indicated for VUR assessment, such as after (recurrent or complicated) UTI, or for assessing complex malformations that involve the urinary tract. The MCUG is the only accepted method of lower urinary tract imaging to demonstrate the urethral anatomy clearly, although perineal US performed during voiding also allows assessment of the urethra. It is essential in boys, where urethral pathology is suspected: for example, in boys with suspected posterior urethral valves (Figs. 4-8 and 4-9), cloacal anomaly, or anorectal anomaly and suspected colovesical fistula (Fig. 4-10). The fistula may not be seen on an MCUG. A distal loopogram (i.e. intubating the distal limb of the colostomy and injecting radio-opaque water-soluble iodine-containing contrast under pressure is the best technique to delineate these connections.

MCUG Technique. A sterile narrow feeding tube is used to catheterise the neonatal urethra, secured with tape. A suprapubic catheter may be used in individual cases, or in-dwelling Foley catheter, provided that the balloon is carefully deflated in order to prevent bladder pathology being obscured, or obstruction to bladder emptying increasing the chance of bladder rupture.[1] Warmed water-soluble iodinated contrast is then dripped from a height of no greater than 60 cm (physiological filling pressure of 30–40 cm water). Rapid bladder filling using a syringe may generate high pressures leading to bladder overextension and artificial VUR, as well as altered bladder capacity values. Bladder capacity increases during the first 8 years of life and normal bladder capacity for children 0–8 years can be estimated using the equation (age + 1) × 30 mL.

Early bladder filling views are obtained with the child supine. Tight coning is important to reduce dose. Oblique views are then obtained to assess the vesicoureteric junction and urethra on voiding. In the first few years of life, cyclical filling is advocated, as there is an increased chance of detecting VUR with consecutive voiding cycles.[1] The bladder is refilled and on the second or third void, the catheter is removed so that a well-distended urethral view is obtained. Prophylactic oral or intravesical antibiotics are used, and MCUG is contraindicated in the presence of a urinary tract infection. In a modified

Indications: febrile and recurrent UTI, particularly in infants, suspected PUV, UT malformation, HN > II° or 'extended criteria'

↓

Preparations: no diet restriction or enema, urine analysis, after AB are completed...
Catheterisation: feeding tube, 4-8Fr or suprapubic puncture, anaesthetic lubricant or coated plaster
Latex precaution: neuro tube defect, bladder exstrophy

↓

Fluoroscopic view of renal fossae and bladder, initial + early filling Bladder filling with radio-opaque contrast medium gravity drip; bottle 30-40 cm above table, watch dripping, AB?

↓

Fluoroscopy: signs of increased bladder pressure, imminent voiding, urge: bilateral oblique views of distal ureters, include catheter, document VUR, include kidney (spot film: intra-renal reflux)

↓

When voiding: remove catheter, unless cyclic VCUG = 3 fillings, 1st y(s) female: 2 spot films of distended urethra (slightly oblique) male: 2–3 spot films during voiding (AP & steep oblique/lateral) include renal fossae during voiding, if VUR→ spot film

↓

After voiding: AP view of bladder and renal fossae assess contrast drainage from kidney if refluxed

Note: VUR staging, minimise fluoroscopy time and spot films; no control film

FIGURE 4-8 ■ **VCUG.** ESPR imaging recommendations for voiding cystourethrography (VCUG). AB = antibiotics, HN = hydronephrosis, PUV = posterior urethral valve, UT = urinary tract, UTI = urinary tract infection, VCUG = voiding cystourethrography, VUR = vesicoureteral reflux. (Adapted from Riccabona M, Avni F E, Blickman J G, et al 2008 Imaging recommendations in paediatric uroradiology: minutes of the ESPR workgroup session on urinary tract infection, fetal hydronephrosis, urinary tract ultrasonography and voiding cystourethrography, Barcelona, Spain, June 2007. Pediatr Radiol 38(2):138–145.[1])

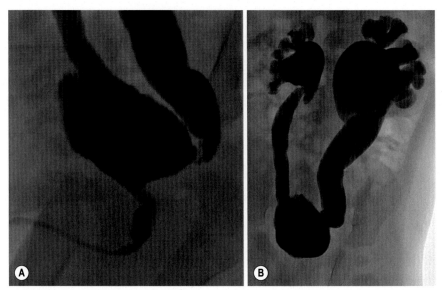

FIGURE 4-9 ■ **Posterior urethral valves on MCUG.** (A) There is acute calibre change in the posterior urethra caused by posterior urethral valves, with a trabeculated bladder note bilateral gross VUR. (B) Bilateral high-grade reflux is demonstrated.

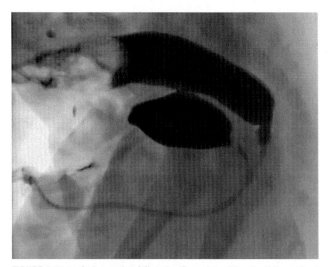

FIGURE 4-10 ■ **Colourethral fistula.** On micturition in this patient with an anorectal malformation, contrast passed retrogradely into the colon via the fistula.

MCUG, the contrast infusion is monitored for stopping or backflow in drip rate, which may represent dysfunctional sphincter or detrusor contractions, indicating functional disturbances.[6,7]

Contrast-Enhanced Ultrasonography (ce-VUS)

Contrast-enhanced voiding urosonography (ce-VUS) is a non-ionising alternative used throughout Europe, but less commonly used in the UK. Recommended indications for ce-VUS presently include screening populations, in girls, bedside investigations and for follow-up, although none of the ce-VUS contrast agents are currently licensed in children. Study recommendations and VUR grading are available (Fig. 4-11).[1,8]

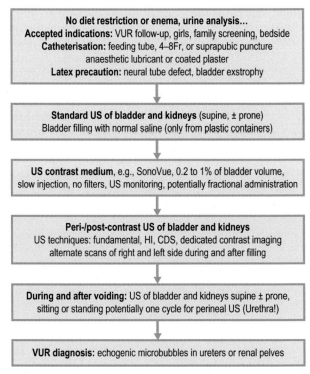

No diet restriction or enema, urine analysis...
Accepted indications: VUR follow-up, girls, family screening, bedside
Catheterisation: feeding tube, 4–8Fr, or suprapubic puncture
anaesthetic lubricant or coated plaster
Latex precaution: neural tube defect, bladder exstrophy

Standard US of bladder and kidneys (supine, ± prone)
Bladder filling with normal saline (only from plastic containers)

US contrast medium, e.g., SonoVue, 0.2 to 1% of bladder volume,
slow injection, no filters, US monitoring, potentially fractional administration

Peri-/post-contrast US of bladder and kidneys
US techniques: fundamental, HI, CDS, dedicated contrast imaging
alternate scans of right and left side during and after filling

During and after voiding: US of bladder and kidneys supine ± prone,
sitting or standing potentially one cycle for perineal US (Urethra!)

VUR diagnosis: echogenic microbubbles in ureters or renal pelves

FIGURE 4-11 ■ **Ce-VUS.** ESPR imaging recommendations for contrast-enhanced voiding urosonography (ce-VUS). CDS = colour Doppler sonography, VUR = vesicoureteral reflux. (Adapted from Riccabona M, Avni F E, Blickman J G, et al 2008 Imaging recommendations in paediatric uroradiology: minutes of the ESPR workgroup session on urinary tract infection, fetal hydronephrosis, urinary tract ultrasonography and voiding cystourethrography, Barcelona, Spain, June 2007. Pediatr Radiol 38(2):138–145.[1] and updated in Riccabona M; Vivier HP; Ntoulj A; Darge K, Avni F; Papadopoulou F; Damasio B; Ording-Mueller LS; Blickman J; Lobo ML; Willi U. (2014) ESPR Uroradiology Task Force—Imaging Recommendations in Paediatric Uroradiology—Part VII: Standardized terminology, impact of existing recommendations, and update on contrast-enhanced ultrasound of the paediatric urogenital tract. Report on the mini-symposium at the ESPR meeting in Budapest, June 2013, Pediatr Radiol submit)

Technique. Typically, SonoVue (Bracco/Italy) at 0.2–1.0% of bladder filling volume is given via urinary catheter as for MCUG by saline drip, following standard renal tract US views. Dedicated low-MI contrast imaging of both kidneys and the bladder including the retrovesical space and the urethra during and after filling is performed, with echogenic microbubbles in the ureters or renal pelvis indicating VUR.

Nuclear Medicine

Direct Radio-Isotope Cystogram (DIC)

A DIC is predominantly used to detect the presence of VUR in baby girls, or as VUR follow-up in baby boys.

Technique. Catheterisation using a 6Fr feeding tube can usually be performed with the baby lying on the Gamma camera, wearing a double nappy. Twenty megabequerels of ^{99m}Tc-pertechnetate is introduced into the bladder followed by warmed saline. The baby is restrained with sandbags and Velcro straps, and bladder filling is performed twice. The baby will spontaneously void when the bladder is full and VUR evaluated. The kidneys are kept in the field of view at all times to detect VUR.

Indirect Radio-Isotope Cystogram

This is a useful, well-tolerated and physiological procedure to assess bladder function and for the presence of VUR. It is performed at the end of dynamic renography in cooperative and toilet-trained children who can void on demand. After a non-diuretic stressed dynamic ^{99m}Tc-MAG3 renogram, the gamma camera is turned vertically Children seated on a commode with their backs to the camera. Boys may stand and void. The acquisition is started just before voiding starts and continues for 30 s after voiding, up to approximately 2 min total acquisition time, if required. The study can be repeated if there is still tracer present in the bladder when bladder emptying is incomplete, or when refluxed tracer re-enters the bladder from the upper renal tract. Bladder dysfunction can be assessed and VUR can be seen on the dynamic study. Guidelines are available from the European Association of Nuclear Medicine.[9]

Static Renal Scintigraphy; ^{99m}Tc-DMSA Scans

Dimercaptosuccinic acid (DMSA) is used as a ^{99m}Tc tracer; it is filtered by the glomeruli and reabsorbed, binding to the proximal convoluted tubules to give a static image over several hours. Approximately 10% of the tracer is excreted in the urine. Routinely, three posteriorly acquired views are obtained (posterior, right and left posterior oblique views), with anterior views used in abnormal renal anatomy (transplants, pelvic and ectopic kidneys) or scoliosis. Anterior and posterior views may then be used to estimate the differential renal function (DRF) by the geometric mean. As renal DMSA uptake relies on sufficient glomerular clearance, sufficient renal function is essential for meaningful results, as well as

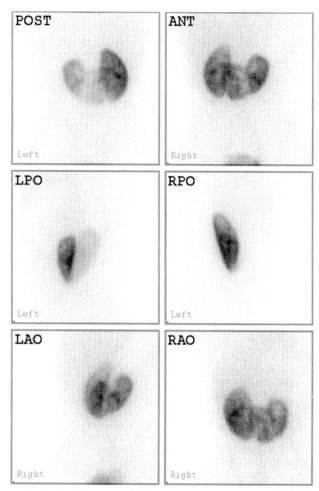

FIGURE 4-12 ■ **Horseshoe kidney.** ^{99m}Tc-DMSA scan of a horseshoe kidney showing fusion at the lower poles in the midline.

sufficient urinary drainage from the renal pelvis to avoid tracer pooling artefacts.

The main use of the ^{99m}Tc-DMSA scan is in the assessment of the DRF and cortical abnormalities, such as renal scarring, fusion defects, ectopic or duplex kidneys and in hypertension (e.g. Fig. 4-12). DRF may also be helpful for pre- and post-transplant assessment and in abdominal tumours, where the renal blood supply may be at risk, or where the kidney lies in the radiotherapy field. All indications are given in Table 4-2. There are no contraindications.

Dynamic Renography

Dynamic renography is used to assess split renal function and drainage from the renal collecting systems in suspected obstruction.[10] In Europe, the most common isotope used in paediatric dynamic imaging is ^{99m}Tc-MAG3, which reflects tubular function. ^{99m}Tc-DTPA is also utilised, and uptake reflects glomerular function; thus, it is more commonly is used to calculate the glomerular filtration rate (GFR) and is the least expensive renal imaging agent capable of dynamic assessment. After intravenous administration, about 50% of the ^{99m}Tc-MAG3 in the blood is extracted by the proximal tubules with each pass through the kidneys. The ^{99m}Tc-MAG3 is

TABLE 4-2   Indications for ^{99m}Tc-DMSA Examination

- Assessment of differential renal function:
  - e.g. Assessment of functioning renal tissue when renal anatomical variants are encountered, such as duplex kidneys, horseshoe kidneys and cross-fused kidneys, as well as ectopic kidneys
- Assessment for focal parenchymal defects, typically 4–6 months following UTI
- Acute DMSA scans may be performed to confirm pyelonephritis
- Differentiating a multicystic dyplastic kidney from a hydronephrotic kidney
- Assessment of which kidney to biopsy in bilateral disease
- Assessment of function in children with cystic renal disease
- Assessment of focal defects in a hypertensive child, particularly prior to catheter angiography
- Assessment of a transplant kidney in those children with an unfavourable bladder who thus may be prone to reflux and silent infection
- Assessment of functioning renal tissue in children with bilateral Wilms' tumours where renal conserving surgery is being contemplated
- Assessment of DRF in children undergoing abdominal radiotherapy where the kidneys are in the therapy field

TABLE 4-3   Indications for ^{99m}Tc-MAG3 Dynamic Renography

- To assess divided renal function and urinary drainage where the collecting system is dilated
- To assess DRF following surgery or procedure, for example post pyeloplasty, or post removal of a double J stent
- Following renal transplant, to assess for urinary leak or possible obstruction

TABLE 4-4   Indications for IVU in Children

- Suspected ureteral and renal trauma, only if CT is not available
- As a delayed KUB view after contrast-enhanced CT (avoiding a second CT)
- In rare settings where CT is impossible, for instance in intensive care
- Urolithiasis, where USS is inconclusive
- Distinct pelvicalyceal or ureteral pathology (e.g. calyceal diverticula, early stages of medullary sponge kidney, ureteral valves)

then secreted into the lumen of the tubule. As ^{99m}Tc-DTPA is filtered by the glomerulus, with only 20% extraction fraction, it is not a good agent to use in neonates, children with impaired renal function or in the presence of significant obstruction.

In ^{99m}Tc-MAG3 studies, if there is dilatation of a collecting system, a diuretic is used such as furosemide at a dose of 1 mg/kg (maximum dose 20 mg). Timing of diuretic administration varies widely, but may be given just after the tracer to try to prevent loss of venous access later in the study, in a distressed child. Time activity curves are generated which demonstrate uptake and excretion. Analogue images in the uptake phase may demonstrate renal scarring, albeit less clearly than on the ^{99m}Tc-DMSA static renal scan. Split renal function can also be calculated—being even more accurate than static renography in a significantly obstructed kidney. The indications are given in Table 4-3. Where VUR is suspected, and the child is toilet-trained, cooperative and continent, an IRC may be performed.

Technique. The children are encouraged to drink plenty so that they are well hydrated upon arrival at the department (which is essential for meaningful results). The administered dose is scaled on a body surface area basis, with a maximum dose of 100 MBq of ^{99m}Tc-MAG3. The child empties the bladder, lies supine on the camera face, distracted by television or a film, and is immobilised with sandbags. Ten- to 20-s frames are acquired for 20 min following isotope injection, imaging the heart, kidneys and bladder. The child then voids again before returning to the gamma camera for images following postural change and micturition, at about 40 min post injection.

The DRF estimation is calculated from the renogram between 60 and 120 s from the peak of the vascular curve, expressed as a percentage of the sum total. The recommended methods to evaluate the DRF are the Patlak–Rutland plot and the integral method. Interpretation of the renogram in a dilated kidney, such as pelviureteric junction obstruction (PUJO) needs to be performed carefully. The shape of the time activity curve, response to furosemide and drainage of the collecting system following a change of posture and micturition are evaluated for significant stasis of tracer. There are four classic drainage patterns, described as normal (I), obstructed (II), dilated unobstructed (IIIa) and equivocal (IIIb). Ideally the renogram should be assessed with the US images available so that the degree of HN and the renal parenchyma can be evaluated. Normal kidneys with DRF below 45% should be monitored using US. If dilatation increases, and a ^{99m}Tc-MAG3 demonstrates stepwise fall in function, pyeloplasty may prevent further deterioration in renal function.

Urography (Plain Radiograph and Intravenous Urogram)

With advances of sophisticated US techniques, and availability of cross-sectional imaging, and widespread use of renal scintigraphy, the use of intravenous urography (IVU) has decreased with very few indications remaining (Table 4-4).[11] Except for urolithiasis, an initial 'control' full radiograph is rarely indicated. The radiation exposure should be minimised, using 1–3 properly timed and coned views (KUB film) based on the individual query.

Computed Tomography

CT urography (CTU) may be performed where specialised ultrasound or MR urography is unavailable.[11] Childhood conditions that may require imaging by CT include three main areas: calculi, tumours and trauma (Table 4-5).

TABLE 4-5   Indications for CT of the Renal Tract in Children

- Diagnosis and follow-up of suspected malignant tumour, although MRI is now regarded as equally reliable in assessing abdominal masses
- Major abdominal trauma with suspicion of serious pelvic injury or fracture, or if haematuria is present or bladder rupture is suspected
- Complicated infection, such as suspected abscess if MRI is unavaible and US is inconclusive
- Less common indications may include a suspicion of chronic renal infection or tuberculosis, or of nephrocalcinosis when a US study is inconclusive
- Large calculi or xanthogranulomatous pyelonephritis (XPG) in an older child where surgery may be planned, and where MRI is not available or detailed stone definition is requested
- CT angiography (CTA) may replace conventional angiography in certain circumstances, discussed further in the section 'Hypertension'

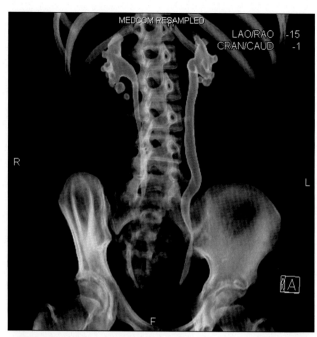

FIGURE 4-13 ■ **CT urography.** This VRT (volume rendered reconstruction) image from a 12 year old shows delineation of the urine within the urinary tract.

Method

Unenhanced CT has almost no role in paediatrics, except for calculi or calcifications,[11] and these are best seen using ultrasound. Thus, standard non-ionic contrast medium (e.g. iohexol 300) is required at an age-adapted dose.[11] Modern imaging techniques using automatic exposure control and low age-adapted kVp and size-based milliampere (mA)s settings will keep the dose to a diagnostic minimum, as will optimal age dependent timing delays and avoiding multiphase acquisitions. In cases of abdominal trauma, topographic delayed imaging after 10–15 min (or a split bolus technique) can be useful in selected cases to detect contrast medium extravasation from the genitourinary tract.[12] Conventional cystography is preferred in suspected urethral injury. Figure 4-13 shows a normal CT urogram.

Magnetic Resonance Imaging

Anatomical MRI is now the imaging modality of choice for abdominal and pelvic masses, as it gives excellent soft-tissue contrast resolution in any imaging plane, decreasing imaging times with modern equipment, improving tissue characterisation without the use of radiation. In most cases, MRI can replace CT, e.g. in the assessment of Wilms' tumour, although thoracic CT may still be required to assess for pulmonary metastases. MRI can also give superior anatomical information to delineate pelvic anatomy, e.g. ambiguous genitalia, or where spinal MRI is needed to evaluate tumoural spread or suspected spinal cord abnormalities (neuropathic bladder). The most common use of MRI/MR urography (MRU) is to evaluate complex urinary tract malformations and urinary tract obstruction, having practically replaced IVU, e.g. Fig. 4-14.[11] MRA is particularly useful to delineate the major renal vessels in preoperative (tumour) imaging, complicated hypertension, or as pre- or post-transplant assessment. The indications are given in Table 4-6.

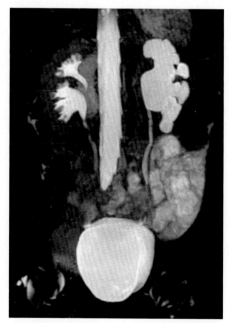

FIGURE 4-14 ■ **MR urography.** Heavily T2-weighted thick-slice coronal MRI image in a 3-year-old girl with right-sided duplex kidney which drains normally, but pelviureteric junction obstruction on the left.

Method

Specific sequences and protocols are now available in most institutions for different clinical scenarios.[13] Axial T1- and T2-weighted imaging are the mainstay of any imaging protocol, and either single-shot coronal heavily T2-weighted imaging or a 3D T2 sequence can give a

TABLE 4-6 Indications for MRI of the Renal Tract in Children

- Diagnosis and follow-up of abdominal or pelvic mass/suspected tumour
- In acute pyelonephritis and its complications, if US inconclusive
- Where spinal imaging is required in children with suspected neuropathic bladder
- Functional MR urography—upper urinary tract obstruction and renal dysplasia
- Contrast-enhanced MRA may have a role in the assessment of hypertension

TABLE 4-7 Indications for Angiography of the Renal Tract in Children

- Hypertension with a high suspicion of renovascular disease, including suspected vasculitis, especially polyarteritis nodosa
- Renal vein sampling for renin values to evaluate which kidney is causing the hypertension
- Before interventional procedures, e.g. embolisation for arteriovenous malformations or balloon dilatation for renal artery stenosis
- Rarely in bilateral Wilms' tumours before surgery
- Testicular vein embolisation for varicocele obliteration

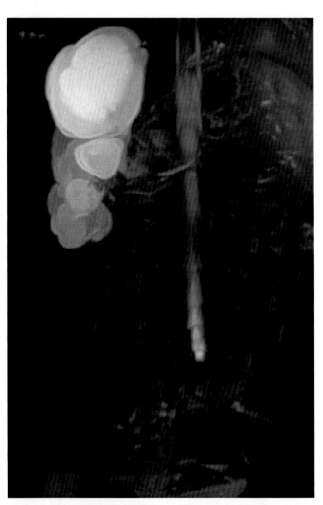

FIGURE 4-15 ■ MR urography. Three-dimensional T2 MRU image demonstrates a grossly dilated collecting system of the right kidney CSF is also demonstrated.

(DWI) is rapidly evolving to give an index of tumour cellularity (but does not differentiate benign from malignant tumours), identifying metastases, and in acute pyelonephritis and tumour treatment response. New techniques such as blood oxygen level-dependent (BOLD) MRI are being assessed to demonstrate changes in oxygenation of the kidney during acute obstructive episodes and in transplant imaging.

Interventional Procedures

Angiography

Angiography is reserved for specific clinical situations (Table 4-7) by an experienced operator. Selective arteriography with magnification and oblique views is necessary to detect lesions in small renal vessels.

Antegrade Pyelogram

This investigation should be carried out by an experienced operator in the radiology department or in theatre, usually before surgery, to provide anatomical detail of the renal pelvis and/or ureter unavailable from US or IVU. Occasionally antegrade studies are combined with pressure flow measurements with or without urodynamic studies to determine the physiological significance of a dilated upper urinary tract (the 'Whitaker test').

Nephrostomy

The placement of a pigtail or J-J catheter in a dilated renal pelvis or ureter should be undertaken by an experienced operator under US guidance, with similar techniques to adults. US-guided needle placement into an appropriate lower pole calyx with contrast injection gives delineation of the collecting system before insertion of the tube. The complications of placing a nephrostomy tube are generally those of catheter placement, extravasation of contrast medium, and leakage of urine; thus, a combined sonographic–fluoroscopic approach is often recommended.

Retrograde Pyelogram

The instillation of dilute contrast medium into a ureter via a catheter inserted into the distal ureteric orifice is usually undertaken by a urologist in the operating theatre. With modern flexible ureteroscopes, the contrast medium

'urogram' overview of the entire urinary system (Fig. 4-15). Serial imaging following contrast enhancement is useful to delineate the enhancement of tumours, or arterial enhancement for anatomy. MRU is the only imaging modality to give detailed functional as well as anatomical detail. Full MRU requires a dedicated protocol, including hydration, sedation, catheterisation and diuresis, with prolonged T1 gradient-echo dynamic sequences demonstrating contrast uptake, elimination and drainage similar to radionuclide renograms. Diffusion-weighted MRI

may be instilled into the upper ureter or even the renal pelvis, to outline the ureter and its drainage.

Renal Biopsy

Many disorders affecting the kidney need a biopsy for histological confirmation or diagnosis, particularly glomerular disease, nephrotic syndrome and IgA nephropathy. Surgical exploration or percutaneous US-guided needle biopsy should be considered, with complications such as subcapsular haematoma and AV fistula being fairly rare. Guidelines have recently been formulated for renal biopsy in children.[14,15]

CONGENITAL ANOMALIES

RENAL ANOMALIES

Renal Agenesis

Unilateral agenesis occurs in approximately 1 in 1250 live births. Antenatal diagnosis is uncommon, suggesting that agenesis may be the result of an involuted multicystic dysplastic kidney.

Most functioning kidneys should be identifiable by US wherever they are located, and either ^{99m}Tc-DMSA or MR can be used to detect poorly functioning kidneys. VUR is more common in a non-functioning kidney, and associated ipsilateral abnormalities, including uterine/seminal vesicle or gonadal abnormalities are common, particularly easier to detect in the neonatal period before these structures involute physiologically.

Abnormal Migration and Fusion of the Kidneys

Appreciating renal embryology will assist in the understanding of the various forms of renal malformation and vascular anomalies. The kidney initially forms from an interaction between the mesonephric duct/ureteric bud and the metanephros at around 4 weeks of gestation. The primitive kidney ascends, rotating 90° from horizontal to medial, taking its blood from the aorta and draining via the inferior vena cava. An ectopic kidney may result from excess, incomplete or abnormal ascent. Abnormalities of fusion may occur if the kidneys touch each other in the process of ascending.

Renal Ectopia

Approximately 1 in 1000 kidneys is ectopic, and 10% are bilateral. The commonest is a pelvic kidney, which normally lies anterior to the sacrum just below the bifurcation of the aorta (Fig. 4-16). The true intrathoracic kidney (entering via the foramen of Bochdalek) is rare. Occasionally the kidney may be a superior ectopic kidney lying below a very thin membranous portion of the diaphragm. The adrenal glands are usually normally sited in the presence of renal ectopia, and there are many adrenal anomalies unrelated to renal variation.

Abnormalities of Renal Fusion

The commonest renal fusion abnormality is the horseshoe kidney. The lower poles of the kidneys are fused in the midline, possibly due to malposition of the umbilical arteries causing the developing nephrogenic masses to come together. The isthmus of the horseshoe commonly lies anterior to the aorta and vena cava, at the level of the inferior mesenteric artery, with malrotated collecting systems lying anteriorly, which may lead to pelviureteric junction obstruction and associated infections or calculi. The abnormal axis of the lower poles of the kidneys in a horseshoe should not be missed on US: if bowel gas obscures the anterior view, the loss of the normal medial renal contour and graded compression is useful, and the kidney itself can be used as a window to visualise the parenchymal bridge. The anterior view of a ^{99m}Tc-DMSA may be helpful to assess functioning renal tissue in a horseshoe. MRI also demonstrates abnormalities of renal and (often associated) vascular anatomy and their complications. The horseshoe kidney may become damaged in a road traffic accident because of the position of the lap belt in relation to the kidney. Power Doppler US provides excellent assessment of small traumatic lesions to a horseshoe kidney rather than resorting to CT. There is an increased risk of Wilms' tumour in horseshoe kidneys and the anomaly may be associated with Edwards' syndrome (trisomy 18) and Turner's syndrome.

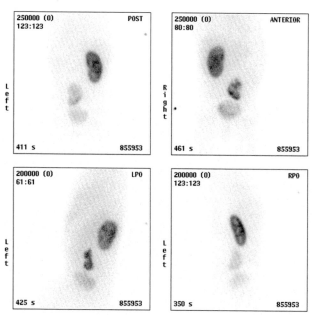

FIGURE 4-16 ■ Ectopic kidney. ^{99m}Tc-DMSA scan of a pelvic ectopic kidney which demonstrates scarring from recurrent UTIs.

Cross Fused Renal Ectopia

Crossed fused renal ectopia is seen in 1 in 7000 post mortem examinations. The crossed ectopic kidney lies on the opposite side to its ureteral insertion into the bladder. The left kidney is more commonly the ectopic kidney and the commonest pattern is fusion of the upper pole of the crossed kidney with the lower pole of the normally positioned kidney, in an L shape (Fig. 4-17). Occasionally the crossed kidney remains unfused. Imaging by US demonstrates a unilateral large mass of renal tissue, with contralateral absence of renal tissue. Because of abnormalities in rotation, PUJO is common and a ^{99m}Tc-MAG3 (or dynamic MRU) study is often helpful in assessment of drainage, and VUR is common. Associated anomalies may be seen (for example, VACTERL association).

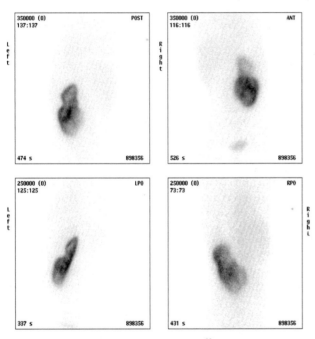

FIGURE 4-17 ■ **Crossed fused ectopia.** ^{99m}Tc-DMSA scan of crossed fused ectopia.

Duplex Kidneys

The commonest renal anomaly (2% of the population) is an uncomplicated duplex kidney. Complete duplication is caused by two separate ureteral buds presenting onto the mesonephric duct. The ureter draining the lower moiety will come to lie more superior to and lateral to the ureter draining the upper moiety, increasing the VUR risk to the lower moiety. The upper moiety ureteric insertion into the bladder usually is more distally and medially, may even be ectopic, or may be associated with an ureterocele, causing varying degrees of dysplasia and obstruction in the upper moiety (Fig. 4-18). Sometimes the upper moiety is difficult to see and if the upper moiety ureter drains ectopically into the vagina in a girl, continuous wetting or recurrent UTIs result. Careful interrogation by US, complemented by MRI, is essential in order to pick up both echogenic and atrophic upper moieties.

Incomplete ureteric duplication ('incomplete duplication') describes ureteric duplication above the bladder. Yo-yo VUR may be demonstrated by dynamic renography with tracer passing down one ureter and back up the partially duplicated second ureter into the respective renal moiety, but the kidney in these children looks the same as in a complete duplication. A 'septated renal pelvis' is the mildest variant of this condition. An ureterocele prolapsing into the vagina may present as a perineal mass in the newborn, or bladder outlet obstruction due to an ureterocele prolapsing into the posterior urethra (mimicking posterior urethral valves).

Imaging

A duplex kidney may be diagnosed by US, with a larger than normal kidney with two distinct collecting systems being separated by a bridge of renal tissue. The appearances of a duplex kidney vary with the pathology of each moiety. The upper moiety is usually dilated, particularly when associated with a ureterocele or ectopic ureteric insertion, or may be atrophic (Figs. 4-19 and 4-20). (Power) Doppler can estimate the degree of dysplasia and may demonstrate the ectopic ureteric jet. The lower

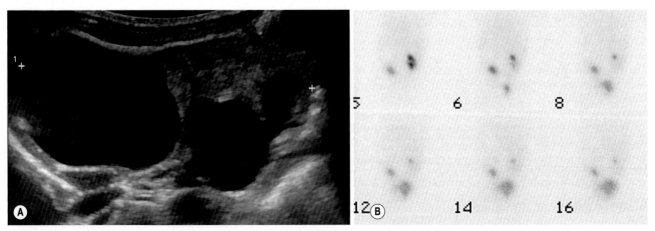

FIGURE 4-18 ■ **Duplex kidney.** (A) US shows grossly dilated upper moiety of the right kidney, with milder dilatation of the lower moiety. (B) Selected images from the MAG3 shows a duplex left kidney with upper moiety obstruction.

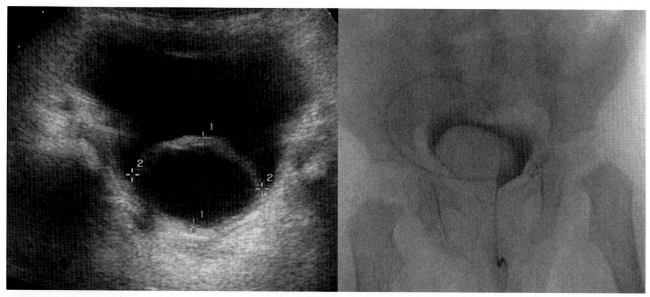

FIGURE 4-19 ■ **Ureterocele.** A large ureterocele is identified on US, clearly visible on the early filling view of the MCUG where contract is seen circumferentially outside the ureterocele within the bladder.

moiety may be dilated in PUJO, or demonstrate scarring and uroepithelial thickening in the collecting system to indicate VUR.

The ^{99m}Tc-MAG3 will be helpful in assessment of renal function, scarring and dysplasia, allowing the relative contribution to function from each moiety to may be calculated. The uncomplicated duplex on a functional study may demonstrate up to 60% DRF compared to a simplex contralateral kidney, giving the false impression of reduced function in the simplex kidney. The axis of the duplex kidney on a DMSA may point towards the ipsilateral shoulder rather than the contralateral shoulder on the image, prompting the radiologist to look carefully on US for the hallmark finding of two separate collecting systems. The ^{99m}Tc-MAG3 renogram is also used to assess function and drainage in a complicated duplex kidney, and an IRC can be used in the toilet-trained child to assess for lower moiety VUR. Correct interpretation and calculations by scintigraphy rely heavily on accurate anatomical knowledge from US or MRI.

An MCUG can be useful both to assess for presence of possible ureterocele and for VUR into the lower moiety. Anatomical MR sequences can delineate the upper and lower poles, and MRU can help distinguish between an obstructed and non-obstructed dilated system. High-resolution isotropic 3D data sets may be reconstructed to clearly demonstrate ectopic insertion of the ureters, provided there is sufficient ureteral distension, dependent upon good hydration and bladder distension.

Anomalies of the Renal Pelvis and Ureter

US may demonstrate calyceal diverticulae or calyceal dilatation due to an infundibular stenosis, either congenital or acquired (secondary to infection or obstruction by

calculi). MRI/MRU may further evaluate these appearances. Megacalycosis is a poorly understood condition where the dysplastic calyces are dilated in the absence of obstruction. It is probably due to underdevelopment of the medullary pyramids or maturation defects (resembling the shape of a pelvic kidney), and there may be an association with a megaureter and renal ectopia. Thus ureteric or pelvicaliceal dilatation does not indicate obstruction, and while the condition may predispose to stone formation, corrective surgery for ureteric dilatation is not beneficial.

Pelviureteric Junction Obstruction

PUJO is the commonest cause of renal tract dilatation, comprising up to 40% of cases. Antenatal and then postnatal US of the renal pelvis is useful in suspected PUJO or pseudo-obstruction. Poorly understood, there may be an anatomical abnormality, which can present early with antenatal unilateral HN, or a crossing vessel causing extrinsic compression, which usually presents later with intermittent pain or infection. Abnormal ureteric peristalsis or VUR (with infections) may lead to ureteric kinking, fibrosis or there may be a delayed recanalisation of the fetal ureter. Secondary PUJO may occur due to scarring after UTI and particularly with high-grade VUR, in elongated tortuous megaureters, as well as with obstructing tumours or retroperitoneal fibrosis.

Imaging

Diagnosis of PUJO is important in order to highlight those severe cases which may progress, causing loss of renal function, which may require surgical intervention. The initial US is performed approximately seven days after birth so that the baby is well hydrated and the degree of renal pelvic dilatation is not underestimated.

Anatomical

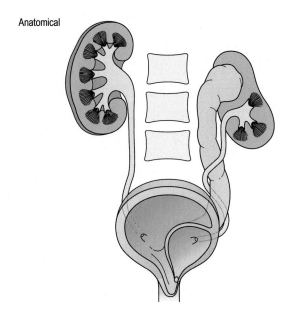

Urographic

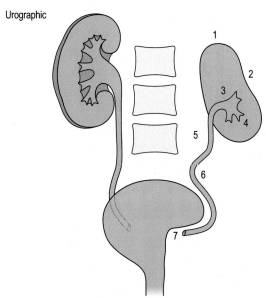

FIGURE 4-20 ■ Duplex kidney. Diagrammatic representation of duplex kidneys with an ectopic ureterocele of the left upper moiety without function. Diagnosis depends on recognition of indirect signs: 1 = increased distance from the top of the visualised collecting system to the upper border of the nephrogram; 2 = abnormal axis of the collecting system; 3 = impression upon the upper border of the renal pelvis; 4 = decreased number of calyces compared to the contralateral kidney; 5 = lateral displacement of the kidney and ureter; 6 = lateral course of the visualised ureter; and 7 = filling defect in the bladder.

The prone transverse view of the renal pelvis is used to assess the AP pelvic diameter: between 7 and 10 mm on antenatal US requires follow-up in the newborn period, and greater than 1 cm thereafter; HN can be graded accordingly.[16] Function and drainage is assessed on the diuretic ^{99m}Tc-MAG3 renogram or fMRU (Fig. 4-21). The study is ideally performed when the baby is over 6–8 weeks of age, preferably over 3 months, when there is some renal maturity.

If renal pelvic dilatation is severe and bilateral, and the significantly thinned renal parenchyma is undifferentiated and echogenic, with reduced vascularity on power Doppler, earlier assessment of function is required. Diuretic sonography with serial measurements after furosemide application may help to differentiate dilated from (partially) obstructed kidneys that then require further imaging. In severe bilateral disease, ^{99m}Tc-DMSA may be used as an assessment of the relative contribution of each kidney to total renal function. The study must be performed with careful attention to detail. The baby must be well hydrated and furosemide should be given immediately or soon after the isotope, although a range of timing protocols are in use.

Following the dynamic renogram, a delayed image, following postural change and micturition (if the bladder emptied) should be performed to assess the contribution of gravity to drainage from the dilated upper urinary tract. The degree of urinary stasis cannot be assessed on the supine imaging alone, and a post-micturition/post-catheterisation view is essential. If there is reduced function in the affected kidney and the degree of renal pelvic dilatation on US is changing, urologists may be more inclined to operate. Less than 25% of cases of antenatally diagnosed PUJO undergo surgery.

Megaureter and Hydroureter

In utero, if the fetal ureter is visualised, then it is dilated: it may indicate a primary megaureter, refluxing megaureter, non-refluxing non-obstructive hydroureter or secondary hydroureter (for example, associated with posterior urethral valves and ureterocele).

Imaging

US is used to assess for a ureterocele, or secondary signs of VUR may be evident (e.g. a laterally positioned or gaping ostium, bladder wall trabeculation and thickening, significant post-voiding residual). Bilateral disease is assessed and extrinsic compression leading to secondary hydroureter is readily seen. An MCUG (or ce-VUS) is performed to assess whether ureteric dilatation is caused by VUR, either causing dilatation or coexisting with megaureter. MRU is used to assess anatomy in more complex situations (Fig. 4-22), as the dynamic sequences may demonstrate ureteric peristalsis, and to assess drainage and function.

Bladder Anomalies

Bladder exstrophy–epispadias–cloacal exstrophy complex represents a spectrum of anomalies, with an incidence of around 1 in 20,000 live births, typically male babies. Absence of the normal bladder or the failure to see bladder filling on antenatal US may suggest bladder exstrophy. This results from a failure of closure of the abdominal wall during fetal development, leading to protrusion of the anterior wall of the bladder through the lower abdominal wall defect, and there may be an associated omphalocele. There is an open defect of the anterior abdominal wall or perineal wall and widening of the

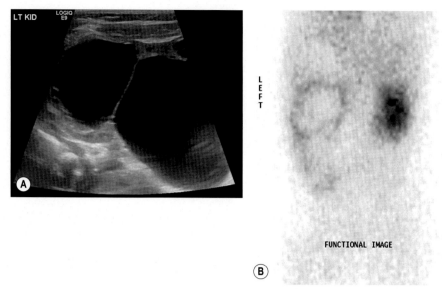

FIGURE 4-21 ■ **Pelviureteric junction obstruction.** An obstructed left kidney on US (A) with diminished function on MAG3 (B).

pubic symphysis, with epispadias in male babies (dorsal cleft in penis exposing the urethral mucosa). Antenatal diagnosis is difficult and the condition most often presents at birth with the exposed bladder. An estimation of the degree of severity of the condition can be found by measuring the extent of pubic symphysis diastasis on fetal US or plain films (Fig. 4-23). This is normally up to 10 mm, and 10–25 mm suggests epispadias with >25-mm bladder exstrophy. The upper renal tracts are initially normal. Treatment involves staged repair of the bladder and genitalia. Following treatment, careful US and ^{99m}Tc-MAG3 is advised as VUR and obstruction are common following bladder closure.

Prune-Belly Syndrome

The combination of absence/hypoplasia of the abdominal wall musculature, urinary tract dilatation and bilateral undescended testes is known as 'prune-belly syndrome', or abdominal musculature deficiency syndrome. The incidence of prune-belly syndrome is approximately 1 in 40,000 live births, predominantly in male babies; female babies cannot have the complete triad, and the urological manifestations may be less severe. The entire spectrum of prune-belly syndrome is difficult to explain but thought to be either a defect of abdominal wall mesoderm formation early in embryogenesis, or severe bladder outlet obstruction leading to overdistension of the abdominal wall and urinary tract.

Clinical presentation is with a lax abdominal wall with thin wrinkled skin and a protuberant abdomen. US may be challenging but will demonstrate dilated ureters with a large-capacity bladder often with little intrarenal dilatation, as well as absent or hypoplasic abdominal wall muscles. The bladder neck is wide with a dilated proximal posterior urethra and more distal conical narrowing, leading to a poor urinary stream through the anterior

urethra ('pseudo-valve'). Prognosis depends on the degree of associated renal dysplasia. These babies are prone to VUR and, consequently, infection. A MCUG is indicated to assess for VUR and the appearances of the urethra. Dynamic diuretic ^{99m}Tc-MAG3 renography may be helpful in long-term follow-up to assess function and drainage in those children without renal compromise.

Functional Bladder Disturbance and Neurogenic Bladder

Children with neurogenic bladder have uncontrolled voiding and incomplete bladder emptying, due to inappropriate detrusor muscle contraction and external sphincter relaxation, e.g. caused by spinal dysraphism, such as a myelomeningocele. Initial spinal US/MRI is essential to rule out spinal abnormality. When no spinal abnormality is found, the term 'non-neurogenic neurogenic bladder' is used: Non-neurogenic voiding disorders or dysfunctional voiding are becoming an increasingly important entity that are identified by modified MCUG or videourodynamics but remain poorly recognised and understood.

Treating neurogenic bladders is aimed towards continence, and preventing deterioration in renal and bladder function. Kidney function deteriorates secondary to poor bladder emptying, leading to HN and VUR, with subsequent complications of infection. Clean intermittent catheterisation, surgical procedures including bladder augmentation, continence procedures and artificial urinary sphincters and medication all have a role in preventing renal damage. Specialised urodynamic clinics are integral in the management of these patients. Regular US of the renal tract with catheterised bladder emptying is necessary to assess renal tract abnormalities. Follow-up dynamic ^{99m}Tc-MAG3 renography with IRC is helpful in

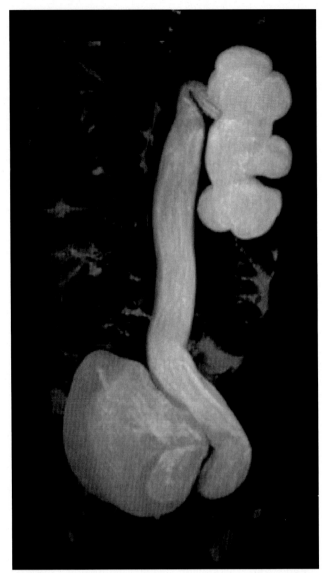

FIGURE 4-22 ■ **Megaureter.** Three-dimensional T2W MRU image/ rotated reconstruction demonstrates a megaureter with an additional kink at the ureteropelvic junction and a markedly dilated collecting system of the kidney.

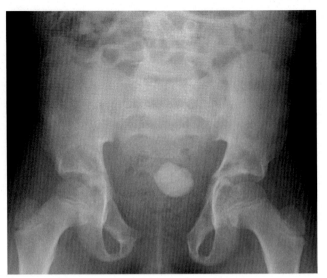

FIGURE 4-23 ■ **Bladder exstrophy.** Abdominal radiograph showing a radio-opaque calculus in a patient with bladder exstrophy with characteristic diastasis of the pubic symphysis.

the assessment of ongoing VUR. MCUG may demonstrate a small-volume trabeculated bladder with diverticula, and VUR into the kidneys; using a modified MCUG protocol or videourodynamic study will give additional functional bladder information. Nonneurogenic bladder and voiding disorders are usually treated by bladder training, often using biofeedback techniques, supported by medications.

URETHRAL ANOMALIES

The urethra is best demonstrated in the oblique lateral projection of the MCUG or by retrograde urethrography. This gives the best view of the bladder neck and posterior urethra, without which an anatomical cause of bladder outlet obstruction cannot be excluded (Fig. 4-9).

Bladder outlet obstruction may be anatomical or functional such as in neurogenic bladder. Anatomical causes of outlet obstruction include posterior urethral valve, ureterocele prolapsing into the posterior urethra causing obstruction, urethral dysplasia, anterior valve/diaphragm/ syringocele, meatal stenosis, paraurethral cysts, urethral diverticula or duplication and post-traumatic or infective urethral strictures as well as (severe) hypospadias. Pelvic tumours or urethral polyps can cause obstruction, as can bladder masses such as haemangioma or neurofibroma. These lesions may be demonstrated by (perineal perimicturitional) US, but MRI will be the imaging of choice for assessment and staging of a pelvic mass.

Posterior Urethral Valves (PUV)

Congenital urethral obstruction creates a spectrum of disease, with the timing and severity determining the presenting symptoms. Boys with high-grade obstruction present as neonates with urosepsis, renal insufficiency and pulmonary hypoplasia with severe respiratory distress, detected on antenatal US exhibiting urinary ascites, oligohydramnios, enlarged bladders and renal dilatation. Less severe obstruction may lead to presentation in childhood with UTI. PUV consist of abnormal folds of mucosa between the wall of the urethra and the verumontanum. There are three types, ranging from type I, slit-like orifice between 2 folds at the verumontanum, to type III, valve with eccentric pinpoint aperture causing the valve to balloon forward on micturition ('wind in the sail' appearance on the MCUG). Type III valve is associated with renal dysplasia, even without significant upper tract dilatation. All newborn boys with significant antenatal HN (grade III or higher) and thick bladder wall, ascites or oligohydramnion should be assessed for the presence of PUV. If valves are suspected, the bladder should be drained suprapubically until valves are ablated; with secondary obstruction at the VUJ, a nephrostomy may

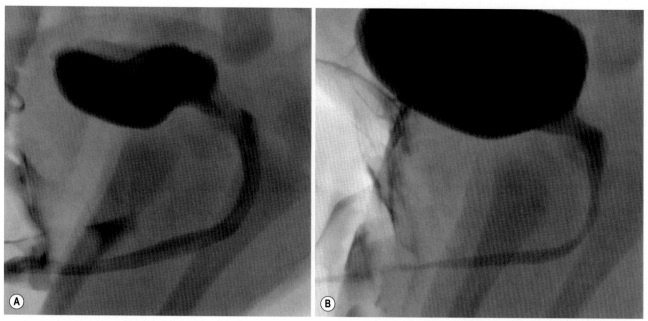

FIGURE 4-24 ■ **Normal urethra.** MCUG demonstrating full-length views of the urethra with a catheter in situ (A) and with the catheter removed (B).

become necessary to ensure sufficient urinary drainage. Note that even with optimal treatment, the associated severe congenital renal dysplasia often still results in renal failure requiring subsequent renal transplantation.

Imaging

In PUV, US may show hydroureteronephrosis, renal dysplasia, or urinomas due to calyceal rupture secondary to increased pressure (the 'pop off' mechanism), and bladder wall thickening with a dilated posterior urethra and hypertrophied bladder neck. If the US is performed before the baby is well hydrated, the degree of hydroureteronephrosis may be underestimated. MCUG is essential (but is contraindicated in acute sepsis). Contrast medium may demonstrate bladder wall trabeculation, a very large (or small) bladder with diverticula, and either unilateral or bilateral VUR, associated with ipsilateral poor renal function. The valve is visualised as an acute-calibre transition on the oblique/lateral urethral projection at micturition. If there is a urethral catheter in situ, a 'catheter out' view when micturating is essential in order to exclude a small valve leaflet compressed by the catheter (Fig. 4-24).

Upper tract drainage by nephrostomy or ureterostomy may be required to preserve renal function. Treatment comprises early cystoscopic valve ablation followed by bladder drainage. A follow-up MCUG after valve ablation may be useful but cystoscopy is required, as remnant valve leaflets may be missed on urethrography. ^{99m}Tc-DMSA is initially used to provide DRF with ^{99m}Tc-MAG3 renography and US follow-up. Antireflux procedures are performed in PUV patients in order to preserve renal function. In boys with severe dysplasia, end-stage renal disease usually occurs in the first 20 years of life.

Anterior Urethral Abnormalities

Anterior urethral valves are around 10 times less common than PUV. The anterior valves may be located anywhere along the anterior urethra, and are often associated with a urethral diverticulum. Severe valves are often diagnosed in the newborn period, but mild valves may present later in childhood. Typical ballooning of the urethra with deviation of the penis may occur during micturition on MCUG. A syringocele is a dilated Cowper's gland or duct that may cause urethral obstruction in the neonate (Figs. 4-25 and 4-26). Sometimes non-specific symptoms of dribbling or haematuria may occur later in childhood. Spontaneous rupture or transurethral incision is curative, but may lead to a urethral stricture.

Urethral Stricture

Strictures may be congenital or acquired and may occur in boys or girls. Seventy-five per cent of male congenital urethral strictures occur in the bulbous urethra (where the embryological proximal urethra merges with the urogenital membrane), and at the urethral meatus in girls. Children with congenital strictures present either as neonates or in the postpubertal period. Early presentation as a neonate may demonstrate significant upper tract dilatation secondary to urethral obstruction. Postpubertal boys present with irritation, urinary dribbling, haematuria and UTI as well as prostatitis or epididymitis. Diagnosis is by MCUG and treatment is usually urethrotomy. Traumatic straddle injuries lead to bulbar strictures. Pelvic trauma and urethral rupture, or catheter induced injuries, tend to cause strictures either at the bladder neck or at the membranous portion of the urethra.

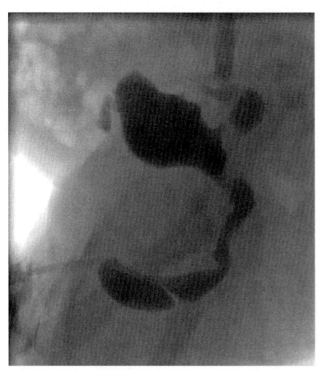

FIGURE 4-25 ■ **Syringocele.** Urethral syringocele demonstrated on MCUG.

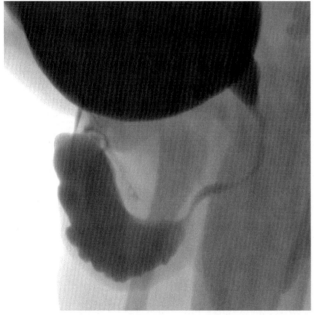

FIGURE 4-26 ■ **Scaphoid congenital megaurethra.** Massive dilatation of the urethra is caused by non-development of the penile erectile tissue, particularly the corpus spongiosum.

Rectourethral Fistula

Rectourethral fistula is usually associated with an imperforate anus and is best demonstrated by a high-pressure loopogram via a distal colostomy which should demonstrate passage of contrast from the bowel to the posterior urethra, or by high-pressure urethrogram/during voiding on a MCUG.

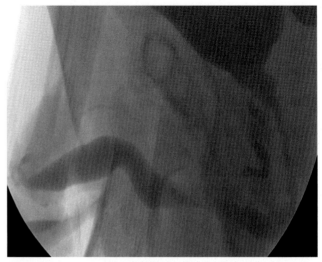

FIGURE 4-27 ■ **Urethal duplication.** There is duplication of the urethra almost from the bladder neck along the whole length of the penis.

Duplication of the Urethra

A rare congenital abnormality usually discovered in childhood with one of the urethras ending as a hypospadias. Duplication of the urethra may be complete and the child presents with a double urinary stream, urinary tract infection, sometimes outflow obstruction and incontinence. The classification of urethral duplication is complex and beyond the scope of this chapter (Fig. 4-27).

UTERUS AND VAGINA

Differentiation of the gonads into ovaries or testes depends on the presence or absence of the Y chromosome. In the absence of hormonal secretion of anti-Müllerian hormone from the fetal testis, the Müllerian ducts meet and differentiate into the uterus, cervix, fallopian tubes and proximal two-thirds of the vagina. The urogenital sinus forms the distal vagina. Uterine development depends on the formation of the Wolffian or mesonephric duct.

Uterovaginal malformations are classified embryologically into either Müllerian agenesis, a developmental defect of the caudal portion of the Müllerian ducts (Mayer–Rokitansky–Küster–Hauser (MRKH) syndrome); disorders of lateral fusion caused by the failure of the two Müllerian ducts to fuse in the midline; and disorders of vertical fusion that are caused by abnormal union between the Müllerian tubercle and urogenital sinus derivatives (leading to disorders of the hymen, cervical agenesis and transverse vaginal septa). Disorders of lateral fusion are heterogeneous and have been classified into six groups. Lateral fusion and vertical fusion abnormalities often coexist and thus congenital vaginal abnormalities can be considered as those with or without obstruction.

Anomalies of the uterus and vagina may present as an abdominal or pelvic mass in the neonatal period. Female genital anomalies are usually suspected on US and diagnosed using MRI, or US genitography using intravaginal saline in centres with experience. Fifty per cent of cases will have an associated renal anomaly and approximately 12% may have associated vertebral segmentation anomalies. Congenital anomalies of the vagina (septation, stenosis, imperforate hymen) often present in pubertal girls with menstrual symptoms but no bleeding due to obstruction (haematometrocolpos; Figs. 4-28, 4-29). Other causes of primary amenorrhoea include Turner's syndrome. MRKH syndrome, which affects 1 in 4000 to 5000 girls, and includes vaginal atresia, uterine anomalies and malformations of the upper urinary tract. Associated renal abnormalities include HN, dysplasia, unilateral ectopia and renal agenesis. Three-dimensional US and MRI are helpful in imaging the spectrum. All girls with genital should have careful US evaluation of the renal tract.

UNDESCENDED TESTIS

Cryptorchidism refers to the absence of a testis in the scrotum, affecting 4% of full-term newborns and 30% of preterm newborns, falling to around 0.8% after the first year. It is usually right-sided, but may be bilateral. During embryogenesis, the testes form beside the mesonephric kidneys and descend via the inguinal canal to the scrotum. This normal process may halt anywhere along its descent, causing an undescended testis, or the testis may become ectopic or absent. Early diagnosis and treatment are important to prevent infertility and a risk of malignancy in the undescended testis. Unilateral testicular agenesis is associated with ipsilateral renal agenesis.

There is current debate regarding whether US can confidently localise undescended testes. US has estimated sensitivity and specificity of around 45 and 80%, respectively, in accurately localising non-palpable testes. US is particularly helpful for testicular locations in the inguinal canal or next to the bladder/close to the abdominal wall—deeper positions are more difficult. US can also detect other scrotal pathology, such as hydrocele or cystic dysplasia of the rete testis, which mimics a testicular tumour and is associated with a multicystic dysplastic kidney. MRI is far superior in localising near-normal, non-palable testes, and is preferable in ambiguous genitalia or hypospadias, but small and dysplastic testes may be indistinguishable from non-specific nodules. The testis is typically hypoplastic with low T2 signal. Diagnostic laparoscopy is the definitive investigation and allows for concurrent biopsy or surgical correction.

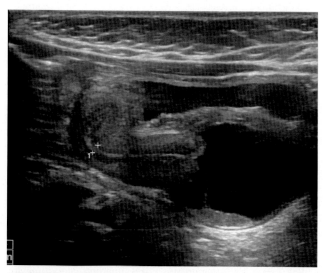

FIGURE 4-28 ■ Haematocolpos. Sagittal US image of thickened endometrium with spill of blood into the obstructed, distended vagina lying behind the normal bladder.

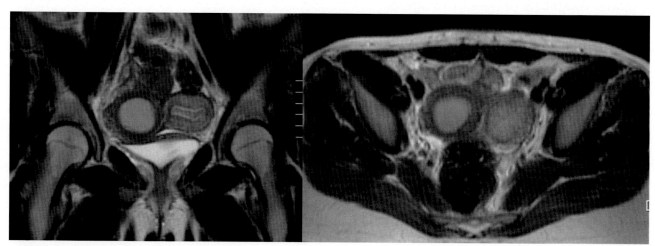

FIGURE 4-29 ■ Haematometrocolpos. Only one, i.e. the right of two uterine cavities in this didelphys uterus, demonstrates haematometrocolpos on coronal and axial MRI.

TABLE 4-8	Differential Diagnosis of Prenatal Hydronephrosis

Unilateral Pathology

Renal pelvic dilatation (RPD)
Vesicoureteric reflux (VUR)
Megaureter (with or without reflux)
Multicystic dysplastic kidney
Complicated duplex kidney
Upper moiety dilatation—either ureterocele or ectopic
  drainage
Lower moiety dilatation—usually VUR but rarely RPD only

Bilateral Pathology

Bilateral renal pelvic dilatation
Bilateral VUR
Bilateral megaureter (with or without reflux)
Bladder pathology, e.g. neurogenic bladder
Bladder outlet pathology (posterior urethral valves)
Bilateral complicated duplex kidneys
Multicystic kidney on one side and cystic dysplastic kidney
  on opposite side

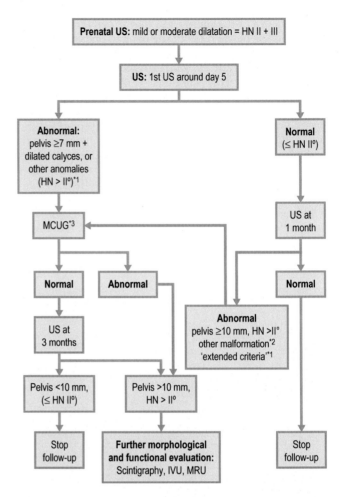

*1 use extended US criteria considering urothelial sign, kidney size & structure, etc.
*2 US genitography: in all patients with single kidney. MCDK, ectopic kidneys. etc.
*3 ce-VUS can be used in girls and for screening populations

FIGURE 4-30 ■ **Hydronephrosis.** ESPR imaging algorithm for mild or moderate fetal hydronephrosis, IVU = intravenous urography, MCDK = multicystic dysplastic kidney, MRU = magnetic resonance urography. (Adapted from Riccabona M, Avni F E, Blickman J G, et al 2008 Imaging recommendations in paediatric uroradiology: minutes of the ESPR workgroup session on urinary tract infection, fetal hydronephrosis, urinary tract ultrasonography and voiding cystourethrography, Barcelona, Spain, June 2007. Pediatr Radiol 38(2):138–145.[1])

ANTENATAL DIAGNOSIS OF HYDRONEPHROSIS

Some anatomical renal abnormalities can now be detected antenatally, which begs the question as to what should be done for the child in the immediate postnatal period? The most obvious abnormalities are anatomical disorders, such as renal agenesis and horseshoe kidneys. The next issue is that of HN (pelvicalyceal dilatation) and hydroureter (ureteric dilatation alone). Imaging should try to distinguish between an obstructed and non-obstructed system; the goal of imaging is to direct treatment to preserve renal function and growth potential. There are many imaging algorithms now developed by the European paediatric radiology community, which have been widely publicised.[1]

Prenatal Diagnosis of Renal/Urological Abnormality and Differential Diagnosis

Newborns with a prenatal US diagnosis of a renal tract abnormality do not form a homogeneous group. Transient renal pelvic dilatation (RPD) is thought to be physiological during fetal development, but persistent or enlarging RPD during the antenatal period will typically be referred for postnatal investigation, although most will be determined to be normal. The differential diagnosis is wide (Table 4-8). Bilateral disease must be distinguished from unilateral disease, as unilateral normal kidney and ureter implies that normal function can be achieved. The most important diagnosis to make immediately (US and MCUG within the first 24 h of life) is that of PUV, potentially causing bilateral obstructive HN and renal damage, so that perinatal surgery can be performed for this indication. For those children with less marked abnormalities, repeating US at

1 and 4–6 weeks of life can often eliminate those in whom the functionally immature system has improved, and no further imaging is required (Fig. 4-30).[1] The urgency of postnatal imaging is heavily dependent on the prenatal US findings and the quality/availability of prenatal US.

Bilateral Renal Pelvic Dilatation

Renal pelvic dilatation (RPD) or hydronephrosis (HN) may be defined as calyceal dilatation plus a renal pelvis of greater than 10–15 mm in its AP diameter with no US evidence of a dilated ureter. This was incorrectly referred to previously as pelviureteric junction (PUJ) obstruction

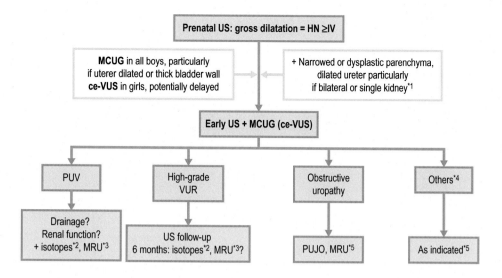

*1 (US) genitography: in patients with single kidney MC1DK, ectopic kidney, suspected genital anomaly
*2 MAG3-better than DMSA in dilated systems and neonates, DMSA usually after 3–6 months, not before 6 weeks;
   + open bladder catheter to avoid VUR-induced errors
*3 MRU-complex anatomy, function, obstructive component, etc.
*4 e.g. MCDK, cystic dysplasia, duplex or horseshoe kidney, other malformations, non-obstructive HN, cysts/cystic tumour, etc.
*5 see relevant algorithm

FIGURE 4-31 ■ Hydronephrosis. ESPR imaging algorithm for postnatally diagnosed severe/high-grade fetal hydronephrosis. MCUG = voiding cystourethrography, ce-VUS = ce-VUS = contrast-enhanced voiding urosonography, PUV = posterior urethral valves, VUR = vesicoureteric reflux, UPUJO = pelviureteric junction obstruction, MRU = MR urography. (Adapted from Riccabona M, Avni F E, Blickman J G, et al; Members of the ESUR paediatric recommendation work group and ESPR paediatric uroradiology work group 2009 Imaging recommendations in paediatric uroradiology, part II: urolithiasis and haematuria in children, paediatric obstructive uropathy, and postnatal work-up of fetally diagnosed high grade hydronephrosis. Minutes of a mini-symposium at the ESPR annual meeting, Edinburgh, June. Pediatr Radiol 39(8):891–898.[17])

or stenosis. The measurement is gestation dependent and equates to approximately 5-mm RPD at 20 weeks' gestation and a 10-mm pelvis in the third trimester. RPD is commonly unilateral but may be bilateral, in which case investigation is essential. Hydronephrosis can be graded according to severity.

High-grade HN or bilateral RPD is frequently associated with severe abnormality, i.e. severe obstructive uropathy and PUV, which may be deteriorate rapidly, and need urgent US and MCUG (Fig. 4-31).[17] The main question in severe HN is whether the child needs early bladder drainage and intervention, after which further imaging work-up may be delayed until physiological maturity of the kidneys occurs.

In mild-to-moderate fetal HN, initial postnatal US is best postponed until after 1 week of age; these US findings should then dictate additional imaging.[1] Treatment and further imaging should then be performed according to the severity of the initial findings (Fig. 4-1). In children with suspected PUJO or ureterovesical junction (VUJ) obstruction (e.g. primary obstructive megaureter, obstructive ureterocele, etc.) a more sophisticated imaging algorithm is proposed (Fig. 4-32),[17] with US findings determining subsequent imaging. MCUG is recommended to differentiate obstructive and refluxing dilatation, and MAG3 renography (increasingly dynamic functional MRU) to assess function and urinary drainage. The exact timing of follow-up will depend on the size of the RPD and DRF: the functionality is much more

important than a simple anatomical abnormality which may have no functional consequence. The results should be used as guidance, as satisfactory grading may be difficult, immaturity of renal function may improve, and there is no convincing benefit of early surgical release of obstruction to improve renal function. Those children with functional impairment clearly require closer follow-up than those with an isolated mild RPD alone. Long-term follow-up is recommended until at least 15–20 years of age.

The largest group of children seen with a prenatal diagnosis of HN will have a normal postnatal US, or only mild residual dilatation. Those with persistent significant dilatation require functional and VUR assessment, using both radionuclide investigation of antegrade function and an MCUG, particularly in boys. However, the use of MCUG is falling out of favour, due to the lack of evidence that low-grade VUR has any consequence on the child's outcome or prevention of renal scarring later in life, and the high incidence of VUR resolving spontaneously. It is important to differentiate these children from the group who present later with UTI, on whom much of the data on VUR and renal scarring are acquired. Both VUR and HN may simply be a marker of unilateral renal dysplasia in these children, which results in abnormal renal function and scarring later in life. The use of prophylactic antibiotics in children with unilateral abnormalities detected antenatally is not evidence based, and it is becoming increasingly difficult to justify

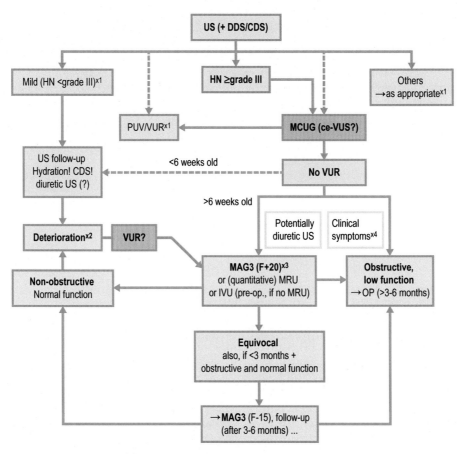

US (+ DDS/CDS)

Mild (HN <grade III)[x1]   HN ≥grade III   Others → as appropriate[x1]

PUV/VUR[x1]   MCUG (ce-VUS?)

US follow-up Hydration! CDS! diuretic US (?)   <6 weeks old   No VUR

>6 weeks old

Potentially diuretic US   Clinical symptoms[x4]

Deterioration[x2]   VUR?   MAG3 (F+20)[x3] or (quantitative) MRU or IVU (pre-op., if no MRU)   Obstructive, low function → OP (>3-6 months)

Non-obstructive Normal function

Equivocal also, if <3 months + obstructive and normal function

→ MAG3 (F-15), follow-up (after 3-6 months) ...

[x1] as appropriate, see also respective algorithms
[x2] imaging criteria for deterioration:
- on US increasing dilatation, decreasing parenchymal width, echotecture, contralateral hypertrophy, decreased vascularisation (on CDS), asymmetrically elevated RI (on DDS or with diuretic stress)
- reduced peristalsis (in MU) or ureteric jet (asymmetrically in unilateral disease)
- on scintigraphy: decreased (split) renal function and drainage, contralateral hypertrophy
[x3] assess drainage pattern and split function
[x4] clinical criteria for deterioration: pain, infection, haematuria (kidney) growth failure, hypertension

FIGURE 4-32 ■ **Urinary obstruction.** ESPR imaging algorithm for suspected obstructive uropathy. (Adapted from Riccabona M, Avni F E, Blickman J G, et al; Members of the ESUR paediatric recommendation work group and ESPR paediatric uroradiology work group 2009 Imaging recommendations in paediatric uroradiology, part II: urolithiasis and haematuria in children, paediatric obstructive uropathy, and postnatal work-up of fetally diagnosed high grade hydronephrosis. Minutes of a mini-symposium at the ESPR annual meeting, Edinburgh, June. Pediatr Radiol 39(8):891–898.[17])

invasive imaging without being able to offer therapeutic treatment.

There is ongoing uncertainty about the management of bilateral RPD. The investigative protocol in this situation should be as for the unilateral RPD dilatation, but should include an MCUG as well as formal sequential glomerular filtration rate (GFR) estimation.

Unilateral Renal Pelvic Dilatation

The natural history of unilateral RPD is a relatively benign condition which frequently resolves spontaneously. True obstruction will typically lead to parenchymal compression and eventually atrophy. If the child has any of these features, assessment of renal function is imperative, although these changes do not predict progressive

renal deterioration. There is no test that will predict which kidney with a prenatal RPD will deteriorate. US assessment within the first 24 h may underestimate RPD due to neonatal dehydration and renal immaturity, and thus US at around 7 days of life should be used to more reliably assess calyceal and pelvic dilatation, measure the transverse diameter of the pelvis and the calyces, assess renal parenchyma and renal volume, and confirm the structural normality of the bladder and opposite kidney.

Megaureter

HN with a dilated ureter is dealt with in the same way as pelvic dilatation above, but suggests that VUR is more likely. The imaging protocol therefore is similar to that of RPD plus a MCUG (ce-VUS) to document or exclude VUR. Careful US of the bladder and VUJ must be performed to exclude a small ureterocele or other bladder abnormality, and ureteric peristalsis. Reimplantation of the ureter into the bladder in a child younger than 1 year of age may result in abnormal bladder function in later life; urodynamics may not be able to clarify this further. In the neonate, a spinal US is useful to exclude spinal cord pathology where a neurogenic bladder may be suspected. Stenting of the ureter or tempory diversion by ureterocutaneostomy may be necessary to preserve renal function, assessed by diuretic ^{99m}Tc-MAG3 drainage studies.

Renal Failure

Acute renal failure in the newborn is a common problem. It may have an antenatal onset, in congenital disease such as renal dysplasia and genetic disorders such as ARPCKD, or hypotensive or hypoxic event at or around delivery, resulting in renal vein thrombosis (RVT), medullary or acute tubular necrosis (ATN), or any combination of these conditions. Ultrasound with Doppler is the first investigation, as all of these disorders result in an echogenic kidney with loss of the normal corticomedullary differentiation. The main task of US is to differentiate between prerenal, intrinsic or postrenal cause of the renal insufficiency.

Renal Vein Thrombosis (RVT)

ATN is typically symmetrical and RVT typically asymmetrical, but can be bilateral. In RVT, swollen echogenic kidneys with prominent interlobular arteries are demonstrated by US. Often no venous flow can be identified at the renal hilum, and echogenic linear streaks of venous thrombi may be seen in the periphery. Seventy-five per cent of RVT is unilateral, starting in the periphery: power Doppler is helpful to depict early stages, around 50% will have IVC involvement, and 10% associated adrenal haemorrhage. Doppler US spectral flow display will show the typical high resistance flow profile with reverse diastolic flow in the affected renal artery. Contrast-enhanced imaging examinations are rarely used in this context; follow-up US (split renal volume assessment) with ^{99m}Tc-DMSA scintigraphy (4–12 months of age) should be performed to assess the long-term effects.

URINARY TRACT INFECTION AND VESICOURETERIC REFLUX

Urinary tract infection (UTI) is a common (bacterial) infection causing illness in infants and children, often with non-specific symptoms. The long-term goal of imaging in UTI is to preserve renal function and growth potential: this is often misinterpreted as (a) identifying VUR on imaging, and (b) minimising future UTIs, although there is limited evidence that these are synonymous.[18]

Many children investigated will be normal; thus, an effort must be made to only image those at high potential clinical risk, and to keep radiation doses to a minimum. Even in those imaged, there is limited evidence to suggest that treatment affects the natural history of renal damage. There is continuing controversy over the significance of VUR in the setting of UTI. In particular, neonatal VUR is now thought to be a transitory condition that, in the majority, diminishes or disappears spontaneously, even in high-grade VUR. There are now in-depth imaging and treatment guidelines both from the ESPR Uroradiology Task Force (Fig. 4-33) and UK National Institute for Clinical Excellence.[1,19]

Clinical Setting

Four per cent of all children under 8 years of age will present with a UTI each year, yet the incidence of children requiring dialysis secondary to pyelonephritis is one child per million age-related population. There is little data to support the belief that hypertension is a complication of mild renal scarring. Most children who respond to antibiotic therapy in the acute setting may not need any imaging. Imaging should be confined to those 'susceptible children' in whom an underlying abnormality may be found. These children may have an atypical UTI presentation, i.e. recurrent infections; clinical signs (poor urinary stream, palpable kidneys, poor response to treatment); unusual organisms (non-*Escherichia coli*) infections; bacteraemia; slow response to antibiotics; or unusual clinical presentation (e.g. older boy).[19] VUR is a radiological sign, not a disease entity (Figs. 4-34 and 4-35) and only 20% of children with VUR show renal damage on DMSA, while scarred kidneys are seen in children where no VUR could be demonstrated by MCUG. Thirty per cent of children with a prenatal diagnosis of HN already have an abnormal kidney at birth; thus VUR may be a marker of dysplasia rather than always reflecting true 'reflux nephropathy'.

Imaging

The aim of imaging is to detect an underlying condition or pyelonephritis. In the acute non-responding UTI, US should be performed to investigate for obstructive uropathy, pyelonephritis and abscess formation in all children. Acute pyelonephritis is best imaged using comprehensive US with power Doppler US, ^{99m}Tc-DMSA or gadolinium-enhanced or inversion recovery (STIR) MRI sequences. European guidelines suggest US imaging in all children following their first upper UTI to exclude anatomical abnormalities which may determine the need for further imaging using MCUG.[1] MCUG is restricted to those younger children with atypical or recurrent upper UTIs, severe infection including pyelonephritis, renal scars or urinary tract anomalies. If there is evidence of obstruction on US then a MAG3 diuretic renogram is required (8 weeks after the UTI). A ^{99m}Tc-DMSA scintigram should be used to detect renal parenchymal defects, not earlier than 4–6 months following the acute infection.

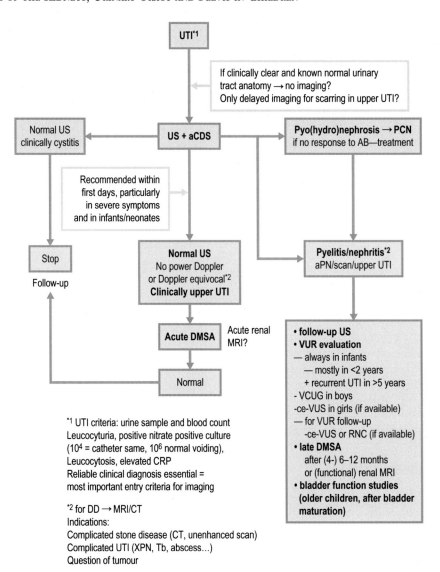

FIGURE 4-33 ■ **Urinary tract infection.** ESPR imaging algorithm for investigation of UTI—aCDS = amplitude-coded colour Doppler sonography, aPN = acute pyelonephritis, CRP = C-reactive protein, DD = differential diagnosis, DMSA = static renal scintigraphy, PCN = percutaneous nephrostomy, RNC = radionuclide cystography, Tb = tuberculosis, XPN = xanthogranulomatous pyelonephritis. (Adapted from Riccabona M, Avni F E, Blickman J G, et al 2008 Imaging recommendations in paediatric uroradiology: minutes of the ESPR workgroup session on urinary tract infection, fetal hydronephrosis, urinary tract ultrasonography and voiding cystourethrography, Barcelona, Spain, June 2007. Pediatr Radiol 38(2):138–145.[1])

In children with recurrent UTI with normal renal appearances on US, the emphasis switches to bladder function: voiding assessment by modified MCUG and (video) urodynamics is more useful than further conventional imaging, allowing assessment of an unstable bladder or destrusor-sphincter dysfunction. The follow-up of children with a damaged kidney and VUR who are on long-term antibiotic prophylaxis is unclear. One approach is to only undertake imaging if it will affect treatment. If surgical intervention has been undertaken to stop VUR, then US and dynamic scintigraphy are essential to exclude obstruction.

Renal Abscess

This complication may follow acute pyelonephritis in a child with a swinging fever with a poor response to antibiotics. Usually the abscess also has a thick wall with heterogeneous internal echogenicity on US. MRI may be helpful, especially if US findings are equivocal or aspiration or drainage is being considered (Fig. 4-36). Lobar nephronia is the term given to focal acute bacterial renal mass without liquefaction, thought to be the stage between acute pyelonephritis and abscess formation, and should not be mistaken for a tumoural mass. Immunodeficient patients may become infected with fungus manifest as 'fungal balls' or fungal abscess formation within the kidney (Fig. 4-37).

Xanthogranulomatous Pyelonephritis

Xanthogranulomatous pyelonephritis (XPN) is a rare chronic inflammatory disease of the kidney in childhood, probably an abnormal inflammatory response to infection

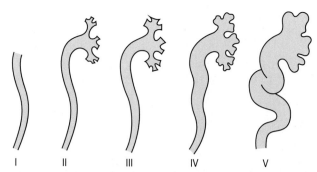

FIGURE 4-34 ■ **Radiographic grading of reflux.** (I) Ureter and upper collecting system without dilatation; (II) mild or (III) moderate dilatation of the ureter and mild or moderate dilatation of the renal pelvis, but minimal blunting of the fornices; (IV) moderate dilatation and/or tortuosity of the ureter with moderate dilatation of the renal pelvis and calyces, and obliteration of the sharp angle of the fornices but maintenance of papillary impression in the majority of calyces; (V) gross dilatation and tortuosity of ureters, renal pelvis, and calyces; papillary impressions are not visible in the majority of calyces. (Reproduced with permission by the American Academy of Pediatrics.)

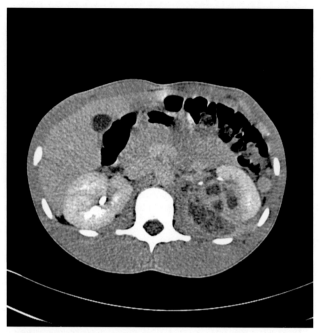

FIGURE 4-36 ■ **Renal abscess.** CT of an adolescent with gross pyelonephritis and abscess cavity formation in the left kidney. This type of image could now be better obtained with MRI.

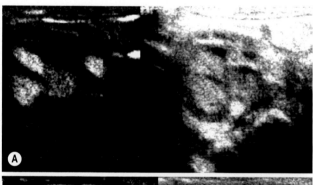
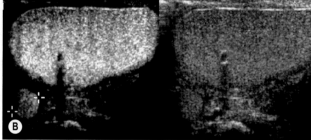

FIGURE 4-35 ■ **VUR using ce-VUS.** (A) Cross-section, upper abdomen/flank during ce-VUS—contrast material depicted in the dilated right renal collecting system in grade IV VUR, easier to see on the dedicated low-MI contrast imaging technique (left image) than on basic US (right image). (B) Cross-section, lower abdomen during ce-VUS—demonstrates contrast material in the dilated distal right ureter retrovesically. VUR is much more conspicuously imaged using a dedicated low-MI contrast imaging technique (left image) than on conventional US (right image).

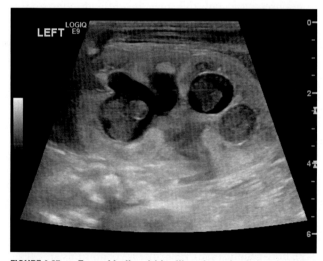

FIGURE 4-37 ■ **Fungal balls within dilated renal calyces.** Longitudinal US of the left kidney in an immunocompromised patient who cultured *Candida* from the urine.

in the presence of a calculus. The clinical presentation is with weight loss, failure to thrive, malaise, anaemia and a renal mass. Urine cultures are positive in 70%, typically for *Proteus* species and *E. coli*. The imaging findings are usually sufficiently characteristic to allow preoperative diagnosis and to avoid confusion with a Wilms' tumour

(Fig. 4-38). The diffuse type of XPN, affecting the entire kidney, is more common in childhood, and focal renal involvement is rare.

Focal XPN tends to manifest with a localised intrarenal mass in an otherwise normal kidney. Plain radiographs reveal an abdominal mass with calculi. US demonstrates general renal enlargement in the diffuse form with hypoechoic areas corresponding to inflammatory masses within the kidney. Calcification can be shown, particularly at the contracted renal pelvis, or within the ureter. ^{99m}Tc-DMSA scintigraphy shows a nonfunctioning kidney or a photon-deficient area. CT after

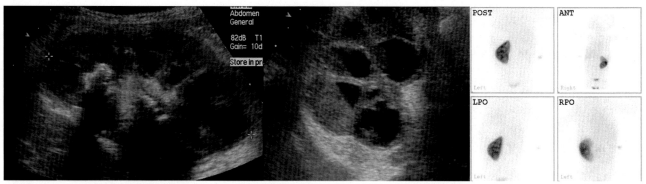

FIGURE 4-38 ■ **Xanthogranulomatous pyelonephritis (XPN).** US demonstrates renal calculi with debris within the right renal collecting system in a hypoechoic, dilated kidney. The DMSA of the same patient shows no function on the right.

intravenous contrast medium characteristically shows global renal enlargement with prominent low-attenuating abscess cavities. The remaining renal parenchyma can often show some rim enhancement due to the perfusion of the inflamed, non-functioning kidney. MRI is preferable, with necrotic areas hyperintense on T2-weighted MRI, with intermediate signal on T1-weighted sequences, which probably represents the high protein content of the cavities. Perinephric extension is common, with hilar or para-aortic adenopathy. The treatment for both types is nephrectomy, but this may be difficult due to the surrounding chronic inflammation. There may be a role for preoperative embolisation to reduce perioperative haemorrhage.

RENAL CYSTIC DISEASE

Antenatal US and fetal MRI have allowed many of the congenital cystic renal diseases to be diagnosed in utero. There is a very wide spectrum of disease with variations in renal involvement both within and between diseases.[20,21] Abnormally large kidneys may be the first indicator of cystic disease prior to the cysts themselves becoming visible: hence the need for accurate age-appropriate renal size assessment. The most widely accepted classification system is based on genetics (Table 4-9); non-genetic cystic renal disease conditions are given in Table 4-10. A careful clinical history must be taken to assess family history of renal disease and a history of diabetes. Consanguinity is a potential risk and evidence of a syndrome should be sought; family members may need to be screened with renal US.

Cystic Dysplasia

The term 'dysplasia' causes confusion when dealing with abnormal kidneys. Dysplasia is a histological diagnosis based on abnormal metanephric differentiation with persistence of fetal kidney tissue associated with primitive ducts. Many clinicians use the term when US demonstrates a small kidney with increased echogenicity, loss of corticomedullary differentiation with or without cysts (Fig. 4-39). If there is associated VUR, the kidney may demonstrate a dilated collecting system and uroepithelial

TABLE 4-9	Genetic Conditions Associated with Renal Cysts

Autosomal Dominant
• Autosomal dominant polycystic kidney disease
• Tuberous sclerosis
• Medullary cystic disease
• Glomerulocystic disease

Autosomal Recessive
• Autosomal recessive polycystic kidney disease
• Juvenile nephronophthisis

Cysts Associated with Syndromes
• Chromosomal disorders
• Autosomal recessive syndromes, mitochrondrial syndromes
• X-linked syndromes, e.g. Alport's syndrome

TABLE 4-10	Non-hereditary Conditions Associated with Renal Cysts

• Cystic dysplasia or dysplasia
• Multicystic dysplastic kidney
• Multilocular cyst
• Multilocular cystic Wilms' tumour
• Localised cystic disease of the kidney
• Parapelvic cyst
• Simple cysts
• Calyceal cyst (calyceal diverticulum)
• Medullary sponge kidney
• Acquired cystic kidney disease (in chronic renal failure)

thickening with a tortuous and dilated ureter, e.g. in boys with dysplastic kidneys secondary to posterior urethral valves or high-grade congenital VUR. The same applies to the so-called 'obstructive dysplasia', probably an early stage of MCDK, with an underlying upper tract obstruction causing the impaired renal development and cyst formation. Care should be taken when interpreting a ^{99m}Tc-DMSA scan in a dysplastic kidney. The appearances of patchy uptake and peripheral photopenic areas may be seen, mimicking renal scarring.

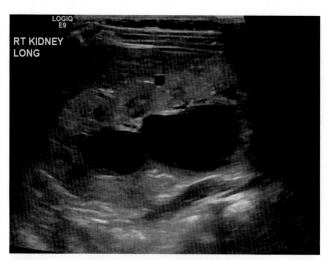

FIGURE 4-39 ■ **Cystic dysplastic kidney secondary to chronic obstruction.** Dilated PC system hyperechoic renal cortex with tiny peripheral hypoechoic cysts in subcapsular distribution.

Multicystic Dysplastic Kidney (MCDK)

MCDK is a developmental abnormality due to failure of union of renal mesenchyme with the ureteric bud. It is a sporadic condition with an incidence of 1 in 2000–4000 and is twice as common in boys. The MCDK is always non-functioning with an atretic ureter. There is usually contralateral but no ipsilateral VUR. Usually there are multiple anechoic cysts of different sizes, often with a peripheral dominant cyst. The key feature for differentiating a MCDK from a PUJO is the position of the residual parenchyma if present: this tends to be central in MCDK, whereas it is peripheral and rim-like in PUJO; it is always echogenic without differentiation, and may (rarely) exhibit some vascular signal on Doppler US.

Most cases of MCDK are detected antenatally, and typically involute if smaller than 5 cm without demonstrable vasculature. Occasionally, they may increase in size or be large enough to interfere with breathing or feeding; rarely they get infected or cause hypertension. Bilateral MCDK is incompatible with life (formerly called 'Potter syndrome'). There is an association with PUJO or ureteric stenosis in the contralateral kidney in up to 30% of babies and VUR is also associated. A ^{99m}Tc-MAG3 renogram or a MRU is indicated where HN or hydroureter is seen in the contralateral kidney. A ^{99m}Tc-DMSA scintigram will show non-function in the MCDK. This is not normally clinically indicated, and in doubtful cases a MRU is preferred.

Simple Cysts

Simple renal cysts are common incidental findings in adults, but cysts are rare in children and should be considered abnormal at any age, requiring investigation. Cysts are more common in children following abdominal radiotherapy and chemotherapy, and should not be confused with an obstructed upper moiety of a duplex kidney. Calyceal cysts or diverticula are rare findings in children that may be indistinguishable from tertiary calyces or simple cysts, requiring more detailed investigation (Fig. 4-40) and may develop calculi within.

Localised Cystic Disease of the Kidney

This condition, segmental cystic nephroma, is recognised as genetically, radiologically and morphologically distinct from ADPKD. The involved segment of the kidney is usually enlarged, containing multiple, small cysts which gradually merge into normal renal tissue and are not sharply demarcated from the adjacent normal parenchyma. The feature which helps differentiate localised cystic disease of the kidney from the multilocular cystic Wilms' tumour is the absence of a surrounding capsule on imaging and histology. There is no familial trait, there are no cysts in the contralateral kidney and the lesions do not progress in the few cases that have been reported and left in situ. Hypertension has been documented but the natural history is unclear.

Acquired Cystic Renal Disease

Cysts commonly develop in patients undergoing dialysis for renal failure, with 90% of patients developing cysts if on dialysis for over 10 years, without an underlying cystic renal disorder. After renal transplantation, the cysts tend to decrease in size. Complications include renal cell carcinoma, haemorrhage, or infection within the cysts.

Genetic Cystic Disease

Table 4-11 compares some of the findings in the more common cystic renal disorders in children.

Autosomal Dominant Polycystic Kidney Disease (ADPKD)

ADPKD most often presents in the third decade of life; however, there is considerable phenotypic variability in the severity of the renal disease, with some affected individuals presenting in childhood or being detected antenatally. Prevalence is approximately 1 in 1000 with two common genetic loci identified. Ninety per cent of families have the gene located on the short arm of chromosome 16 (*PKD1*). The second gene is on chromosome 4 (*PKD2*). In *PKD1* families, 64% of children <10 and 90% aged <20 years will have cysts. There may be no family history, as spontaneous mutation accounts for approximately half of cases, and phenotypes vary within families.

The extrarenal manifestations of ADPKD include cysts in the liver, pancreas and/or spleen. These are, otherwise, unusual in children and become more common with age. Subarachnoid haemorrhage due to associated intracranial aneurysm is also rare in childhood, but there may be a familial link. Screening for extrarenal manifestations is usually confined to high-risk adults, such as those with strong family history or warning symptoms. Congenital hepatic fibrosis is generally associated with autosomal recessive PKD (ARPKD; see below) and rarely with ADPKD.

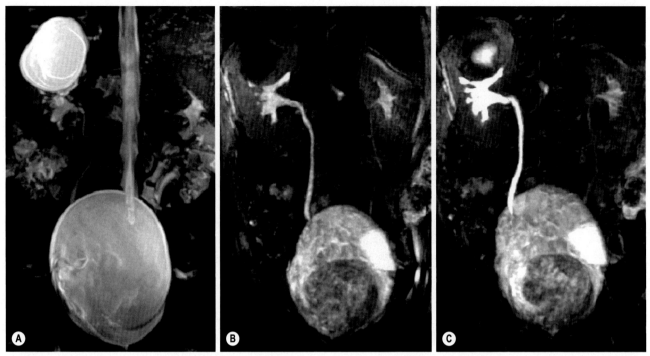

FIGURE 4-40 ■ **Diagnostic use of MRU to evaluate a renal cyst.** (A) Three-dimensional T2W MRU image demonstrates a large 'cystic' structure on the upper pole of the right kidney; note the disturbance from other fluid-filled structures in this rendered 3D image. (B) Three-dimensional contrast-enhanced T1 GRE MRU in the early excretory phase (10 min, rendered image). Both collecting systems are well visualised; there is no contrast in the 'cyst'. (C) Three-dimensional contrast-enhanced T1 GRE MRU in the delayed excretory phase (45 min, rendered image): this shows obvious contrast influx into the cyst, connecting to the somewhat clubbed and displaced upper calyx, suggesting that this structure is in fact a large calyceal diverticulum.

TABLE 4-11   Comparison of Features of Renal Cystic Disease

	ADPKD	Tuberous Sclerosis	ARPKD	MCDK	Simple Cyst
Inheritance	D	D	R	None	None
Uni- or bilateral	Bilateral unequal	Bilateral	Bilateral equal	Uni- or bilateral	Unilateral
Kidney size	Normal or large	Normal or large	Very large > 90th centile	Small or large	Normal
Extrarenal manifestations	Hepatic and pancreatic cysts, cerebral and aortic aneurysms	Cardiac rhabdomyomas, intracranial tubers	Congenital hepatic fibrosis (biliary dysgenesis)	None	None
Age at presentation	Third decade	Often <18 months	Neonate and childhood	Antenatal, rare in childhood	Onset in adult life
Cyst size	Visible cysts of variable size	Similar to ADPKD, ± angiomyolipomas	Generally small, related to collecting ducts	Large then often involute	Variable
Diagnosis	US, genetic	US, cardiac echo, cranial MRI	US, IVU, liver biopsy	US, MAG3	US, IVU
Malignancy risk	No	Yes	No	Rare	No

ADPKD = autosomal dominant polycystic kidney disease; ARPKD = autosomal recessive polycystic kidney disease; D = autosomal dominant; MCDK = multicystic dysplastic kidney; R = autosomal recessive.

Imaging

In the prenatal period, US may demonstrate highly reflective kidneys similar to that in ARPKD. In infancy the US appearances vary, from a normal kidney to a few isolated cysts, to a kidney packed full of cysts (Fig. 4-41). Typically the cysts are scattered throughout both the cortex and medulla with asymmetrical involvement of the two kidneys, which are usually enlarged. The intervening renal parenchyma appears normal. When found in the young child (younger than 5 years of age) with no family history, a diagnosis of tuberous sclerosis (TS) must also

be considered and actively excluded. MRI can help, especially to identify fatty tissue in an angiomyolipoma in TS, or for a baseline assessment prior to treatment.

Tuberous Sclerosis

TS is one of the neurocutaneous disorders, an autosomal dominant condition with a prevalence of 1 in 10,000. It is characterised by multiple hamartomas in the brain, skin, heart, kidneys, liver, lung and bone, and cysts are also seen in the kidneys. Two per cent of children with

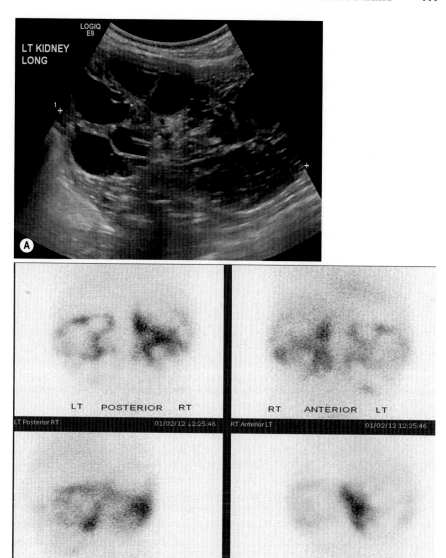

FIGURE 4-41 ■ ADPKD. (A) Enlarged kidneys with multiple large cysts in a 3-year-old with no family history of renal disease. (B) ^{99m}Tc-DMSA shows bilateral photopenic areas representing the cysts.

TS have ADPKD, with TS genetically linked to chromosome 9 in about one-third of families, and to chromosome 16 in the same region as the ADPKD1 gene.

Fifty to 75% of TS patients have renal manifestations, most commonly angiomyolipomas, with or without cysts (Fig. 4-42). Renal cysts are found less frequently (20–50%) and occur in younger patients. No imaging modality can currently differentiate cysts in TS from ADPKD. US may demonstrate multiple cysts, or multiple small rounded echogenic foci throughout the renal parenchyma due to multiple angiomyolipomas. Angiomyolipomas greater than 4 cm in diameter are at risk of haemorrhage from abnormal renal vasculature, and some advocate prophylactic embolisation. Renal cell carcinoma may also occur later in life.

Autosomal Recessive Polycystic Kidney Disease

ARPKD is a rare genetic disorder with an incidence of approximately 1 in 55,000 live births. The parents are

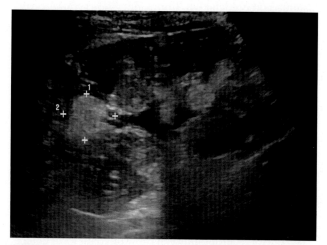

FIGURE 4-42 ■ Angiomyolipoma. Oblique US shows hyperechoic mass within the kidney in a patient with known tuberous sclerosis.

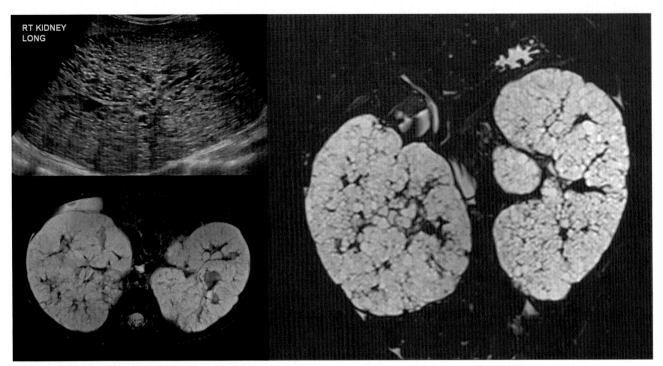

FIGURE 4-43 ■ **ARPKD.** US shows bilateral enlarged hyperechoic kidneys which retain their reniform shape with multiple tiny hypoechoic cysts in a 5-year-old boy, confirmed on axial and coronal T2W MR sequences.

always unaffected. The gene for ARPKD has been located on chromosome 6. All patients with ARPKD have some degree of congenital hepatic fibrosis, the severity of which is usually inversely proportional to the severity of renal disease: early presentation (perinatal/neonatal) has more severe renal involvement, whereas in older children (infantile and juvenile type) the liver disease predominates.

Prenatal diagnosis with US has been reported as early as 14–17 weeks' gestation. However, as bilateral highly reflective kidneys during the fetal period is not specific to ARPKD, caution is necessary before suggesting this diagnosis on prenatal US. Both kidneys are symmetrically involved and markedly enlarged, measuring > 95th centile in early infancy. The characteristic appearance is increased echogenicity in the cortex and medulla, although variations, with the medulla much brighter than the cortex, may be seen (Fig. 4-43). Using high-frequency US probes, 1- to 2-mm cysts may be detected in the medulla ('pepper and salt' kidney). In some cases these may evolve into larger cysts of different sizes with an appearance very similar to ADPKD in older children (Table 4-11).

In the young child (and sometimes even in the neonate) the liver is enlarged with increased periportal echogenicity from bile duct proliferation and fibrosis. Ectatic, dilated and cystic biliary ducts may be indistinguishable from Caroli's disease. A large spleen and evidence of portal hypertension should be excluded in older children. ^{99m}Tc-DMSA scintigraphy can show bilateral focal defects in enlarged kidneys with a high background activity; this combination of US and DMSA appearances is characteristic of ARPKD.

Functional imaging of the liver may be helpful in children with ARPKD. US may fail to show biliary duct

dilatation. Children with ARPKD may present in childhood with ascending cholangitis. Liver imaging is performed over the age of 1 year, either using a hepatobiliary agent such as ^{99m}Tc-HIDA, or comprehensive MR evaluation.

Juvenile Nephronophthisis/Medullary Cystic Disease

These are two different terms for conditions that have a different inheritance, different age of onset and different associations, but a similar renal morphology and imaging. Both present with slowly progressive renal failure.

Juvenile nephronophthisis (JN) has an autosomal recessive inheritance, presenting in childhood as chronic renal failure. It is characterised by an early concentrating defect with polyuria and polydipsia, growth retardation, anaemia, and causes end-stage renal disease <25 years of age. Medullary cystic disease (MCD) shows an autosomal dominant inheritance and presents up to the fourth decade of life.

Imaging

The characteristic finding on US is normal or near-normal-sized kidneys with globally increased echogenicity. Corticomedullary cysts are not present until late in the disease. In the early stages of the disease when the tubules are affected to a greater degree than the glomeruli, the ^{99m}Tc-DMSA scintigram may fail to show the kidneys, as the tracer is taken up by the proximal tubules. A ^{99m}Tc-DTPA scintigram may be almost normal as the tracer is filtered by the glomerulus. The diagnosis can only be made on biopsy. Extrarenal manifestations

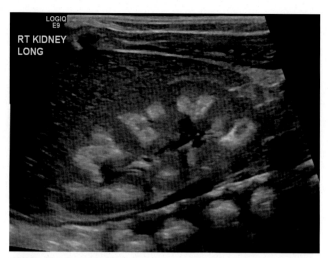

FIGURE 4-44 ■ **Nephrocalcinosis.** Concentric medullary nephrocalcinosis on US consistent with stage II of medullary nephrocalcinosis.

TABLE 4-12   Causes of Increased Medullary Echogenicity in Children

- Nephrocalcinosis (primary hyperoxaluria, cystinuria, xanthinuria)
  - Non-iatrogenic, e.g. idiopathic hypercalcaemia in Williams' syndrome, absorptive hypercalciuria
  - Iatrogenic, e.g. treatment for hypophosphataemic rickets or furosemide for bronchopulmonary dysplasia or cardiac failure in a premature infant
- Tubulopathies, e.g. renal tubular acidosis
- Protein deposits giving transient increased medullary echogenicity in newborns
- Vascular congestion, e.g. sickle cell anaemia
- Infection, e.g. candidiasis and cytomegalovirus
- Metabolic disease, e.g. urate deposits as in Lesch–Nyhan syndrome. Also seen in tyrosinaemia and glycogen storage disease
- Cystic medullary renal disease, e.g. autosomal recessive polycystic kidney disease

reported in JN include skeletal abnormalities, congenital hepatic fibrosis and mental retardation.

No such association has been reported in MCD.

NEPHROCALCINOSIS

Nephrocalcinosis may be a complication of metabolic disorders or genetic diseases, or may be seen in (pre-term) infants following diuretic treatment. Early diagnosis and treatment are essential in order to exclude a progression in nephrocalcinosis, which may lead to deterioration in renal function.

US is much more sensitive in the detection of early calcium deposition in the kidneys than plain radiography of the abdomen. Increased medullary echogenicity of the kidneys in children, while non-specific on US, may be an unexpected finding and indicative of underlying metabolic disease (Fig. 4-44). It always requires a clinical explanation, although there is a wide range of causes (Table 4-12). Iatrogenic nephrocalcinosis (diuretics, vitamin D) is the most common cause in children for an increased echogenicity of the medullary pyramids. Other common causes include idiopathic hypercalciuria and hyperoxaluria, distal tubular acidosis and rare causes include hyperthyroidism and hyperparathyroidism. The differentiation on US among medullary, cortical and global nephrocalcinosis may be important in terms of aetiology, and also to detect complications such as secondary stone formation or papillary necrosis. US can be used for grading medullary nephrocalcinosis, but cannot distinguish between calcium phosphate (nephrocalcinosis) and calcium oxalate (oxalosis) deposition.

RENAL CALCULI

Renal calculi are often asymptomatic in the paediatric population. Older children may present with UTI, pain or haematuria, as in adults, but small children may have non-specific abdominal pain, vomiting or isolated haematuria. Adult standard imaging protocols cannot be directly applied to children because of higher incidence of poorly calcified stones (e.g. cystinuria, infectious stones), and very little fat surrounding a child's small ureter.

US is best used to investigate echogenic foci, dilatation of the ureter and pelvicalyceal system, and increased renal echogenicity and size (Fig. 4-45).[17] An acoustic shadow is not a reliable sign in children, as stones may be too small (<4 mm) or low in calcium content. The twinkling artefact on CDS may enhance the suspicion or diagnosis of urinary calculi. Most stones are found in the pelvicalyceal system or in the proximal (PUJ) and/or the distal (VUJ) ureter, well visualised by US with adequate hydration and bladder distension. In larger patients and with less experienced operators, US may miss mid-ureteral stones (10–20% overall), but as most of these will cause proximal obstruction or frank HN. Stones may also form within ureteroceles or calyceal diverticulae (Fig. 4-46).

A KUB may be necessary for stone localisation prior to lithotripsy, or as a baseline study for follow-up evaluation in selected cases in older children. Ninety per cent of stones contain calcium, and should be visible on an abdominal radiograph. A limited IVU (2–4 images total) is still used by some in the diagnostic imaging of paediatric urolithiasis, especially if CT is not available or access to it is limited. There are very limited data available on the diagnostic accuracy of low-dose CT in children.

One diagnostic algorithm is that if US is negative and there is a low clinical suspicion, a watchful waiting approach may be preferable to further imaging. At present, CT may be complementary in cases with non-diagnostic or equivocal US findings that do not correlate with the clinical findings, or in high suspicion with a negative US examination, or in complex cases. MRI and MR urography for stone imaging needs to be fully evaluated.

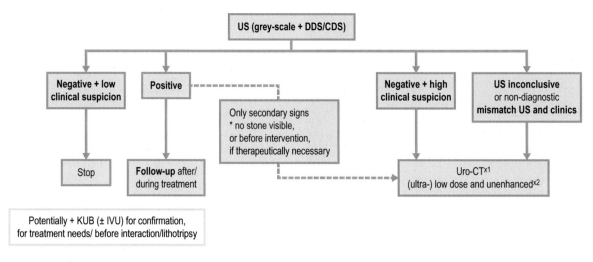

FIGURE 4-45 ■ **Urolithiasis.** ESPR imaging algorithm for suspected urolithiasis. (Adapted from Riccabona M, Avni F E, Blickman J G, et al; Members of the ESUR Paediatric Recommendation Work Group and ESPR Paediatric Uroradiology Work Group 2009 Imaging recommendations in paediatric uroradiology, part II: urolithiasis and haematuria in children, paediatric obstructive uropathy, and postnatal work-up of fetally diagnosed high grade hydronephrosis. Minutes of a mini-symposium at the ESPR annual meeting, Edinburgh, June. Pediatr Radiol 39(8):891–898.[17])

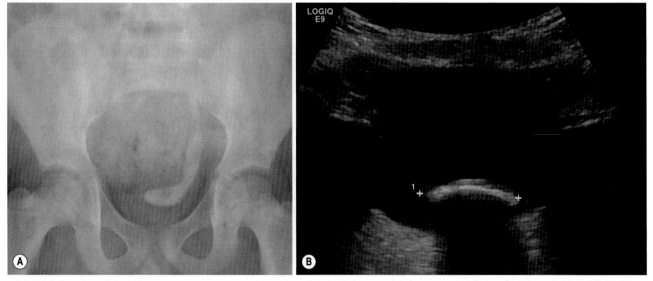

FIGURE 4-46 ■ **Stone in large ureterocele.** Abdominal radiograph of a J-shaped stone (A) which has formed in a large ureterocele, confirmed on US (B) and cystoscopy.

TUMOURS

BENIGN TUMOURS

Nephroblastomatosis

Benign tumours of the paediatric kidney are more common than initially perceived. Nephrogenic rests (NR) are abnormally persistent nephrogenic cells (metanephric blastema, or embryonic renal parenchyma) within the kidney. These may be focal (NR) or diffuse, whence termed 'nephroblastomatosis'. Nephrogenic rests are regarded as precursors of Wilms' tumour (nephroblastoma): nephroblastomatosis occurs in 41% of

unilateral Wilms' tumours, 94% of metachronous bilateral Wilms' tumours and 99% of synchronous bilateral Wilms' tumours.[22] They are associated with many syndromes which predispose to Wilms' tumour, such as Beckwith–Wiedemann syndrome, hemihypertrophy and aniridia. However, NR are found in around 1% of tissues at autopsy, and only a minority of nephrogenic rests develop into Wilms' tumour; thus the malignant potential of any individual lesion is uncertain.

Nephroblastomatosis may be unifocal, multifocal or diffuse. Individual foci are usually homogeneous and of low echogenicity on US, although lesions smaller than

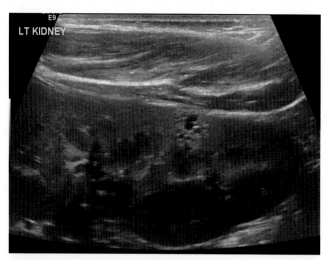

FIGURE 4-47 ■ **Nephrogenic rest.** High-frequency US of this left kidney shows a small echogenic and cystic mass, in a patient with Beckwith–Wiedemann syndrome; difficult to differentiate form a segmental cystic nephroma.

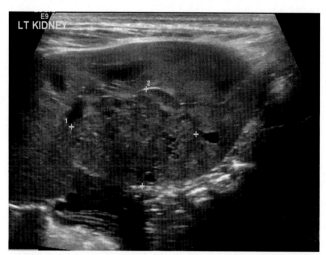

FIGURE 4-48 ■ **Nephrogenic rests.** Larger, more heterogeneous area of nephrogenic rests within the left kidney of a patient who had contralateral Wilms' tumour. Appearances are similar to that of Wilms' tumour.

1 cm may be difficult to depict using US alone; CDS and ce-US, however, improve detection rates (Figs. 4-47 and 4-48). MRI shows homogeneous lesions of low signal intensity; typically they do not enhance with contrast medium due to poorer perfusion than the relatively vascular renal cortex. Diffuse nephroblastomatosis may present as a thick rind of reduced echogenicity on US. Multifocal disease may be difficult to identify as small nephrogenic rests, may resemble normal renal cortex on all modalities, or present as slightly nodular or plaque-like lesions. They are typically identified as small homogeneous lesions in the context of an individual with a Wilms' tumour or genetic predisposition. The differential diagnosis of diffuse nephroblastomatosis on US mainly includes renal lymphoma or leukaemia. Despite the known malignant risk, regular US or MRI surveillance may be chosen in preference to biopsy of individual lesions.

Mesoblastic Nephroma

Mesoblastic nephroma is the most common renal neoplasm in the first 3 months of life, presenting as a neonatal abdominal mass, and accounting for 3–10% of all paediatric renal tumours. The mass is typically solid and homogeneous, with a hypoechoic vascular ring around the periphery. Heterogeneity suggests cystic change or necrosis. Neither US nor CT can reliably distinguish mesoblastic nephroma from Wilms' tumour: the former show uptake of ^{99m}Tc-DMSA. Mesoblastic nephroma does not invade the vascular pedicle, nor does it usually metastasise. Local recurrence may result from incomplete removal or capsular penetration, but complete excision carries an excellent prognosis. US is usually sufficient for diagnosis.

Multilocular Cystic Nephroma (MCN)

Multilocular cystic nephroma is an uncommon cystic renal mass, derived from metanephric blastema, occasionally seen in children. There is a bimodal distribution, seen more commonly in boys under 4 years and in women in the fifth or sixth decade. The child will present with an abdominal mass and US will show a multilocular renal mass with multiple cysts and hyperechoic septations. On cross-sectional imaging, the mass typically has well-defined margins or capsule, multicystic architecture and enhancing septae. It may herniate into the collecting system. Unfortunately, imaging is unable to differentiate the histological spectrum from completely benign (multilocular renal cyst) to malignant (multilocular cystic Wilms' tumour). Typically, the lesion is non-functioning on isotope imaging. (Partial) nephrectomy is curative and is recommended because of the malignant potential.

Angiomyolipoma

Angiomyolipoma (see section above on TS; Fig. 4-42) is rarely encountered as an isolated phenomenon in children but more usually represents one of the renal manifestations of tuberous sclerosis.

MALIGNANT TUMOURS

Wilms' Tumour

Wilms' tumour (nephroblastoma), first described by German surgeon Dr Max Wilms, accounts for up to 12% of all childhood cancers with a peak incidence at around 3 years of age.[23] It commonly presents with an asymptomatic abdominal mass, or haematuria following minor trauma; pain, fever, or hypertension are unusual. Microscopic haematuria is present in 25% of cases. There is equal gender distribution, with the highest incidence being in the black population in the USA and Africa. Around 10% of Wilms' tumours are bilateral, of which two-thirds are synchronous and one-third metachronous.

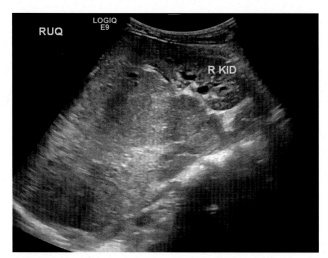

FIGURE 4-49 ■ **Wilms' tumour.** Large heterogeneous mass on US arising from the upper right kidney with inferior displacement of the lower renal pole.

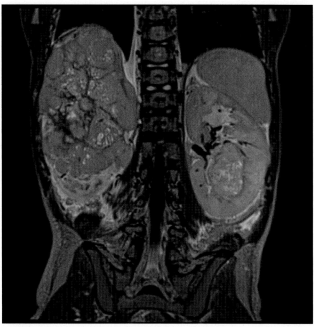

FIGURE 4-50 ■ **Bilateral Wilms' tumour.** MRI is now the gold standard for assessment of bilateral disease. Here, a small mass in the left kidney may be overlooked by the large right-sided mass.

Whereas 75% of Wilms' tumours occur in otherwise normal children, there are associated anomalies in around 15%, including cryptorchidism and horseshoe kidney. Certain syndromes have a predisposition to Wilms' tumour, including aniridia (absence of ophthalmic iris), Beckwith–Wiedemann (macroglossia, exomphalos, gigantism), hemihypertrophy, Denys–Drash (pseudohermaphroditism), Sotos' (cerebral gigantism), Bloom's (immunodeficiency and facial telangiectasia) and Perlman's syndromes. In Denys–Drash syndrome, for example, most but not all patients will develop a Wilms' tumour, the median age at presentation being 18 months, and 20% of cases are bilateral. Routine US screening to detect tumours at an early stage is controversial, because despite 3-monthly US studies large interval tumours may occur (Fig. 4-49).

Wilms' tumours are mostly solid lesions with a fibrous pseudocapsule and variable areas of haemorrhage and necrosis or cysts. The tumour may invade the renal vein and IVC with tumour thrombus extending superiorly, often to the right atrium. Metastases to local para-aortic lymph nodes and haematogenous spread to the lungs, liver or bone are seen.

The (post-surgical) staging of Wilms' tumour according to the North American National Wilms' Tumor Study Group is summarised below:
• Stage I (43%)—tumour confined to the kidney without capsular or vascular invasion.
• Stage II (23%)—tumour extends beyond the renal capsule, vessel infiltration, biopsy performed before resection or intraoperative tumour rupture.
• Stage III (23%)—positive abdominopelvic lymph nodes, peritoneal invasion or residual tumour at surgical margins/unresectable elements.
• Stage IV (10%)—haematogeous spread (typically lung, liver, bone or brain) or metastatic disease outside the abdomen or pelvis.
• Stage V (5%)—bilateral tumours at original diagnosis (Fig. 4-50).

The International Society of Paediatric Oncology (SIOP) in Europe generally uses the same staging system with the exception of masses that have been biopsied regarded as Stage I disease when later excised.

As with all abdominal masses, US must be the first radiological method of assessment. The tumour typically is large, with a mixture of solid hyperechoic masses and relatively cystic areas; often the cystic components predominate. Normal native renal tissue can be difficult to detect and may be stretched at the periphery of the lesion (Fig. 4-49). The renal vein, IVC, liver, contralateral kidney and lymph nodes should be carefully assessed for spread of disease.

US is the best way to assess renal vein and IVC tumour invasion/thrombus, and movement of the mass separate from adjacent organs such as the liver (suggesting a lack of direct invasion).

Contrast-enhanced CT or MRI is necessary for further delineation of tumour extent. Although MRI is the imaging modality of choice, as it can be easily repeated and does not involve ionising radiation, chest CT may still be needed to exclude pulmonary metastases. Wilms' tumours are typically heterogeneous with areas of low attenuation. Calcification is unusual (<10%) and the lesions enhance less than normal renal parenchyma. A 'claw' or 'beak' of normal renal tissue may be seen to stretch around the periphery. Cross-sectional imaging helps to assess the contralateral kidney, and to exclude localised lymphadenopathy, peritoneal or liver lesions, and bone metastases. Small superficial or intrarenal nephroblastomatosis lesions are often not identified, even with high-resolution CT images. Wilms' masses on MRI are generally hypointense on T1, variably hyperintense on

T2, and enhance heterogeneously, and often poorly, with gadolinium contrast administration. Gadolinium is required to assess the contralateral kidney for nephroblastomatosis or another Wilms' mass, and to guide biopsy.

The value of chest CT at initial diagnosis remains controversial, as the commonly used staging systems are based on chest radiographs alone. The presence of (small) metastases on chest CT which are not apparent on chest radiographs is currently of uncertain prognostic significance.

The typical North American treatment practice is initial surgical removal followed by adjuvant chemotherapy as dictated by the staging at surgery. European oncologists favour initial chemotherapy after biopsy confirmation with later resection. It is not surprising, therefore, as tumour response to chemotherapy is often dramatic, that preoperative chemotherapy increases the percentage of Stage I and II patients. The prognosis for Wilms' tumour patients is excellent, irrespective of approach taken. The 4-year overall survival (presumed cure) rate ranges between 86 and 96% for Stages I–III disease, 83% for Stage IV and 70% for Stage V (bilateral) disease. Patients with the diffuse anaplastic Wilms' tumours have a much poorer outcome, with 4-year survival rates of 45% for Stage III and only 7% for Stage IV disease.

Clear Cell Sarcoma of the Kidney

Clear cell sarcoma of the kidney is a rare tumour with marked male preponderance, but perhaps one of the most common with an 'unfavourable' histology (Fig. 4-51). There are no known genetic associations and no reports of bilateral tumours; it does not have an association with nephrogenic rests. The peak age of incidence is similar to that of Wilms' tumour. There are no specific radiological features to help distinguish clear cell sarcoma of the kidney from a Wilms' tumour; the distinction is purely histological. Only 5% of patients present with metastases, but metastases to bone first: hence, the alternative name was 'bone metastasising renal tumour BMRT'. ^{99m}Tc-MDP bone scintigraphy is used for staging. The presence of bone lesions but absence of lung lesions with a presumed Wilms' tumour should raise the possibility of a clear cell sarcoma.

Rhabdoid Tumour of the Kidney

Rhabdoid tumour of the kidney is the most aggressive malignant renal tumour in childhood and accounts for 2% of paediatric renal neoplasms. They are characterised by early metastases and resistance to chemotherapy, with survival rates of only 20–25%. Most cases are diagnosed in the first year of life, but indistinguishable from Wilms' tumour on imaging. Metastases to the lungs, liver and brain have been reported. There is also an association with synchronous primitive neuroectodermal tumours, usually in the posterior fossa. Hypercalcaemia is a recognised finding in rhabdoid tumour but it is not specific, found occasionally in mesoblastic nephroma.

Renal Cell Carcinoma

Renal cell carcinoma (RCC) rarely presents in the first two decades of life, with less than 1% of all cases in children, with mean paediatric presentation age 9 years. Abdominal mass or flank pain is more common than haematuria at presentation. A typically solid intrarenal mass cannot be distinguished from a Wilms' tumour; the age of the patient is a better discriminating factor. Histologically RCCs are characteristically high-grade, high-stage, papillary tumours with numerous ring-like calcifications. Metastases to the lungs, liver, skeleton or brain are present in 20% of patients at diagnosis. A third of RCCs are associated with other diseases, such as tuberous sclerosis, neuroblastoma, Saethre-Chotzen syndrome, chronic renal failure or inherited disorders.

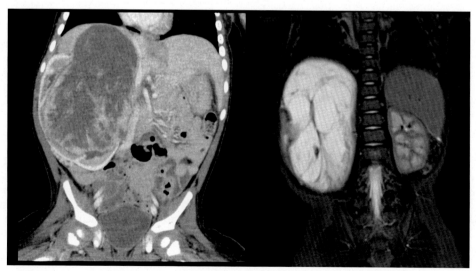

FIGURE 4-51 ■ **Clear cell sarcoma.** Coronal CT and MRI STIR sequences show a large heterogeneous mass arising from the right kidney.

Lymphoma and Leukaemia

Renal involvement with or without retroperitoneal adenopathy is seen in 12% of children with non-Hodgkin's lymphoma, most commonly B-cell Burkitt's lymphoma. Multiple, usually bilateral, nodules are typical, although diffuse renal infiltration may be seen. There is generally widespread disease elsewhere. Renal enlargement on US with altered echo texture is characteristic of both renal lymphoma and leukaemia. The changes in the kidneys can be quite subtle on CT and may be more conspicuous on contrast-enhanced MRI. US is recommended in all children with leukaemia/lymphoma before starting chemotherapy to detect tumour infiltration or calyceal dilatation. Before and during initial chemotherapy, a large fluid load is administered, which, in addition to the excretion of tumour metabolites, may result in renal obstruction or uric acid nephropathy.

Rhabdomyosarcoma

Rhabdomyosarcoma is the most common malignant neoplasm of the pelvis in children. The genitourinary tract is the second most common site of rhabdomyosarcoma in children after head and neck locations. Although the term suggests a mesenchymal tumour derived from striated muscle, the tumour frequently arises in sites lacking striated muscle. The two major cell types are embryonal (commoner, better prognosis) and alveolar. Five per cent are a botryoid subtype of embryonal rhabdomyosarcoma, characterised macroscopically by the presence of grape-like polypoid masses which classically occur in the vagina, rarely metastasise and have a good prognosis.

In general, pelvic tumours may be very large at presentation and present as abdominal masses. Prostate tumours may cause urinary obstruction and manifest with marked bladder distension or acute retention. The mass is typically solid but heterogeneous on US, with variable vascularity. Regional lymph nodes must be evaluated.

MRI is recommended in general for all pelvic tumours. Coronal or sagittal T1-weighted imaging without contrast can often be the most useful sequences for follow-up. Staging includes chest CT (10% of rhabdomyosarcomas have pulmonary metastases) and ^{99m}Tc-MDP skeletal scintigraphy.

Rhabdomyosarcomas in favourable sites such as the vagina have up to 94% 3-year survival (Fig. 4-52). Prostatic tumours commonly infiltrate locally into the perivesical tissues and bladder base, and have a worse prognosis with a 3-year survival of approximately 70%. The goal of therapy for bladder or bladder/prostate tumours (as it is frequently very difficult to tell the exact organ of origin) is survival with an intact bladder.

INFLAMMATORY DISEASES OF THE SCROTUM

The more common causes of acute pain and/or swelling in the scrotum include testicular torsion, torsion of the testicular appendages, epididymitis with or without orchitis, trauma, acute hydrocele, incarcerated hernia and

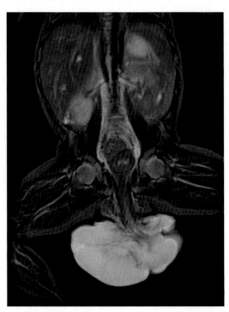

FIGURE 4-52 ■ **Rhabdomyosarcoma.** Coronal MRI shows an exophytic vaginal mass, subsequently found to be a vaginal rhabdomyosarcoma.

acute scrotal oedema. US is the imaging modality of choice, although Doppler examination in the very young child may be limited as even modern high-resolution linear array transducers may be not reliably detect very slow flow in small testes.

Testicular torsion is a surgical emergency; if suspected clinically, the scrotum should be explored without delay. Torsion shows ipsilateral increased echogenicity with absence of intratesticular flow (always perform spectral analysis and compare to contralateral side—any asymmetry is suspicious, e.g. for partial or intermittent torsion), occasionally with surrounding fluid. Following the vessels into the inguinal canal may reveal a corkscrew-like appearance, proving torsion. The main differential is epididymitis or orchitis, where there is normal or increased testicular colour flow. The other entity is torsion of testicular appendices, where the testis is normal with a swollen appendix, with scrotal fluid. Acute scrotal oedema presents clinically with abrupt onset of a swollen, painful, red scrotal sac, with normal underlying structures on US. In children with recurrent epididymitis, always consider an associated urinary tract anomaly.

SCROTAL MASSES

Intratesticular benign and malignant tumours are relatively common neoplasms in children. Primary testicular neoplasms include germ cell tumours (teratomas, most common and often with calcification), endodermal sinus tumour and embryonal carcinoma. The testes are also secondary sites of disease in children with leukaemia, lymphoma and neuroblastoma, although much less frequently than in adults.

Paratesticular rhabdomyosarcoma includes tumours arising in the spermatic cord, testis, epididymis and penis.

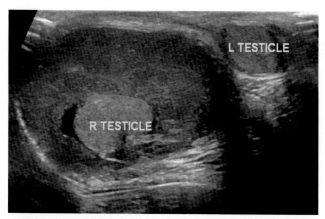

FIGURE 4-53 ■ **Paratesticular rhabdomyosarcoma.** US confirms a large homogeneous mass surrounding the right testis, which is lying centrally and appears normal otherwise.

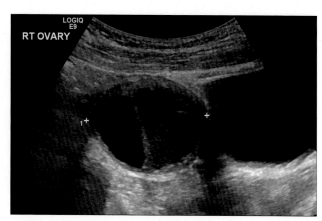

FIGURE 4-55 ■ **Haemorrhagic ovarian cyst.** The medial aspect of the cyst demonstrates a blood/fluid level on US.

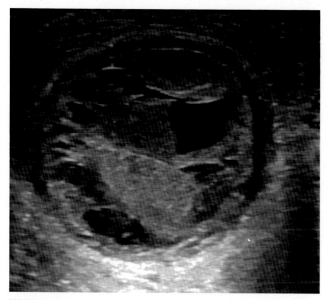

FIGURE 4-54 ■ **Paratesticular haematoma.** Following localised trauma during a football match, this US confirms a multiseptated hypoechoic mass surrounding a testis with patchy appearances. This patient made a full recover with integrity of vascular supply to the testis.

US is the first-line examination to evaluate scrotal disease (Figs. 4-53 and 4-54). A heterogeneous appearance within the testis with increased flow on Doppler may mimic infection, but may have presented with a palpable mass rather than infection. Cross-sectional imaging (CT or MRI) is essential to assess for lymphatic spread to the para-aortic nodes, as retroperitoneal lymph node dissection may be necessary. Paratesticular rhabdomyosarcoma has a good prognosis in young children, with a >90% 5-year survival.

OVARIAN MASSES

Ovarian Cysts

Simple ovarian cysts are large follicles and represent the majority of ovarian masses. In the neonate they usually present as abdominal masses, and the differential may include mesenteric cysts, intestinal duplication and urachal cysts. In pubertal girls, ovarian cysts result from continuous growth of a follicle after failed ovulation, or when it does not involute after ovulation. Most follicular cysts are 3–10 cm in size and contain clear fluid. Corpus luteal cysts contain serous or haemorrhagic fluid, and, as with follicular cysts, usually involute spontaneously. Most ovarian cysts are asymptomatic, but when complications such as haemorrhage (Fig. 4-55), torsion, or rupture occur, patients present with acute abdominal pain, nausea, vomiting and leucocytosis. Torsion of the ovaries and Fallopian tubes results from partial or complete rotation of the ovary on its vascular pedicle. US can demonstrate a fluid–debris level or septa, which can indicate haemorrhage or infarction. A more specific sign of torsion is the presence of multiple follicles in the cortical portion of a unilaterally enlarged and hyperechoic ovary. As there is dual blood supply to the ovary, a lack of Doppler signal is a much less reliable sign than in testicular torsion. Physiological or pathological cysts may be found coincidentally in patients with lower abdominal or pelvic pain. Repeating the US study at a different phase of the menstrual cycle is useful, and may detect more adult-type pathology such as endometriosis.

Ovarian Tumours

Ovarian neoplasms account for 10% of all childhood tumours, and 10–30% of these are malignant, commonly malignant germ cell tumours. Tumours include dysgerminoma, immature teratoma, embryonal carcinoma, endodermal sinus tumour and choriocarcinoma. The differentiation between tumour and ovarian torsion may be difficult, requiring MRI and serum markers. Tumours can occur at any age, but typically present as abdominal pain or mass after puberty. Mature teratomas and dermoid cysts account for two-thirds of paediatric ovarian tumours and have a wide spectrum of imaging characteristics (Fig. 4-56). Usually, US shows a low reflectivity mass with an echogenic mural nodule, with fat–fluid levels and calcification. Cystadenomas represent 20% of ovarian tumours in children and are of epithelial origin; they are

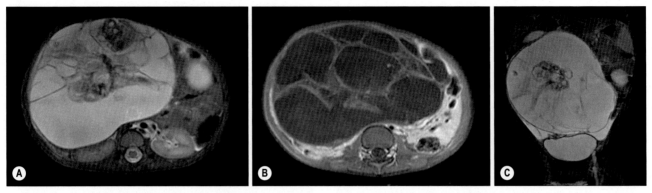

FIGURE 4-56 ■ **Ovarian teratoma.** (A) Axial STIR, (B) axial contrast-enhanced and (C) coronal STIR MRI show a multiseptated mass arising from the pelvis with peripheral enhancement.

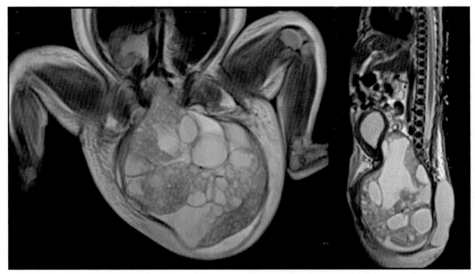

FIGURE 4-57 ■ **Sacrococcygeal teratoma.** Coronal and sagittal MRI show the large presacral mass which protrudes outside the perineum. These masses are sometimes large enough to obstruct vaginal delivery of the baby. Normal appearances to the spinal cord.

large tumours, with loculations. Imaging cannot differentiate between malignant and benign cystadenomas. Leukaemia, lymphoma and neuroblastoma are among the primary tumours that metastasise to the ovaries in children.

PRESACRAL MASSES

Sacrococcygeal germ cell teratomas are the most common presacral tumour and the most common solid tumour in neonates. These lesions occur more frequently in girls, are mostly non-familial, and are classified according to the degree of intrapelvic or extrapelvic involvement.[24] Sacrococcygeal teratomas have solid components, and are attached to the sacrum, with the internal component best depicted on sagittal MRI sequences (Fig. 4-57), allowing differentiation from an anterior sacral meningocele. Benign teratomas are usually cystic, with calcification and fat. Malignant teratomas are predominantly solid and may invade adjacent structures. All sacrococcygeal teratomas are removed due to the potential for malignant

transformation. Other presacral lesions include anterior myelomeningocele and neuroenteric cyst, and forms of spinal dysraphism associated with a sacral defect. Neuroblastoma, ganglioneuroma and lymphoma in the pelvis are less common.

HYPERTENSION

Renovascular hypertension is rare in children. However, unlike in adults, renovascular is more common than idiopathic hypertension: renal disease is the cause of hypertension in over 90% of children after 1 year of age. The more severe the hypertension and the younger the child, the more likely it is to be secondary hypertension. Any abnormal kidney may produce renin and so generate hypertension. Renal scarring and glomerular disease are the most common causes, and occasionally PUJ obstruction, neuroblastoma, or Wilms' tumours present with hypertension.

Renovascular disease accounts for approximately 10% of cases, with fibromuscular dysplasia being the most common cause. Other associations are neurofibromatosis, idiopathic hypercalcaemia of infancy, an arteritic illness or middle aortic syndrome. Phaeochromocytomas, albeit uncommon in childhood, are seen and are often both multiple and extra-adrenal in origin. Essential hypertension is usually encountered in milder cases, often with a positive family history of hypertension.

Optimal imaging and managing children with suspected renovascular hypertension remains controversial (Fig. 4-58).[12] Angiography with vascular intervention offers the highest diagnostic accuracy, with the option of simultaneous treatment. MRA is feasible in older children and is relatively sensitive for significant stenoses of the main renal artery, but less sensitive in smaller children and for the more peripheral interlobar and arcuate arteries due to the lower temporal and spatial resolution. The use of non-invasive CT angiography (CTA) is particularly controversial.

US may demonstrate a small kidney, a severely scarred kidney, significant HN, and both renal and most adrenal tumours. Doppler US of the aorta and intrarenal arteries may reveal aortic narrowing or renal artery stenosis. However, Doppler findings and flow parameters have not been widely or adequately evaluated for diagnostic

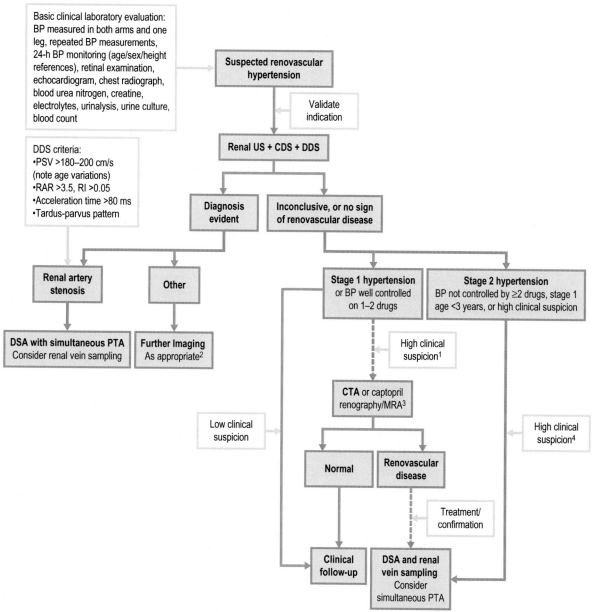

FIGURE 4-58 ■ **ESPR imaging algorithm for suspected renovascular hypertension.** BP = blood pressure, CDS = colour Doppler sonography, CTA = computed tomography angiography, DDS = spectral duplex Doppler, DSA = digital subtraction angiography, PSV = peak systolic velocity, RAR = renal-aortic ratio, δ-RI = resistive index difference. (Adapted from Riccabona M, Lobo M L, Papadopoulou F, et al 2011 ESPR uroradiology task force and ESUR paediatric working group: imaging recommendations in paediatric uroradiology, part IV: Minutes of the ESPR uroradiology task force mini-symposium on imaging in childhood renal hypertension and imaging of renal trauma in children. Pediatr Radiol 41(7):939–944.[12])

performance in childhood renal arterial stenosis (RAS). It is unclear whether adult criteria (e.g. a peak systolic velocity >180–200 cm/s) are applicable to children. Only the typical distal pulsus tardus and parvus waveforms, and the direct visualisation of the stenosis on CDS (turbulent flow at increased velocity causing aliasing) are reliable predictors for childhood RAS. The current recommendation, although not evidence based, is that children with a high pre-test probability of renovascular disease and positive Doppler US findings should be referred for catheter angiography with renal vein sampling, potentially with simultaneous endovascular treatment (Fig. 4-59).[25] Further non-invasive imaging by CTA or MRA currently has no significant benefit in these children as it cannot demonstrate intrarenal vasculature stenoses adequately, but this may improve in the future.

TRAUMA

Children have a higher risk of renal damage from trauma than adults following blunt abdominal trauma. This is due to increased organ mobility and less body fat protection of the kidneys. Haematuria is common, but the degree of haematuria does not necessarily correlate with the presence or severity of possible renal injury; therefore, every child with haematuria after abdominal trauma should undergo renal imaging.

CT is considered the imaging modality of choice in severe abdominal trauma; its use at first-line evaluation is unequivocally accepted in haemodynamically stable children, especially in suspected spinal or pelvic trauma, and suspected rupture of the urinary bladder. CT is the safest, most reliable and most widely available method to exclude significant urinary tract injuries. However, CT encompasses transporting an injured patient to the scanner, a significant radiation dose and the need for intravenous iodinated contrast medium. Some authors feel that a comprehensive US examination, including power, colour and spectral Doppler analysis, may be sufficient to reliably exclude major renal injury when performed by an experienced examiner. US will undoubtedly miss some subtle lesions that will be identified by CT, although the clinical significance of this is limited. US is therefore the imaging modality of choice in minor or moderate paediatric trauma, and CT should be considered where the US is limited, inconclusive, discordant with worsening clinical findings, or warrants further investigation. There is no role for following up renal lesions or severe urinary tract trauma with CT, even if initially evaluated by CT. US should be used, and MRI used wherever possible, if further cross-sectional imaging is needed (Fig. 4-60).[12]

RENAL TRANSPLANTATION

In the UK in 2009 the prevalence of patients (both adult and child) receiving renal replacement therapy was 794 per million population. It is well recognised that mortality is much higher in dialysed children than in those who have received a transplant, and that results are better in those transplanted before dialysis. Unlike adults, the majority of children with chronic renal failure are suitable candidates for renal transplantation. Live donation is increasingly being used in the paediatric population, with better outcomes than with cadaveric transplants. ABO-incompatible kidney transplantation is now possible following desensitisation by using plasmapheresis and immunoabsorption. The three most common causes of end-stage renal disease leading to transplantation are renal dysplasia, glomerular disease and pyelonephritis.

Pre-Transplantation

Ultrasound of the kidneys and abdominal vessels is essential in prerenal transplantation assessment. US of the abdominal, pelvic and femoral vessels is all that may be needed if the child has not had previous venous access; otherwise an MR venogram and MR angiogram are warranted. Intravenous gadolinium is contraindicated in patients with renal failure, and therefore non-enhanced 'time of flight' or 'fresh blood techniques' are used. Patients needing to undergo haemodialysis may require arm venography or vascular US pre-fistula formation. Follow-up US for fistula complications such as stenosis or thrombus in the fistula circuit may be required. Donor imaging of adult patients is not covered in this chapter.

Post-Transplantation

Following transplantation, an initial US scan in theatre or in the recovery area is advised, particularly using CDS to assess renal perfusion. This may be particularly helpful if there were several renal arteries to anastomose or if any renal vessels were sacrificed (Fig. 4-61). Collections may also be assessed (Fig. 4-62). Regular follow-up US are performed, or when complications such as haemorrhage following biopsy may occur (Fig. 4-63).

If the child has an unfavourable bladder (unused, or thick walled and non-compliant), the chance of pyelonephritis is high, with additional VUR up the short transplant ureter. An early ^{99m}Tc-DMSA scan is performed at 4–6 weeks following surgery to give baseline imaging in case scarring develops. ^{99m}Tc-DTPA or ^{99m}Tc-MAG3 studies are no longer routinely used in post-transplant imaging unless obstruction or urinary leak is suspected. As no single technique allows specific diagnosis of graft dysfunction, often a direct biopsy is required. The role of MRI in post-transplant assessment is being developed.

Complications of immunosuppressive therapy after transplant include post-transplant lymphoproliferative disorder. A diagnosis of PTLD is made by having a high index of suspicion in the appropriate clinical setting; histopathological evidence of lymphoproliferation on tissue biopsy; and the presence of EBV DNA, RNA or protein in tissue. Most cases of PTLD are observed in the first post-transplant year. The more intense the immunosuppression used, the higher the incidence of PTLD and the earlier it occurs. Successful treatment of PTLD involves reduction or withdrawal of immunosuppression, which

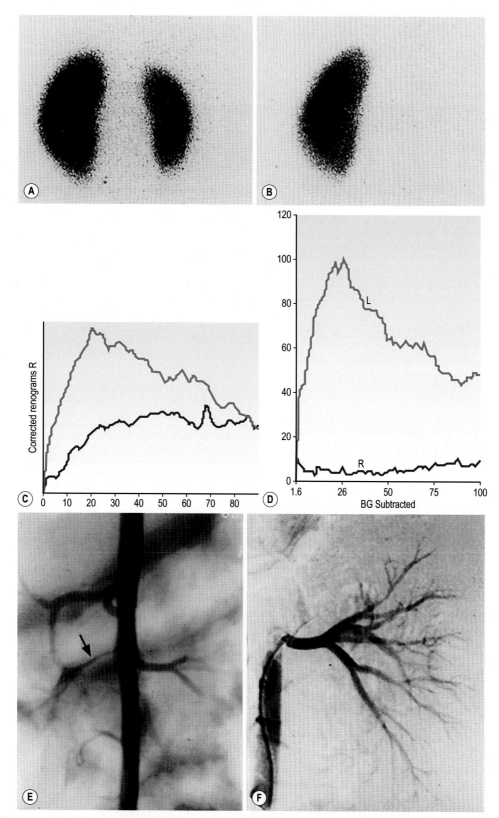

FIGURE 4-59 ■ **Hypertension.** A 7-year-old boy presented with left facial nerve palsy, a well-recognised presenting feature of hypertension in paediatrics. (A) A ^{99m}Tc-DMSA scintigram at outset shows a smaller unscarred right kidney contributing only 31% to overall function. US was unremarkable. (B) Repeat ^{99m}Tc-DMSA scintigraphy 1 month later following oral captopril ingestion shows absent function in the right kidney while the left kidney remains normal. (C) The ^{99m}Tc-DTPA renogram curves after background subtraction show a normal left kidney (L); the right kidney (R) shows a decreased uptake of radionuclide with a poor renogram. (D) Following oral captopril the ^{99m}Tc-DTPA renal curves reveal no change on the left, and a very abnormal right curve. (E) Free-flush aortic angiogram. The aorta is normal; the right renal artery shows narrowing from its origin all the way to the renal hilum (arrow). The left renal artery looks normal apart from narrowing at the origin of the artery inferiorly. (F) Selective left renal arteriogram reveals a normal intra-arterial supply within the left kidney.

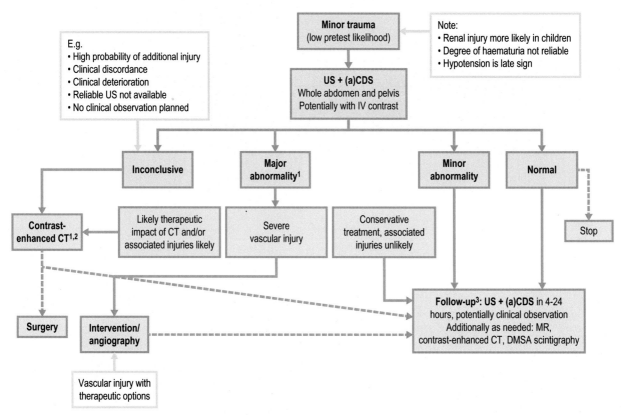

FIGURE 4-60 ■ **Trauma.** ESPR imaging algorithm for mild paediatric urinary tract trauma. DMSA = Dimercaptosuccinic acid static renal scintigraphy, CT = computed tomography, MRI = magnetic resonance imaging, US = ultrasound. (Adapted from Riccabona M, Lobo M L, Papadopoulou F, et al 2011 ESPR uroradiology task force and ESUR paediatric working group: imaging recommendations in paediatric uroradiology, part IV: Minutes of the ESPR uroradiology task force mini-symposium on imaging in childhood renal hypertension and imaging of renal trauma in children. Pediatr Radiol 41(7):939–944.[12])

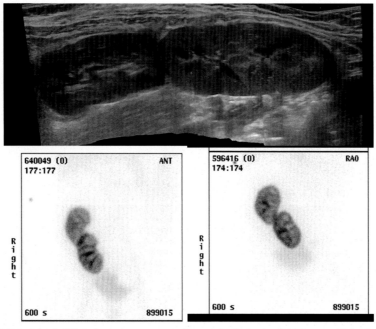

FIGURE 4-61 ■ **En bloc renal transplant.** Often from very young donors, both (paired) kidneys will be transplanted in the recipient. Normal appearances on US and DMSA.

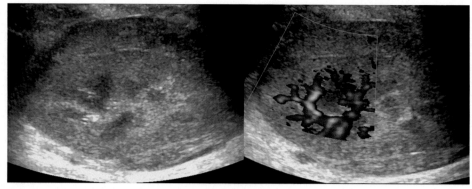

FIGURE 4-62 ■ There is a non-vascular subcapsular haematoma which may be easily overlooked, but can cause significant compression of the kidney.

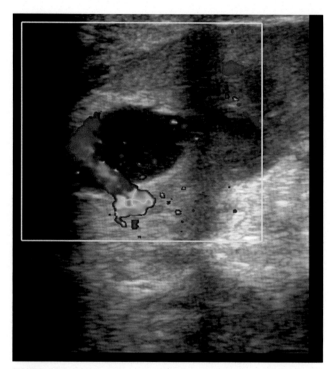

FIGURE 4-63 ■ **Arteriovenous fistula.** US shows high-flow AV fistula following biopsy of a renal transplant for suspected rejection.

inherently carries the risk of allograft dysfunction or loss. US imaging is useful in the search for lymphadenopathy or solid organ infiltration, and cross-sectional imaging with CT or MRI may be needed to plan the biopsy and to stage the lymphoproliferative disease.

REFERENCES

1. Riccabona M, Avni FE, Blickman JG, et al. Imaging recommendations in paediatric uroradiology: minutes of the ESPR workgroup session on urinary tract infection, fetal hydronephrosis, urinary tract ultrasonography and voiding cystourethrography, Barcelona, Spain, June 2007. Pediatr Radiol 2008;38(2):138–45.
2. Daneman A, Navarro OM, Somers GR, et al. Renal pyramids: focused sonography of normal and pathologic processes. Radiographics 2010;30(5):1287–307.
3. Kiechl-Kohlendorfer U, Geley TE, Unsinn KM, Gassner I. Diagnosing neonatal female genital anomalies using saline-enhanced sonography. Am J Roentgenol 2001;177(5):1041–4.
4. Riccabona M. Potential role of 3DUS in infants and children. Pediatr Radiol 2011;41(S1):S228–37.
5. Agrawalla S, Pearce R, Goodman TR. How to perform the perfect voiding cystourethrogram. Pediatr Radiol 2004;34:114–19.
6. Riccabona M. Imaging if the neonatal genito-urinary tract. Eur J Radiol 2006;60:187–98.
7. Riccabona M. Functional disorders of the lower urinary tract in childhood: an update. Pediatr Radiol 2012;42(Suppl. 3):S403–578.
8. Darge K, Riedmiller H. Current status of vesicoureteral reflux diagnosis. World J Urol 2004;22(2):88–95.
9. Gordon I, Colarinha P, Fettich J, et al; Paediatric Committee of the European Association of Nuclear Medicine. Guidelines for indirect radionuclide cystography. Eur J Nucl Med 2001;28(3):BP16–20.
10. Gordon I, Piepsz A, Sixt R; Auspices of Paediatric Committee of European Association of Nuclear Medicine. Guidelines for standard and diuretic renogram in children. Eur J Nucl Med Mol Imaging 2011;38(6):1175–88.
11. Riccabona M, Avni FE, Dacher JN, et al; ESPR uroradiology task force and ESUR paediatric working group. ESPR uroradiology task force and ESUR paediatric working group: imaging and procedural recommendations in paediatric uroradiology, part III. Minutes of the ESPR uroradiology task force minisymposium on intravenous urography, uro-CT and MR-urography in childhood. Pediatr Radiol 2010;40(7):1315–20.
12. Riccabona M, Lobo ML, Papadopoulou F, et al. ESPR uroradiology task force and ESUR paediatric working group: imaging recommendations in paediatric uroradiology, part IV: Minutes of the ESPR uroradiology task force mini-symposium on imaging in childhood renal hypertension and imaging of renal trauma in children. Pediatr Radiol 2011;41(7):939–44.
13. Grattan-Smith JD, Little SB, Jones RA. MR urography in children: how we do it. Pediatr Radiol 2009;28(Suppl. 1):S3–17.
14. Barnacle AM, Roebuck DJ, Racadio JM. Nephro-urology interventions in children. Tech Vasc Interv Radiol 2010;13(4):229–37.
15. Riccabona M, Willi U. Renal biopsy in children. Pediatr Radiol 2012;42(S3):S471.
16. Fernbach SK, Maizels M, Conway JJ. Ultrasound grading of hydronephrosis: introduction to the system used by the Society for Fetal Urology. Pediatr Radiol 1993;23:478–80.
17. Riccabona M, Avni FE, Blickman JG, et al; Members of the ESUR paediatric recommendation work group and ESPR paediatric uroradiology work group. Imaging recommendations in paediatric uroradiology, part II: urolithiasis and haematuria in children, paediatric obstructive uropathy, and postnatal work-up of fetally diagnosed high grade hydronephrosis. Minutes of a mini-symposium at the ESPR annual meeting, Edinburgh, June. Pediatr Radiol 2009;39(8):891–8.
18. Moorthy I, Easty M, McHugh K, et al. The presence of vesicoureteric reflux does not identify a population at risk for renal scarring following a first urinary tract infection. Arch Dis Child 2005;90:733–6.
19. National Institute for Clinical Evidence. Urinary tract infection: diagnosis, treatment and long term management of urinary tract infection in children. London: Department of Health; 2007.

20. Avni FE, Garel C, Cassart M, et al. Imaging and classification of congenital cystic renal diseases. Am J Roentgenol 2012;198(5): 1004–13.
21. Riccabona M, Avni F, Damasio B, et al. ESPR Uroradiology Task Force / ESUR Paediatric Working Group—Imaging recommendations in Paediatric Uroradiology, Part V: Childhood cystic kidney disease, childhood renal transplantation, and contrast-enhanced ultrasound in children. Pediatr Radiol 2012;42:1275–83.
22. Beckwith JB, Kiviat NB, Bonadio JF. Nephrogenic rests, nephroblastomatosis, and the pathogenesis of Wilms' tumor. Pediatr Pathol 1990;10:1–36.

23. Strouse PJ. Pediatric renal neoplasms. Radiol Clin North Am 1996;34:1081–100.
24. Kocaoglu M, Frush DP. Pediatric presacral masses. Radiographics 2006;26(3):833–57.
25. Deal JE, Snell MF, Barratt TM, et al. Renovascular disease in childhood. J Pediatr 1992;121:378–84.

CHAPTER 5

Skeletal Radiology in Children: Non-traumatic and Non-malignant

Amaka C. Offiah

CHAPTER OUTLINE

CONSTITUTIONAL DISORDERS OF BONE

LOCALISED DISORDERS OF THE SKELETON

NEUROCUTANEOUS SYNDROMES

NON-INFLAMMATORY DISORDERS

METABOLIC AND ENDOCRINE DISORDERS

TOXIC DISORDERS

HAEMOGLOBINOPATHIES

INFECTION OF THE BONES AND JOINTS

CONSITUTIONAL DISORDERS OF BONE

Nomenclature

The constitutional disorders of bone include osteochondrodysplasias and dysostoses.

Osteochondrodysplasias consist of dysplasias (abnormalities of bone and/or cartilage growth) and osteodystrophies (abnormalities of bone and/or cartilage texture). Abnormalities in the osteochondrodysplasias are intrinsic to bone and cartilage,[1] and because of gene expression will continue to evolve throughout the life span of the individual.

Dysostoses occur as a result of altered blastogenesis in the first 6 weeks of intrauterine life. In contrast to the osteochondrodysplasias, the phenotype is fixed, and previously normal bones will remain so. However, more than one bone may be involved.

Inevitably there is some overlap and, from the radiological point of view, when establishing a diagnosis it is useful to consider them together. Most are genetically determined but some malformation syndromes are the result of environmental effects. In addition to making a diagnosis, radiologists are required to identify complications of the condition itself and complications of medical (see Fig. 5-1) and/or surgical intervention.

The 2011 international nosology and classification of genetic skeletal disorders[1] includes 456 different conditions subdivided into 40 groups defined by molecular, biochemical and/or radiographic findings. Of these 456 conditions, 316 are associated with one or more of 226 different genes. Major conditions are summarised in Table 5-1.

While the international classification lists only those conditions with a proven genetic basis, there are currently over 2000 malformation syndromes, many of which are associated with skeletal abnormalities. In this chapter, only an approach to diagnosis can be given and only the more common conditions are used as illustrative examples.

Prevalence

Although individually rare, collectively malformation syndromes and skeletal dysplasias form a large group, which is expensive in both medical resources and human care and commitment. The prevalence of affected patients is difficult to ascertain. As a rough estimate, approximately 1% of live births have clinically apparent skeletal abnormalities. This figure does not take into account the large numbers of spontaneous abortions or elective terminations, many of which have significant skeletal abnormalities. Nor does it include those dysplasias presenting only in childhood, or those relatively common conditions that may never present for diagnosis because they are mild, e.g. hypochondroplasia and dyschondrosteosis, both of which merge with normality in individual cases. At orthopaedic skeletal dysplasia clinics in England and Scotland, approximately 10,000 patients are seen; 6000 of whom will require repeated hospitalisation for surgical procedures and some will require more prolonged admissions.

Diagnosis

Arriving at an accurate diagnosis requires a multidisciplinary approach with combined clinical, paediatric, genetic, biochemical, radiological and pathological (molecular, cellular and histopathological) input.

Rapid advances are being made in the field of gene mapping, with many conditions being localised to abnormalities at specific loci on individual chromosomes. Identification of genetic mutations allows 'families' of conditions to be recognised, with some common clinical and radiological features. One example of this is the recently described TRPV4 group of disorders, consisting of autosomal dominant brachyolmia, spondylometaphyseal dysplasia-type Kozlowski and metatropic dysplasia. Although classification based on genetic mutations is of value in determining an underlying causative defect, this diagnostic approach does not necessarily arrive at a precise clinical diagnosis, with prediction of natural history, morbidity and mortality, and in individual cases may be conflicting and indeterminate.

The international classification of skeletal dysplasias recognises the radiological features as being paramount in accurate diagnosis. Whilst clinical features, such as cleft palate, deafness and myopia, are of diagnostic

Text continued on p. 135

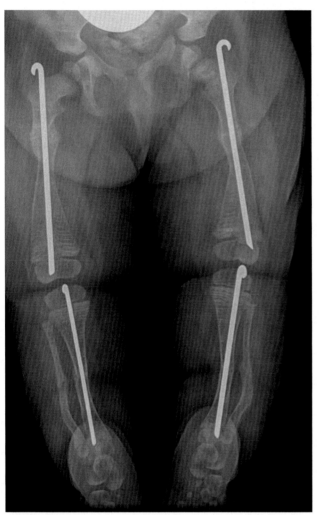

FIGURE 5-1 ■ **Osteogenesis imperfecta.** Bilateral femoral and tibial intramedullary nails. Note multiple bisphosphonate lines (see also Fig. 5-17F).

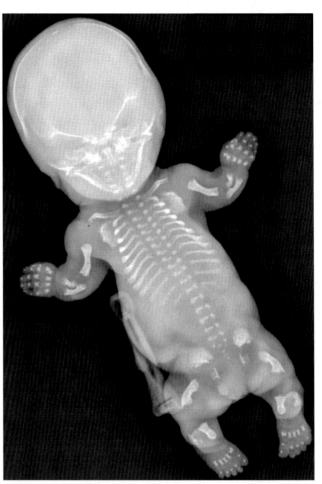

FIGURE 5-2 ■ **Thanatophoric dysplasia type 1.** Micromelia with bowed femora and metaphyseal spurs. Short ribs with a small thorax. Platyspondyly. Trident acetabula.

TABLE 5-1   Clinical and Radiographic Features of Selected Osteochondrodysplasias and Dysostoses

	Clinical Features	Radiological Features
Group 1 (FGFR3 Chondrodysplasia Group)		
Thanatophoric dysplasia (Fig. 5-2)	Most common lethal neonatal skeletal dysplasia Short markedly curved limbs Respiratory distress, small thoracic cage Inheritance: Sporadic AD mutation Gene: *FGFR3*	Short ribs with wide costochondral junctions Severe platyspondyly 'Trident acetabula': horizontal roofs with medial spikes Marked shortness and bowing of the long bones ('telephone receiver femora') Irregular metaphyses Short broad tubular bones of the hands and feet Small scapulae Type 1—Normal skull Type 2—'Clover leaf' skull

TABLE 5-1   **Clinical and Radiographic Features of Selected Osteochondrodysplasias and Dysostoses (Continued)**

	Clinical Features	Radiological Features
Achondroplasia (Fig. 5-3)	Common Short limbs, short trunk Narrow thorax with respiratory distress in infancy Bowed legs Prominent forehead with depressed nasal bridge Hydrocephalus and brainstem and spinal cord compression Inheritance: AD Gene: *FGFR3*	'Bullet-shaped' vertebral bodies Decrease of the interpedicular distance of lumbar spine caudally (in older child and adult) Short vertebral pedicles Posterior vertebral body scalloping (in older child and adult) Squared iliac wings with small sciatic notch Flat acetabular roofs Short ribs Short wide tubular bones Relative overgrowth of fibula Large skull vault, relatively short base Small foramen magnum Dilatation of lateral cerebral ventricles V-shaped notches In growth plates ('chevron deformity') 'Trident' hands
Hypochondroplasia	Variable short stature Prominent forehead Inheritance: AD Gene: *FGFR3*	Absence of normal widening of the interpedicular distance of the lumbar spine caudally Short, relatively broad long bones Elongation of the distal fibula and of the ulnar styloid process Variable brachydactyly
Group 2 (Type 2 Collagen Group)		
Spondyloepiphyseal dysplasia congenita (Fig. 5-4)	Short stature with short trunk at birth Cleft palate Myopia Maxillary hypoplasia Thoracic kyphosis and lumbar lordosis Barrel-shaped chest Inheritance: AD Gene: *COL2A1*	Oval, 'pear-shaped' vertebral bodies Irregular-sized vertebral bodies with L5 smaller than L1 in infancy, 'anisospondyly' Odontoid hypoplasia and cervical spine instability Short long bones Absent ossification of epiphyses of knees, shoulders, talus and calcaneus at birth Pubic and ischial hypoplasia at birth Severe coxa vara developing in early childhood Horizontal acetabulum Relatively normal hands
Group 8 (TRPV4 Group)		
Metatropic dysplasia (Fig. 5-5)	Short limbs Relatively narrow chest Small appendage in coccygeal region ('tail') Progressive kyphoscoliosis Progressive change from relatively short limbs to relatively short trunk (hence name, 'metatropic') Inheritance: AD Gene: *TRPV4*	Short long bones with marked metaphyseal widening ('dumb-bell') Platyspondyly with relatively wide intervertebral disc spaces Flat acetabular roofs Short iliac bones Short ribs with anterior widening Progressive kyphoscoliosis Hypoplastic odontoid peg
Group 9 (Short Rib Dysplasias (with or without Polydactyly) Group)		
Ellis–van Creveld (Fig. 5-6)	Short stature Short limbs, more marked distally Polydactyly Hypoplasia of the nails and teeth Ectodermal dysplasia with sparse hair Congenital cardiac defects (ASD, single atrium) Fusion of upper lip and gum Inheritance: AR Gene: *EVC1, EVC2*	Short ribs (in infancy) Short iliac wings; horizontal 'trident' acetabula (pelvis becomes more normal in childhood) Premature ossification of proximal femoral epiphyses Laterally sloping proximal tibial and humeral epiphyses Polysyndactyly; carpal fusions (90% cases) Cone-shaped epiphyses of middle phalanges Exostosis of upper medial tibial shaft
Asphyxiating thoracic dysplasia—Jeune (Fig. 5-7)	Often lethal Respiratory problems with long narrow thorax Short hands and feet Nephronophthisis in later life in survivors Inheritance: AR Gene: *IFT80, DYNC2H1*	Small thorax with short ribs, horizontally orientated Widened costochondral junctions High clavicles Short iliac bones Trident acetabula Premature ossification of proximal femoral epiphyses Cone-shaped epiphyses of phalanges Polydactyly (10% cases)

Continued on following page

TABLE 5-1   Clinical and Radiographic Features of Selected Osteochondrodysplasias and Dysostoses (Continued)

	Clinical Features	Radiological Features
Group 10 (Multiple Epiphyseal Dysplasia and Pseudoachondroplasia Group)		
Pseudoachondroplasia (Fig. 5-8)	Short limbs with normal head and face Accentuated lumbar lordosis Genu valgum or varum Joint hypermobility <u>Inheritance</u>: AD <u>Gene</u>: *COMP*	Platyspondyly with 'tongue-like' anterior protrusion of the vertebral bodies Biconvex upper and lower vertebral end plates Atlantoaxial dislocation Small proximal femoral epiphyses Short iliac bones Wide triradiate cartilage Irregular acetabulum Small pubis and ischium Pointed bases of the metacarpals Short tubular bones with expanded, markedly irregular metaphyses Small irregular epiphyses with delayed bone age Wide costovertebral joints Relatively long distal fibula
Multiple epiphyseal dysplasia (Fig. 5-9)	Joint stiffness ± limp Early osteoarthritis Mild limb shortening <u>Inheritance</u>: AD <u>Gene</u>: *COMP, MATN3, COL11, COL9A1, COL9A2, COL9A3*	Delayed ossification and irregularity of the epiphyses of the tubular bones Delayed bone age of carpus and tarsus Short tubular bones of the hands and feet Only mild irregularity of the vertebral bodies Mild acetabular hypoplasia Early osteoarthritis *Multilayered patella only seen in autosomal recessive MED due to mutations in the *DTDST* gene (Group 4, sulphation disorders)
Group 11 (Metaphyseal Dysplasias)		
Metaphyseal chondrodysplasia type Schmid (Fig. 5-10)	Short limbs, short stature presenting in early childhood Waddling gait Genu varum <u>Inheritance</u>: AD <u>Gene</u>: *COL10A1*	Metaphyseal flaring Irregular widened growth plates, most marked at hips Increased density and irregularity of metaphyses, especially of hips and knees Large proximal femoral epiphyses Coxa vara; femoral bowing Anterior cupping of ribs Normal spine
Group 18 (Bent Bone Dysplasias)		
Campomelic dysplasia (Fig. 5-11)	*Neonatal* Respiratory distress Cleft palate Prenatal onset of bowed lower limbs Pretibial dimpling *Survivors* Short stature Learning difficulties Recurrent respiratory infections Kyphoscoliosis <u>Inheritance</u>: AD (sex reversal) <u>Gene</u>: *SOX9*	11 pairs of ribs Hypoplastic scapulae Angulation of femora (junction of proximal third and distal two-thirds) Angulation of tibiae (junction of proximal two-thirds and distal third) Short fibulae Progressive kyphoscoliosis Dislocated hips Deficient ossification of the ischium and pubis Hypoplastic patellae
Group 21 (Chondrodysplasia (CDP) Group)		
Chondrodysplasia punctata (Fig. 5-12)	Flat nasal bridge, high arched palate Cutaneous lesions, e.g. ichthyosis Asymmetrical or symmetrical shortening of long bones Joint contractures Cataracts <u>Inheritance</u>: XLD, XLR, AR, AD <u>Gene</u>: XLD—*EPP, NHDSL* XLR—*ARSE* AR—*LBR, AGPS, DHPAT, PEX2* AD—Unknown (also some AR types)	Stippled calcification in cartilage, particularly around joints and in laryngeal and tracheal cartilages. Disappears later on in life Shortening, symmetrical or asymmetrical of the long bones Short digits in some types Coronal cleft vertebral bodies Punctate calcification is also seen in some chromosomal disorders, fetal alcohol syndrome, mucolipidoses (Fig. 5-20), neonates of mothers with autoimmune disorders, Pacman dysplasia, warfarin embryopathy and Zellweger syndrome

TABLE 5-1   **Clinical and Radiographic Features of Selected Osteochondrodysplasias and Dysostoses (Continued)**

	Clinical Features	Radiological Features
Group 22 (Neonatal Osteosclerotic Dysplasias)		
Caffey disease (infantile cortical hyperostosis)	Usually present in the first 5 months of life Hyperirritability Soft-tissue swelling <u>Inheritance:</u> AD, AR <u>Gene:</u> AD—*COL1A1* AR—Unknown	Commonly affects mandible, clavicle, ulna May be asymmetrical Periosteal new bone and cortical thickening Abnormality limited to diaphyses of tubular bones Proximal pointing of 2nd to 5th metacarpals
Group 23 (Increased Bone Density without Modification of Bone Shape)		
Osteopetrosis (Fig. 5-13)	Several types Enlargement of liver and spleen Bone fragility with fractures Cranial nerve palsies Blindness Osteomyelitis Anaemia <u>Inheritance:</u> Severe types—AR Milder/delayed types—AD <u>Gene:</u> AR—*TCIRG1, CLCN7, RANK, RANKL* AD—*LRP5, CLCN7*	Generalised increase in bone density Abnormal modelling of the metaphyses, which are wide with alternating bands of radiolucency and sclerosis 'Bone-within-bone' appearance Rickets Basal ganglia calcification (in the recessive form associated with carbonic anhydrase deficiency)
Pyknodysostosis (Fig. 5-14)	Short limbs with a propensity to fracture Respiratory problems Irregular dentition <u>Inheritance:</u> AR <u>Gene:</u> *CTSK*	Multiple Wormian bones Delayed closure of fontanelles Generalised increase in bone density Straight mandible (reduced mandibular angle) Prognathism Deficient ossification of terminal phalanges Re-absorption of lateral clavicles Pathological fractures
Osteopoikilosis (Fig. 5-15)	Often asymptomatic May be associated with skin nodules (Buschke-Ollendorff syndrome) <u>Inheritance:</u> AD <u>Gene:</u> *LEMD3*	Sclerotic foci/bone islands, particularly around pelvis and metaphyses
Melorheostosis (Fig. 5-16)	Sclerodermatous skin lesions over affected bones Asymmetry of affected limbs Vascular anomalies Abnormal pigmentation Muscle wasting and contractures <u>Inheritance:</u> Sporadic	Dense cortical hyperostosis of affected bones with 'dripping candle wax' appearance Long bones most commonly affected
Group 24 (Increased Bone Density Group with Metaphyseal and/or Diaphyseal Involvement)		
Diaphyseal dysplasia (Camurati–Englemann disease)	Muscle weakness Pain in the extremities Gait abnormalities Exophthalmos <u>Inheritance:</u> AD <u>Gene:</u> *TGFβ*	Sclerotic skull base Progressive endosteal and periosteal diaphyseal sclerosis Narrowing of medullary cavity of tubular bones <u>Isotope bone scan:</u> Increased uptake
Group 25 (Osteogenesis Imperfecta and Decreased Bone Density Group)		
Osteogenesis imperfecta (Fig. 5-17)	See Table 5-5 <u>Inheritance:</u> Types I & V—AD Types II, III and IV—AD, AR <u>Genes:</u> Type I—*COL1A1, COL1A2* Type II—*COL1A1, COL1A2, CRTAP, LEPRE1, PPIB* Type III—As for type II plus *FKBP10, SERPINH1* Type IV—*COL1A1, COL1A2, CRTAP, PKBP10, SP7* Type V—Unknown	See Table 5-5

Continued on following page

TABLE 5-1   **Clinical and Radiographic Features of Selected Osteochondrodysplasias and Dysostoses (Continued)**

	Clinical Features	Radiological Features
Group 27 (Lysosomal Storage Diseases with Skeletal Involvement (Dysostosis Multiplex Group))		
Mucopolysaccharidoses (Figs. 5-18 and 5-19) This group of conditions is characterised by an abnormality of mucopolysaccharide and glycoprotein metabolism. Differentiation between the types is dependent upon laboratory analysis (of urine, leucocytes and fibroblastic cultures)	Typically present in early childhood Variable clinical manifestations Short stature Distinctive coarse facies Intellectual impairment (in some) Corneal opacities (in some) Joint contractures Hepatosplenomegaly Cardiovascular complications <u>Inheritance</u>: AR, except for MPS type 2 which is XLR <u>Gene</u>: Hurler/Scheie (type 1H/1S)—*IDA* Hunter (type 2)—*IDS* Sanfilippo (type 3)—*HSS, NAGLU, HSGNAT, GNS* Maroteaux–Lamy (type 6)—*ARSβ* Sly (type 7)—*GUSβ*	Macrocephaly Thick skull vault with 'ground-glass' opacification Elongated 'j-shaped' sella turcica Wide ribs, short wide clavicles, poorly modelled scapulae Ovoid, hook-shaped vertebral bodies with hypoplastic vertebral body(ies) and gibbus at thoracolumbar junction Odontoid hypoplasia Flared iliac wings with constricted bases of iliac bones Small irregular proximal femoral epiphyses Coxa valga Poorly modelled long bones with thin cortices Coarse trabecular pattern Short wide phalanges with characteristic proximal pointing of 2nd to 5th metacarpals Neurological changes include hydrocephalus, leptomeningeal cysts and a variety of abnormalities best demonstrated by MRI
Morquio syndrome (MPS type 4) (Fig. 5-19)	Normal intelligence Joint laxity Knock knees Short stature Corneal opacities <u>Inheritance</u>: AR <u>Gene</u>: *GALNS, GLβ1*	Hypoplastic/absent odontoid peg (cervical instability may lead to cord compression) Platyspondyly with posterior scalloping of vertebral bodies Anterior 'beak' or 'tongue' of vertebral bodies Flared iliac wings with constricted bases of the iliac bones Progressive disappearance of the femoral heads Coxa valga and genu valgum Irregular ossification of metaphyses of long bones Small irregular epiphyses Proximal pointing of 2nd to 5th metacarpals
Mucolipidoses type II (I-cell disease) (Fig. 5-20)	Symptoms may be apparent in neonatal period Craniofacial dysmorphism Gingival hyperplasia Joint stiffness <u>Inheritance</u>: AR <u>Gene</u>: *GNPTα/GNPTβ*	Osteopenia with coarse trabeculae Periosteal cloaking Pathological fractures Stippled/punctate calcification Metaphyseal irregularity Flared iliac wings Broad ribs Ovoid vertebral bodies
Group 29 (Disorganised Development of Skeletal Components Group)		
Multiple cartilaginous exostoses (Fig. 5-21)	Multiple bony prominences, particularly at the ends of long bones, ribs, scapulae and iliac bones Secondary deformity and limitation of joint movement Ulnar deviation of wrist <u>Inheritance</u>: AD <u>Gene</u>: Type 1—*EXT1* Type 2—*EXT2* Type 3—Unknown	Multiple flat/protuberant, polypoid/sessile exostoses Secondary joint deformities Reverse Madelung deformity (short distal ulna) Iliac crest and scapulae may be involved Vertebral bodies rarely involved Skull vault spared
Enchondromatosis (Ollier) (Fig. 5-22)	Asymmetrical limb shortening Expansion of affected bones Occasional pathological fracture Absence of vascular malformation (Ollier) Presence of vascular malformation (Maffucci) Malignancy rare in Ollier Malignancy relatively common in Maffucci (at least 15%) <u>Inheritance</u>: Non-genetic <u>Gene</u>: Non-genetic (*PTHR1* and *PTPN11* mutations found in a few patients— significance unknown)	Typically asymmetrical Shortening of affected long bones Rounded/streaky radiolucencies, particularly in metaphyses Expansion of bone with cortical thinning Areas of calcification within lesions Pathological fractures Joint deformity Reverse Madelung deformity (short distal ulna) Calcified phleboliths within vascular malformations (in Maffucci, but not usually seen until adolescence)

TABLE 5-1   **Clinical and Radiographic Features of Selected Osteochondrodysplasias and Dysostoses (Continued)**

	Clinical Features	Radiological Features
Fibrous dysplasia (Fig. 5-23)	Pain and deformity of involved bones Monostotic—only one bone involved Polyostotic—multiple bones involved McCune–Albright syndrome consists of polyostotic fibrous dysplasia, patchy café au lait skin pigmentation and precocious puberty (usually in girls) Inheritance: Sporadic Gene: *GNAS1* (polyostotic)	Asymmetrical thickening of skull vault, with sclerosis of the base; multiple rounded opacities Obliteration of the paranasal air sinuses Marked facial deformity ('leontiasis ossea') 'Ground glass' or radiolucent areas of trabecular alteration in the long bones associated with patchy sclerosis and expansion, with cortical thinning and endosteal scalloping Pathological fractures and deformities due to bone softening e.g. 'shepherd's crook' femoral necks Localised or asymmetrical overgrowth Secondary spinal stenosis
Neurofibromatosis type 1 (Fig. 5-24)	See Table 5-6 Inheritance: AD Gene: *NF1*	See Table 5-6

Group 32 (Cleidocranial Dysplasia and Isolated Cranial Ossification Defects Group)

	Clinical Features	Radiological Features
Cleidocranial dysplasia (Fig. 5-25)	Macrocephaly Large fontanelle with delay in closure Multiple supernumerary teeth Excessive shoulder mobility Narrow chest Inheritance: AD Gene: *RUNX2*	Frontal bossing Wide sutures of the skull with persistently open anterior fontanelle Multiple Wormian bones Prominent jaw with supernumerary teeth Variable hypoplasia/pseudoarthrosis of the clavicle Small scapulae Absent or delayed pubic ossification

Group 33 (Craniosynostosis Syndromes)

	Clinical Features	Radiological Features
Pfeiffer syndrome (Figs. 5-26A and 5-26B)	Craniofacial dysmorphism Broad, medially deviated thumbs and 1st toes Soft-tissue syndactyly of fingers and toes Inheritance: AD Gene: *FGFR1, FGFR2*	Sagittal/coronal craniosynostosis Squamous temporal craniosynostosis ('clover leaf skull') Dysplastic proximal phalanges of 1st toes Medial deviation of thumbs and 1st toes Hypoplastic or absent middle phalanges $\frac{2}{3}$ and/or $\frac{3}{4}$ soft-tissue syndactyly of fingers and toes Carpal fusions
Apert syndrome (Fig. 5-26C)	Craniofacial dysmorphism present from birth Proptosis High arched/cleft palate Bifid uvula 'Mitten/sock deformity' of hands/feet Inheritance: AD Gene: *FGFR2*	Coronal craniosynostosis Bony and soft-tissue syndactyly of hands and feet Progressive carpal and tarsal fusions Progressive symphalangism Progressive fusion of cervical spine (commonly C5/C6) Progressive fusion of large joints Hypoplastic glenoid fossae Dislocated radial heads

Group 35 (Dysostosis with Predominant Vertebral with or without Costal Involvement)

	Clinical Features	Radiological Features
Spondylocostal dysostosis	Short thorax with respiratory distress More or less symmetrical chest Protuberant abdomen Kyphoscoliosis (mild, non-progressive) Inheritance: Types 1 to 4—AR 　　　　　Type 5—AD 　　　　　Others—AD/AR Gene: Type 1—*DLL3* 　　　Type 2—*MESP2* 　　　Type 3—*LFNG* 　　　Type 4—*HES7* 　　　Type 5 and others—Unknown	Vertebral segmentation defects affecting 10 or more contiguous vertebral bodies 'Pebble beach' appearance of vertebrae in early childhood Kyphoscoliosis Intrinsic rib anomalies (malalignment, broadening, intercostal fusions, bifid ribs, missing ribs)
Spondylothoracic dysostosis	Short thorax with respiratory distress (≥50% infant mortality) Symmetrical chest Protuberant abdomen Kyphoscoliosis (mild or absent) Inheritance: AD Gene: *MESP2*	Vertebral segmentation defects affecting 10 or more contiguous vertebral bodies 'Tramline' appearance (on AP projection) of prominent vertebral pedicles in early childhood 'Sickle cell' appearance of vertebral bodies on lateral projection Ribs regularly aligned Posterior fusion of ribs at their costovertebral origins, fanning out in a 'crab-like' appearance No intercostal fusions

AD = autosomal dominant; AR = autosomal recessive; XLD = X-linked dominant; XLR = X-linked recessive.

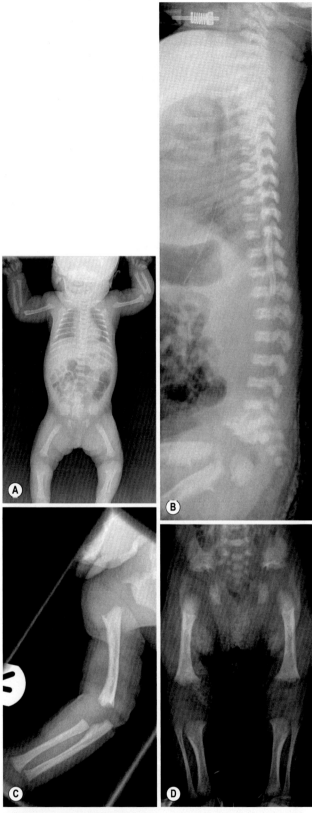

FIGURE 5-3 ■ **Achondroplasia in a neonate.** Narrow interpedicular distances of the lumbar spine and posterior scalloping of the vertebral bodies develop with age. (A) Micromelia, short ribs with a small thorax, sloping metaphyses. (B) Platyspondyly and bullet-shaped vertebral bodies. (C) Sloping metaphyses of proximal and distal humerus. (D) Small square iliac wings, short sacrosciatic notches, horizontal trident acetabula, sloping metaphyses, relatively long fibula.

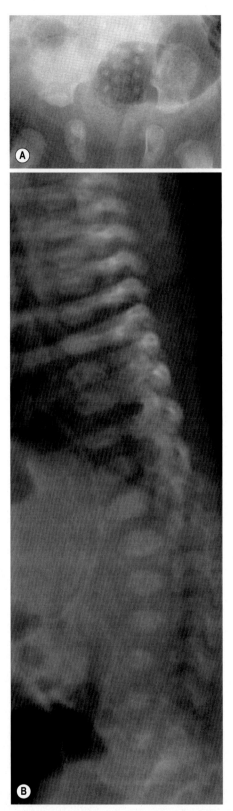

FIGURE 5-4 ■ **Spondyloepiphyseal dysplasia congenita in a 3-week-old infant.** (A) Hypoplastic superior pubic rami. (B) Anisospondyly (varying shape and size of the vertebral bodies). L5 is smaller than L1 (may be more subtle than in this example).

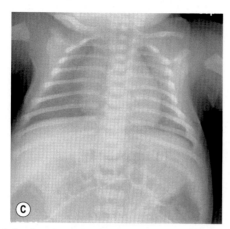

FIGURE 5-4, Continued ■ (C) Small chest with delayed appearance of the proximal humeral epiphyses.

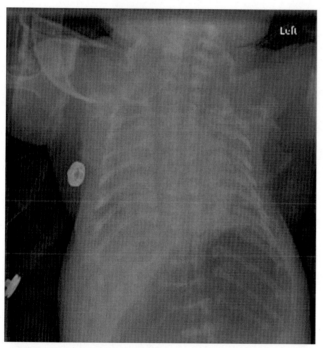

FIGURE 5-5 ■ **Metatropic dysplasia.** Narrow thorax, short ribs with prominent anterior ends and marked platyspondyly. Expanded metaphyses (seen here of the right proximal humerus) with narrow diaphyses gives rise to the so-called 'dumb-bell' appearance of the long bones.

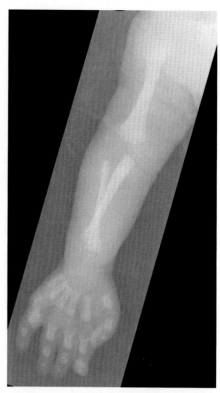

FIGURE 5-6 ■ **Ellis–van Creveld syndrome.** Postaxial polydactyly, short middle and terminal phalanges, cupped metaphyses (the epiphyses will be cone-shaped when they ossify) and sloping of the proximal humeral metaphysis.

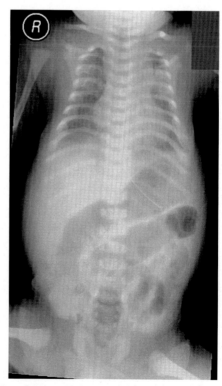

FIGURE 5-7 ■ **Jeune asphyxiating thoracic dystrophy.** Short ribs, trident acetabula. No platyspondyly.

importance, the onus is still on the radiologist to evaluate the wealth of findings on the radiographic skeletal survey by careful observation and accurate interpretation, and thereby arrive at an accurate diagnosis. An approach to the radiological interpretation of skeletal surveys performed in the context of suspected dysplasia is available.[2]

Because of the large number of relatively rare conditions, it is difficult or impossible for an individual radiologist to be familiar with every feature of every disorder. In addition, many of these conditions may have

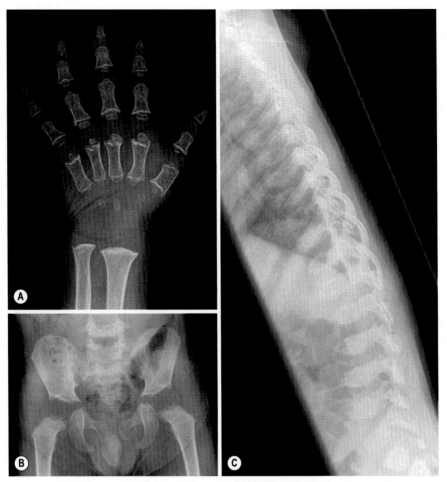

FIGURE 5-8 ■ **Pseudoachondroplasia in a 3 year old.** (A) Short tubular bones of the hand, small epiphyses with delayed bone age, pointed bases of the metacarpals with pseudoepiphyses, irregular metaphyses, flared metaphyses of distal radius and ulna. (B) Irregularity of acetabula and proximal femoral metaphyses, delayed ossification of femoral heads with short femoral necks, wide triradiate cartilages. (C) Mild platyspondyly with anterior protrusions of the vertebral bodies.

age-dependent features such that the radiological findings evolve or even resolve with time.

Examples of this temporal change include:
1. Spondyloepiphyseal dysplasia congenita (SEDC). Radiological features in the neonate (Fig. 5-4) include absent ossification of the pubic rami and short femoral necks. However, by the age of 10 to 12 years, the pubic rami will have ossified and there will usually be some degree of coxa vara.
2. Morquio disease (mucopolysaccharidosis, MPS type 4) in which the capital femoral epiphyses are well ossified at the age of 2 years, but at 8 years are small and flattened, and by 10 years have typically disappeared (see Fig. 5-19D).

Each radiologist's personal experience of the individual conditions will be limited because of the vast numbers of conditions involved. Textbooks are also of limited value because of the necessarily restricted number of illustrations and obsolescence. For these reasons, skeletal dysplasias and malformation syndromes as a group lend themselves to computer and web-based applications.

Computer assistance may take the form of menu-driven databases of clinical and radiological features. A number of findings in a particular case can be matched and a group of conditions selected from the database for further consideration before arriving at a diagnosis, e.g. the Winter Baraitser Dysmorphology Database.[3] This approach is really an automated method for cross-referencing gamuts. An alternative method is by means of a knowledge-based expert system in which experts in the field lead the user (the general radiologist) with a series of questions through a differentiation strategy to arrive at a diagnosis. Either system can be linked to a computerised image database capable of illustrating many thousands of images. Web-based resources include those that allow individuals to refer cases to a group of experts, e.g. the European Skeletal Dysplasia Network (ESDN)[4] or those that allow individuals to attempt to make a diagnosis themselves, e.g. the digital Radiological Electronic Atlas of Malformation Syndromes (dREAMS).[5]

A specific diagnostic label should only be attached to a patient when it is secure. An inaccurate diagnosis may have a profound effect upon the family in terms of genetic counselling, and upon the patient in terms of management and outcome. There may be a need to monitor and re-evaluate the evolution of radiological findings over

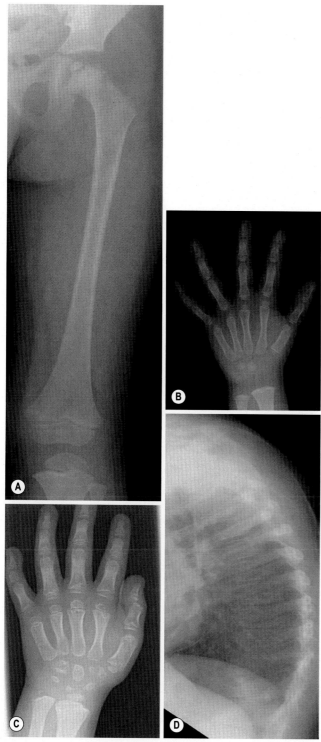

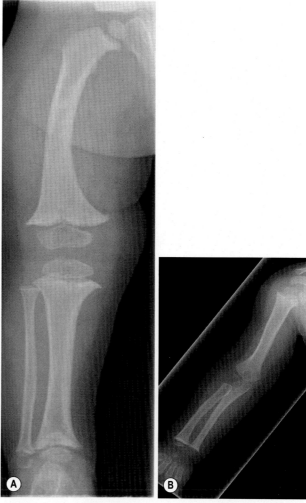

FIGURE 5-10 ■ **Metaphyseal chondrodysplasia type Schmid.** Bowed femur and coxa vara (A) and irregular cupped metaphyses of upper (B) and lower (A) limbs are shown. Bone density is normal.

FIGURE 5-9 ■ **Multiple epiphyseal dysplasia.** (A) Small proximal femoral epiphysis with irregularity of the metaphysis. Flattened epiphyses of the knee. (B) Delayed bone age (chronological age of 4 years) with small carpal bones. (C, D) Another child with proven *COMP* mutation. Small irregular carpal bones, metaphyseal irregularity, cone-shaped epiphyses (C). Mild irregularity of vertebral end plates and narrow intervertebral disc spaces (D). Relative sparing of the spine differentiates this from pseudoachondroplasia (Fig. 5-8).

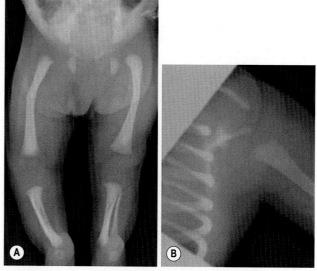

FIGURE 5-11 ■ **Campomelic dysplasia.** (A) Narrow iliac wings, flared iliac bones, mesomelic shortening and characteristic angulation of the femora (although usually affected, the tibiae in this child are not angulated). (B) Hypoplastic scapula.

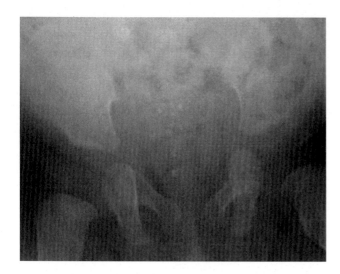

FIGURE 5-12 ■ **Chondrodysplasia punctata.** Punctate stippling of sacrum and coccyx.

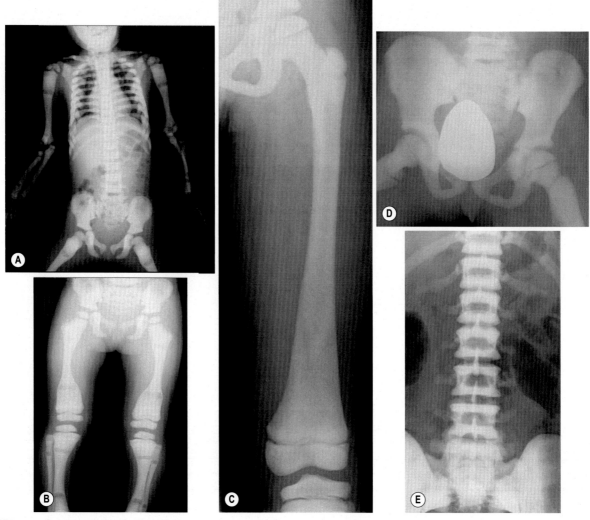

FIGURE 5-13 ■ **Osteopetrosis.** (A, B) Infantile/autosomal recessive. Generalised increase in bone density with radiolucent metaphyseal bands. Abnormal modelling with broad metaphyses. (C–E) Juvenile/autosomal dominant. Generalised increase in bone density. Broad distal femoral metaphysis. Sclerotic vertebral end plates ('rugger-jersey' spine).

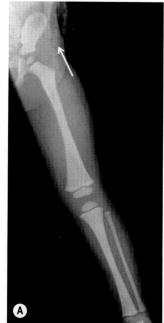

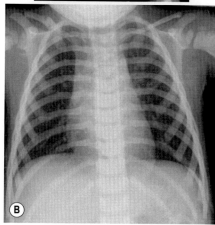

FIGURE 5-14 ■ **Pyknodysostosis.** (A) Generalised increase in bone density. Slender overmodelled long bones. Hypoplastic terminal phalanges of the left hand can just be appreciated on the edge of the radiograph (arrow). (B) Increased bone density. Fracture of the right clavicle. Mild narrowing of the thorax.

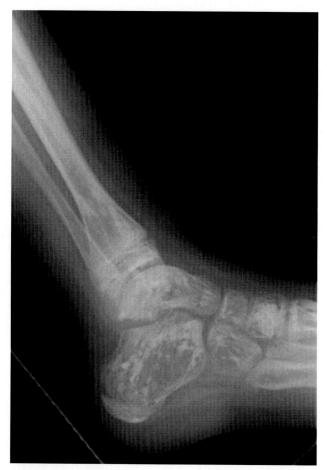

FIGURE 5-15 ■ **Osteopoikilosis.** Multiple sclerotic bone islands.

TABLE 5-2	Clinical Data Used in the Diagnosis of Skeletal Dysplasias and Malformation Syndromes

Stature—proportionate, disproportionate, asymmetry
Abnormal body proportion—short trunk, short limbs, macrocephaly, microcephaly
Abnormal limb segments—rhizomelic, mesomelic, acromelic
Local anomalies and deformities—cleft palate, polydactyly
Facies—dysmorphology
Other—hearing, sight, learning difficulties
Temporal changes
Pedigree

time before establishing a diagnosis. A significant proportion of cases (approximately 30%) are unclassifiable because the combination of findings does not conform to any recognised condition. It is important that data, both clinical (Table 5-2) and radiological, and specimens, such as bone, tissue and blood, are stored and that the information can be widely disseminated. Only in this way will it be possible to 'match' conditions and to establish the natural history of a disorder.

Prenatal Diagnosis

In the UK, almost all pregnant women now undergo prenatal US screening at between 14 and 18 weeks' gestation. All neonatally lethal skeletal dysplasias may be diagnosed at this stage by demonstrating short limbs, bowed limbs (Fig. 5-2), or a narrow thorax. Where there has been a previously affected sibling, specific malformations such as polydactyly, polycystic kidneys, or micrognathia may be assessed. Skeletal US findings are highly significant but are not very specific, and in general it is unwise to offer a precise diagnosis on the basis of US findings alone. Pregnancy terminations offered on the grounds of such US findings should subsequently have radiological and histopathological evaluation to determine the precise diagnosis, and before genetic counselling is offered.

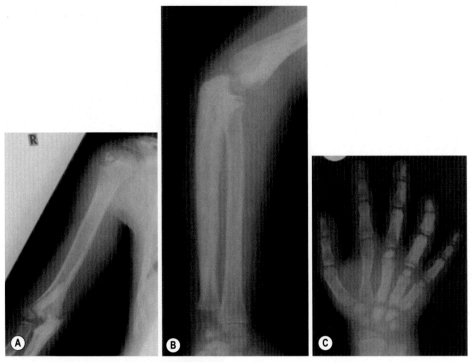

FIGURE 5-16 ■ **Melorheostosis (same patient as in Fig. 5-15).** Dense cortical bone ('dripping candle wax') in a ray distribution affecting (A) the right humerus, (B) the ulna and (C) the medial three digits and their associated carpal bones.

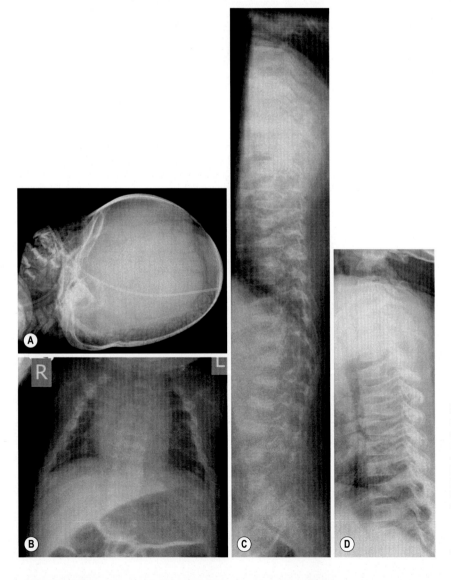

FIGURE 5-17 ■ **Osteogenesis imperfecta (OI).** (A) OI type III. Turricephaly, platybasia (but no basilar invagination) and multiple Wormian bones. (B, C) OI type III 4-week-old child: (B) reduced bone density, broad ribs with multiple healing fractures, platyspondyly; and (C) multiple vertebral compression fractures with reduced bone density. (D) OI type III aged 4 years and 7 months (same child as depicted in (B, C)). Improved bone density on bisphosphonate therapy. Multiple vertebral wedge fractures.

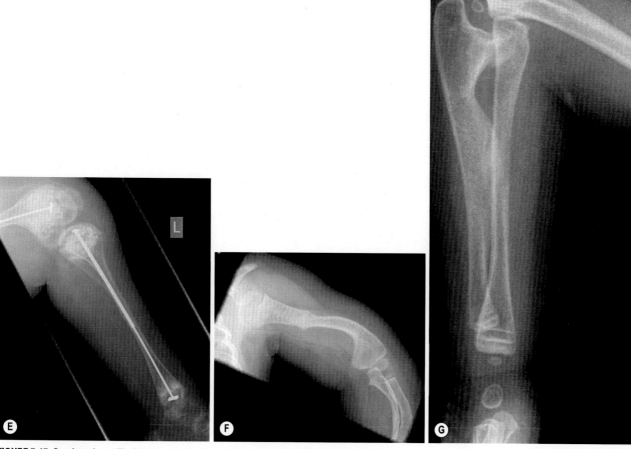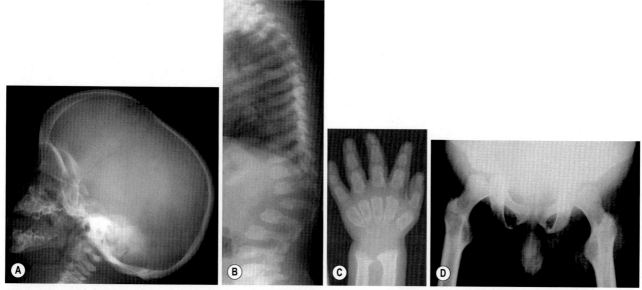

FIGURE 5-17, Continued ■ (E) OI type III. Reduced bone density. 'Popcorn' calcification of the metaphyses. Intramedullary rodding of femur and tibia. (F) OI type III. Bowing deformity of the bones. Healing shaft fractures of the humerus and ulna. Multiple bisphosphonate lines of the proximal humerus. See also Fig. 5-1. (G) OI type V. Ossification of the interosseous membrane. Dislocated radial head.

FIGURE 5-18 ■ **Mucopolysaccharidosis type 1H/1S (Hurler/Scheie).** (A) Macrocephaly, ground-glass appearance, elongated 'j-shaped' sella turcica. Mild hypoplasia of the odontoid peg. (B) Hypoplastic L2 vertebral body with a kyphosis at this level. Anterior beaking of vertebral bodies. Mild posterior scalloping of the upper lumbar vertebral bodies. Broad ribs. (C) Undermodelled tubular bones of the hand with proximal pointing of the second to fifth metacarpals. Short terminal phalanges. Undermodelling of the distal radius and ulna with a reduced carpal angle. (D) Flared iliac wings, elongated femoral necks with small proximal femoral epiphyses.

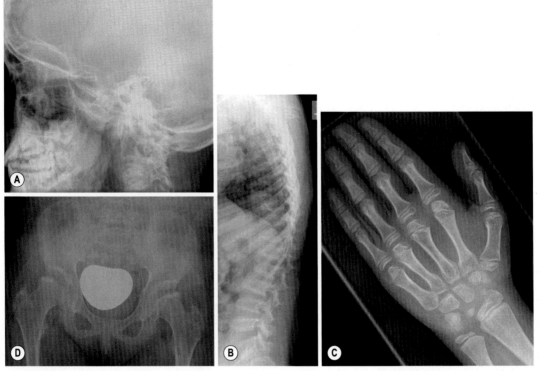

FIGURE 5-19 ■ **Mucopolysaccharidosis type 4 (Morquio) in a girl aged 10 years and 8 months with corneal clouding and normal intelligence.** (A) Hypoplastic odontoid peg. (B) Platyspondyly, anterior beaking and posterior scalloping of the vertebral bodies. (C) Flattened metacarpal heads and irregular carpal bones. (D) Small (nearly absent) and sclerotic femoral heads (progressive fragmentation over the preceding few years), irregular acetabula.

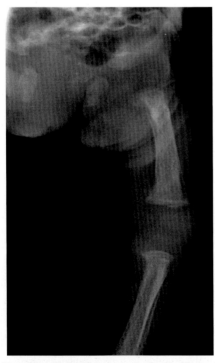

FIGURE 5-20 ■ **Mucolipidosis type II (I-cell disease).** Coarse trabeculation and periosteal cloaking of the long bones. Stippling of the lower spine and at the knee.

Many non-lethal conditions which may present at birth can also be ascertained on prenatal US. Fetal anomaly US examinations are offered to parents of previous babies who have had congenital dysplasias or malformation syndromes, and to at-risk parents with high maternal or paternal ages, or with specific environmental exposures (including certain medications).

Occasionally, other imaging techniques may help to confirm a suspected prenatal diagnosis. Maternal abdominal radiographs are now almost obsolete; the poor diagnostic quality does not justify the radiation risk to either fetus or mother, particularly as the fetus may be normal or have the potential to survive with a good quality of life.

Low-dose prenatal CT is being successfully performed in some centres for the evaluation of skeletal anomalies.[6]

Magnetic resonance imaging (MRI) is increasingly used for in utero evaluation of specific anomalies, particularly of the central nervous system but more recently of other systems including the musculoskeletal[7] and for the assessment of lung volumes.[8]

Chorionic villus sampling can be used for biochemical evaluation of fetuses at risk from storage disorders when a previous pregnancy has been affected. Fetal chromosomal analysis from skin biopsy can be assessed when a sibling or carrier parent is affected.

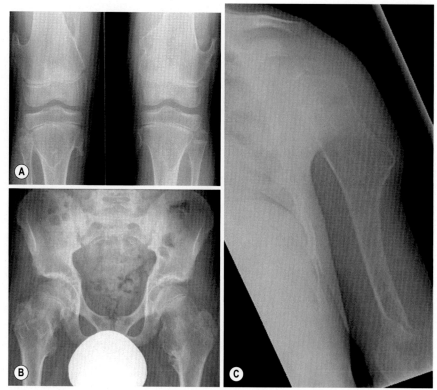

FIGURE 5-21 ■ **Multiple cartilaginous exostoses.** (A) Multiple exostoses around the knee. Note that they point away from the growth plates. (B) Exostoses causing broadening of the femoral necks. (C) A large sessile exostosis of the proximal humerus—again pointing away from the nearest growth plate.

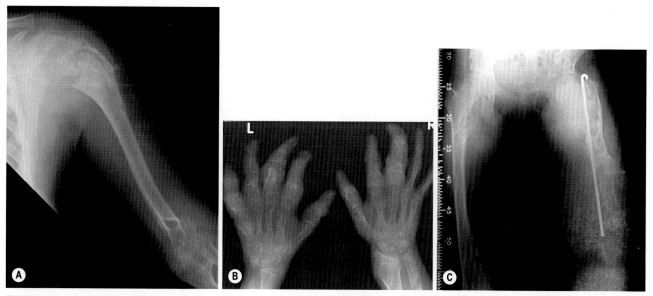

FIGURE 5-22 ■ **Multiple enchondromatosis (Ollier's disease).** (A) Enchondromata of the proximal humerus appear as metaphyseal striations and stippled calcification. Bowing deformity of proximal humerus. (B) Multiple expansile lytic lesions with associated soft-tissue swelling of some fingers. Short left distal ulna (reverse Madelung deformity). (C) Characteristic asymmetrical involvement with severe involvement of the left femur and tibia and milder involvement of the right femur.

Imaging

Making the Diagnosis

In addition to prenatal US, a skeletal survey should be performed on any pregnancy termination resulting from a US diagnosis of short-limbed dwarfism or significant malformation. Also, a skeletal survey should be performed on any stillbirth. Although this may involve anteroposterior (AP) and lateral 'babygrams' of the entire infant, ideally additional views of the extremities should

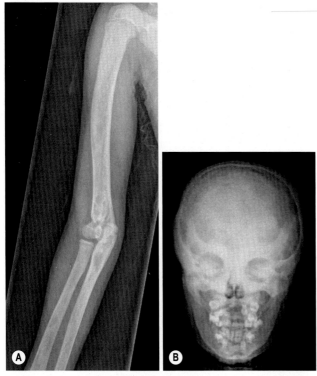

FIGURE 5-23 ■ **Fibrous dysplasia.** (A) Expansile radiolucent lesions, some with a sclerotic margin ('rind' appearance). Some cortical scalloping. (B) Patchy sclerosis of the skull vault and facial bones.

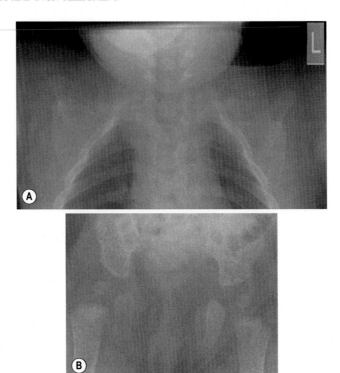

FIGURE 5-25 ■ **Cleidocranial dysplasia.** (A) Hypoplastic lateral ends of the clavicles. (B) Hypoplastic pubic rami. Bilateral coxa valga.

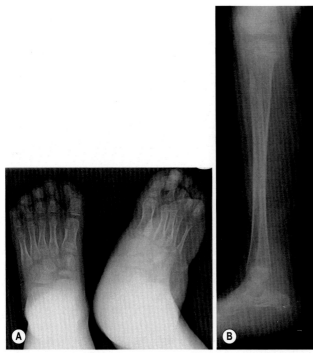

FIGURE 5-24 ■ **Neurofibromatosis.** (A) Soft-tissue and bony overgrowth of the right foot. (B) Soft-tissue overgrowth of the right leg. Thickened heel pad with characteristic erosion of the calcaneum.

be performed. Spontaneous abortions should also have a radiographic skeletal survey. However, this can rarely be achieved.

After birth, a standard full skeletal survey is indicated when attempting to establish a diagnosis for short stature or for a dysmorphic syndrome. This should include:

- AP and lateral skull (to include the atlas and axis)
- AP chest (to include the clavicles)
- AP pelvis (to include the lumbar spine and symphysis pubis)
- lateral thoracolumbar spine
- AP one lower limb
- AP one upper limb
- posteroanterior (PA) one hand (usually the left; allows bone age assessment).

Occasionally, additional views will be required, particularly with specific clinical abnormalities, and these may include views of the feet, e.g. if polydactyly is present, or views of the cervical spine if cervical instability is suspected with specific diagnoses, or both upper and lower limbs if asymmetry or deformity is a clinical feature.

If a diagnosis cannot be established, then (limited) follow-up imaging is indicated (e.g. at 1 and 3 years), to evaluate progression and evolution of radiographic appearances.

Occasionally a technetium radionuclide skeletal scintigram showing the photon-deficient area of avascular necrosis (AVN) may be of value in differentiating bilateral Perthes disease from the small fragmented capital femoral epiphyses of multiple epiphyseal dysplasia. In this regard, contrast-enhanced MRI is also useful.

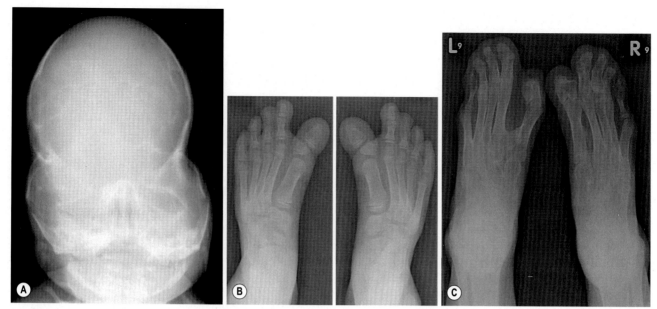

FIGURE 5-26 ■ **Acrocephalosyndactyly syndromes.** (A) Pfeiffer syndrome. Craniosynostosis with a clover-leaf skull. Prominent sutural markings and wide anterior fontanelle. (B) Pfeiffer syndrome. Characteristic hypoplastic trapezoid proximal phalanges of broadened great toes, which are medially deviated. Significant hypoplasia of all middle phalanges, bilateral two-thirds soft-tissue syndactyly. (C) Apert syndrome. Single dysplastic phalanx of broadened great toes and only two phalanges for second to fifth toes. Fusion of the metatarsophalangeal joints of second to fourth toes. Fusion of metatarsal bases. Bony bar between first and second metatarsals bilaterally (left more prominent). Soft-tissue syndactyly of second to fifth toes ('sock foot').

Conditions with decreased bone density may be assessed and monitored by means of dual-energy X-ray absorptiometry (DEXA).

Assessing Complications

When a confident diagnosis is established, further imaging is essential to monitor the progress of potential complications. Complications may result as part of the natural evolution of the condition, but may also be iatrogenic.

Radiography and MRI of the cervical spine in flexion and extension will monitor instability; AP and lateral views of the spine will monitor kyphosis and scoliosis. Long limb radiographic views or (increasingly) computed tomography (CT) scannograms will help to assess asymmetry, genu varum and genu valgum, and to monitor progression of limb length discrepancy. CT or MRI may monitor the development of hydrocephalus or the presence of neuronal migration defects and structural defects, such as the absence of the corpus callosum. CT may also demonstrate encroachment on the cranial nerve foramina and both CT and MRI are of value in assessing spinal cord compression.

US can demonstrate associated organ anomalies, e.g. cystic disease of the kidneys or hepatosplenomegaly, and echocardiography may reveal associated intracardiac abnormalities.

Arthrography, US, CT and MRI are of value in the assessment of joint problems, particularly when surgical intervention is proposed or following surgery.

Technetium skeletal scintigrams are occasionally used to determine the extent of bony involvement in specific disorders, e.g. asymptomatic lesions identified in chronic recurrent multifocal osteomyelitis. However, in patchy disorders such as fibrous dysplasia, radiographically affected areas may not demonstrate abnormal uptake of radionuclide.

Postoperative Imaging

US has a place in assessing the development of new bone formation following osteotomies and limb-lengthening procedures and plain radiography and CT in confirming the correct alignment in this situation. CT is also of value for the assessment of hip reduction in developmental hip dysplasia (see Fig. 5-30F). All imaging investigations are brought into play in the assessment of a patient following bone marrow transplantation.

Management

Only when an accurate diagnosis has been established can the prognosis and natural history be given. For example, myopia can be corrected and retinal detachment prevented in Stickler syndrome (hereditary arthro-ophthalmopathy); cord compression can be prevented in conditions with instability of the cervical spine (Table 5-3) or with progressive thoracolumbar kyphosis and spinal stenosis, as in achondroplasia. Various imaging techniques have a role in evaluating the cervical spine.[9]

In some conditions, cure may be achieved, e.g. in the severe form of osteopetrosis (which is lethal in childhood unless treated), by means of a compatible bone marrow transplant in the first 6 months of life. Not only do the radiographic changes revert to normal but also the

TABLE 5-3	Disorders with Instability in the Cervical Spine

Cervical Spine Instability with Odontoid Peg Absence or Hypoplasia

Achondroplasia
Chondrodysplasia punctata
Diastrophic dysplasia
Dyggve–Melchior–Clausen disease
Hypochondrogenesis
Infantile hypophosphatasia
Kniest dysplasia
Metaphyseal chondrodysplasia, type McKusick
Metatropic dysplasia
Morquio disease (MPS type 4) and other mucopolysaccharidoses (MPS)
Mucolipidoses (MLS)
Multiple epiphyseal dysplasia
Neurofibromatosis type 1
Opsismodysplasia
Pseudoachondroplasia
Pseudodiastrophic dysplasia
Spondyloepiphyseal dysplasia congenita
Trisomy 21

Cervical Spine Instability with Cervical Kyphosis (C2/C3)

Diastrophic dysplasia
Spondyloepiphyseal dysplasia congenital

Lethal

Atelosteogenesis
Campomelic dysplasia

TABLE 5-4	Asymmetric Shortening or Overgrowth

Beckwith–Wiedemann syndrome
Chondrodysplasia punctata (Conradi–Hünermann)
Dysplasia epiphysealis hemimelica
Epidermoid nevus syndrome
Hereditary multiple exostoses
Hypomelanosis of Ito
Klippel–Trénaunay syndrome
Maffucci syndrome
McCune–Albright syndrome
Melorheostosis
Neurofibromatosis
Ollier's disease (multiple enchondromatosis)
Polyostotic fibrous dysplasia
Silver–Russell syndrome
Sturge–Weber syndrome

predisposition to fractures resolves, cranial nerve compression is arrested and life expectancy improved.

Bone marrow transplantation has also been used with some success in treating selected patients with mucopolysaccharidoses. Although this treatment has resulted in iatrogenic manipulation of the natural history of the mucopolysaccharidoses (skeletal abnormalities persist), with the associated improved quality of life and increased life expectancy, later complications, often the result of spinal cord compression, are now being recognised.

In many conditions, orthopaedic procedures are invaluable in maintaining or improving mobility. For example, osteotomies prevent or correct dislocations or long bone bowing deformities. Patients with osteogenesis imperfecta may require multiple osteotomies to correct severe deformities, as well as intramedullary rodding to reduce fractures, maintain alignment and provide support and stability (see Fig. 5-1). These patients suffer from basilar invagination, resulting in compression of the brainstem. Surgical intervention may prevent severe neurological impairment. Spinal deformities, kyphosis and scoliosis are common in the constitutional disorders of bone. Prevention and treatment consists of spinal bracing and timely arthrodeses or laminectomies for cord compression. Joint replacements may be necessary, especially in those dysplasias, such as multiple epiphyseal dysplasia, in which major involvement of the epiphyses may result in premature osteoarthritis. In some conditions, limb-lengthening procedures may be appropriate to improve mobility. This is usually offered in disorders with asymmetric shortening (Table 5-4), but is sometimes offered

to selected patients with achondroplasia (Fig. 5-3) or other short-limbed dysplasias for cosmetic reasons. Achondroplasia has proved particularly amenable to limb-lengthening procedures because redundant soft tissues are a feature of this dysplasia and insufficient soft tissue has proved to be a limiting factor in lengthening procedures in other conditions. An increase of approximately 30% in the length of the long bones may be achieved in achondroplasia, compared with 15% in other disorders.

Only with an accurate diagnosis in those conditions presenting at birth can those that are likely to be lethal be predicted. The diagnosis of a lethal dysplasia can prevent unnecessary and distressing prolongation of life, help to reduce parental expectations and anguish and help save on economic resources.

Termination of pregnancy may be offered with prenatally diagnosed lethal conditions, or where there is intra-uterine evidence of short limbs. When a sibling has suffered from a disabling condition associated with particular malformations, these may be specifically looked for prenatally in subsequent pregnancies. This practice is leading to a change in the incidence of certain conditions formerly presenting at birth.

With the identification and localisation of specific chromosomal abnormalities associated with particular disorders, the development of gene therapy for clinical use poses many challenges and offers great potential for the future.

Growth hormone therapy is used in selected disorders to influence final height. Growth hormone stimulates Type I collagen production and is being used, in particular, to augment growth rate in children with osteogenesis imperfecta (see Table 5-5).

Bisphosphonates are pyrophosphate analogues that inhibit osteoclast function. They have been used in osteogenesis imperfecta to improve bone density, and have also been used to treat bone pain and osteopenia in a variety of rheumatological and dermatological conditions. The radiological hallmark of bisphosphonate therapy, so-called 'bisphosphonate lines', are now well recognised (see Figs. 5-1 and 5-17F).

TABLE 5-5   Osteogenesis Imperfecta Clinical (Based on the Sillence Classification) and Radiological Findings

	I	II	III	IV	V[a]
Clinical Findings					
Incidence	1:30,000	1:30,000	Rare	Unknown (rare)	Unknown (rare)
Severity	Mild	Lethal	Severe	Mild/moderately severe	Moderate
Death	Old age	Stillborn	By 30 years	Old age	Old age
Sclerae	Blue	Blue	Blue, then grey	White	White
Hearing impairment	Frequent	—	Rare	Rare	Rare
Teeth	IA normal	—	DI[b]	IVA normal	Normal
	IB DI	—		IVB DI	
Stature	Normal	—	Short	Normal/mildly short	Normal/mildly short
Radiological Findings					
Fractures at birth	<10%	Multiple	Frequent	Rare	Rare
Osseous fragility	Moderate/mild	Severe	Moderate/severe	Moderate/mild	Moderate
Deformity	Mild	—	Severe	Variable	Moderate/severe

[a]Other radiological findings in type V OI include dense metaphyses in the paediatric age range, healing of fractures with hyperplastic callus formation, ossification of the interosseous membrane and dislocated radial head.
[b]DI = dentinogenesis imperfecta.

TABLE 5-6   Clinical and Radiographic Features of Neurofibromatosis[28,29]

Clinical Features	Radiographic Features
Focal gigantism (soft-tissue overgrowth or plexiform neurofibroma)—Fig. 5-24	Neuromas and/or fibromas (with enlarged cranial foramina[30]), schwannomas and neurofibrosarcomas[29]
Macrocrania	Aplasia/hypoplasia of the sphenoid wings (empty orbit)
Axillary freckling	Dumb-bell neurofibromas/lateral meningoceles
Multiple café au lait macules	Hypoplasia of posterosuperior orbital wall (pulsatile exophthalmos)
Molluscum fibrosum	Mesodermal dysplasia (calvarial defects)
Anteromedial bowing of tibia	Angular kyphoscoliosis
	Posterior scalloping of the vertebral bodies (dural ectasia)
	'Ribbon' ribs (mesodermal dysplasia), rib notching
	Pseudoarthroses of the tibia, fibula or clavicle
	Fibrous cortical defects (multiple and large)
	Intraosseous cysts

Genetic Counselling

When an accurate diagnosis has been made, meaningful genetic counselling can be given, both to the parents and to the affected individual. Most conditions are inherited in an autosomal dominant (AD) or autosomal recessive (AR) manner. In conditions with an AD inheritance, the affected individual has a one in two chance of passing the same abnormality on to his/her offspring. However, many of these conditions arise as a spontaneous mutation, which means that the parents of the affected individual, who are themselves normal, have an extremely low risk of having another affected child. In AR conditions, both the parents are carriers of the disorder, but are not affected, and they have a one in four chance of having another affected child.

Other important, although uncommon, modes of inheritance are the result of somatic or gonadal mosaicism or uniparental disomy. Mosaicism is the presence of at least two cell lines in a single individual or tissue that derive from a single zygote. Somatic mosaicism for AD conditions results in asymmetric or patchy disorders (Table 5-4). It is thought that when not a mosaic, these disorders are lethal. Clinical evidence of somatic mosaicism includes asymmetry, localised overgrowth, pigmentation and haemangiomas. In uniparental disomy, both copies of a chromosome or part of a chromosome are inherited from one parent, e.g. paternal uniparental disomy 14 (patUPD14). Imprinting refers to the situation where a gene's expression depends on the parent of origin: hence, paternal UPD15 leads to Angelman syndrome, while maternal UPD15 causes Prader–Willi syndrome.

Osteochondrodysplasias

The clinical and radiographic features of selected osteochondrodysplasias and dysostoses are described in Tables 5-1, 5-5 and 5-6.

Chromosomal Disorders

Trisomy 21 (Down's Syndrome)

Craniofacial abnormalities include brachycephaly, microcephaly, hypertelorism and relatively small facial bones. The iliac wings are flared with relatively sloping acetabula. Frequently there are 11 pairs of ribs and the ribs themselves are gracile. There are often two ossification

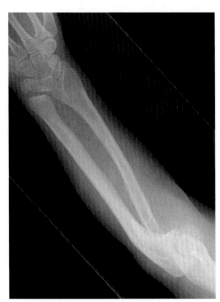

FIGURE 5-27 ■ **Dyschondrosteosis (Léri–Weill syndrome).** Premature fusion of the ulnar half of the distal radial epiphysis with sloping of the distal radius and reduced carpal angle. Dislocation of the radial head.

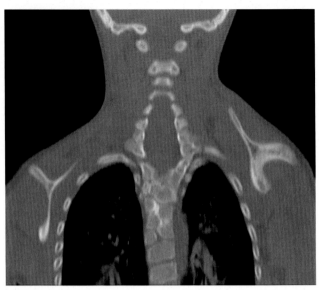

FIGURE 5-28 ■ **Klippel–Feil syndrome.** Coronal CT of the thorax on bone windows showing a high-riding left scapula and segmentation defects of the upper thoracic spine.

centres in the manubrium sterni. Atlantoaxial subluxation and instability with hypoplasia of the odontoid process are a frequent cause of myelopathy. There is generalised joint laxity. The vertebral bodies are relatively tall. The hands are short, with fifth finger clinodactyly due to a hypoplastic middle phalanx. Congenital heart lesions include endocardial cushion defects and intra- and extracardiac shunts. Duodenal atresia, duodenal stenosis, Hirschsprung's disease and anorectal anomalies are associated.

45XO (Turner's Syndrome)

Short stature and lymphoedema may be clinically obvious. Important radiological findings include short fourth metacarpals, a reduced angle between the distal radial and ulnar metaphyses similar to that seen in dyschondrosteosis (Madelung deformity; Fig. 5-27; see also Fig. 5-29 below), flattening of the medial tibial condyle with a transitory exostosis, osteoporosis, scoliosis, coarctation of the aorta, and increased occurrence of urinary tract anomalies, such as horseshoe kidneys.

LOCALISED DISORDERS OF THE SKELETON

Sprengel Deformity (Congenital Elevation of the Scapula)

This is the most common congenital abnormality of the shoulder. There is failure of the normal descent of the scapula from its initial mid-cervical to its final mid-thoracic position. This descent should occur between the sixth and eighth weeks of gestation. Males and females are affected equally. It may affect one or both sides.

When unilateral, the left shoulder is more often involved. It may occur in isolation or in association with fusions of the cervical spine (Klippel–Feil syndrome). The scapula is elevated and rotated with the inferior edge of the glenoid pointing towards the spine. The superomedial angle is high and prominent, and the affected scapula is larger than the normal one. An autosomal dominant inheritance has been suggested.

An omovertebral bone (bony or fibrous connection between the superomedial angle of the scapula and the spinous process, lamina or transverse process of a vertebral body between C4 and C7) occurs in approximately 50% of cases. Both MRI[10] and CT (Fig. 5-28) are useful for depicting the deformity, associated vertebral segmentation defects and the omovertebral bone (when present).

Madelung Deformity

This condition results from abnormality (premature fusion) of the medial half of the distal radial epiphysis. The radii are short and bowed. There is reduction of the carpal angle, with wedging of the carpal bones between the distal radius and ulna. Madelung deformity may be inherited when it occurs as an autosomal dominant mesomelic dysplasia (dyschondrosteosis) or it may present as an isolated disorder, for example following trauma or infection (Fig. 5-29A).

In reverse Madelung deformity, there is bowing of the forearm bones, in association with a short (abnormal) ulna. Causes of reverse Madelung include trauma, multiple cartilaginous exostoses and multiple enchondromatosis (Fig. 5-29B).

Developmental Dysplasia of the Hip

This may occur as an isolated disorder (increased female incidence, breech presentation, first-born children, oligohydramnios, and when there is a positive family history) or in association with other conditions (e.g. sternomastoid tumour, torticollis, talipes calcaneovalgus, arthrogryposis multiplex and trisomy 21). The incidence in the UK approaches 1 in 400 live births, while in the USA it is 3–4 in 1000.

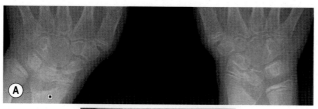

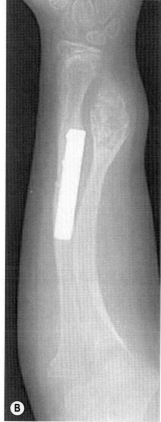

FIGURE 5-29 ■ Compare the bilateral Madelung deformity (long ulna) in dyschondrosteosis (A) with the reverse Madelung deformity (short ulna) in a patient with multiple enchondromatosis (B).

Although guidelines may vary slightly, both in the UK and the USA, static and dynamic US examination is performed on all newborn infants with a positive Ortolani and/or Barlow test, breech presentation, or positive family history. US should usually be performed when the infant is about 6 weeks old. A high-frequency linear probe is used to obtain a coronal view of the hip joint. Measurements and their interpretation are summarised in Figs. 5-30A, B and in Table 5-7. The various imaging appearances of developmental dysplasia of the hip (DDH) are illustrated in Figs. 5-30C–G.

When ossification of the proximal femoral epiphysis renders US examination difficult, then radiographs are useful for follow-up and monitoring the response to treatment. CT is useful for assessing the position of the femoral head following operative reduction (Fig. 5-30F). Screening programmes[11] for at-risk infants have led to earlier detection and treatment, and cases such as those with bilateral dislocation and formation of pseudoacetabulae are now less common. When it occurs, osteonecrosis secondary to surgical treatment for DDH is a relatively benign complication, not significantly affecting general physical function or quality of life.[12]

Femoral Dysplasia (Idiopathic Coxa Vara/Proximal Focal Femoral Deficiency Spectrum)

The spectrum of femoral dysplasia encompasses all conditions from the mild idiopathic coxa vara, through moderate forms with deficiency of the proximal femur (Fig. 5-31), to severe forms in which only the distal femoral condyles develop.

Idiopathic Coxa Vara

In this condition, there is coxa vara (reduction of femoral neck/shaft angle). A separate fragment of bone (Fairbank's triangle)—from the inferior portion of the femoral neck—is characteristic. If the neck/shaft angle is less than 100°, then without surgical intervention the varus deformity will progress.

Proximal Focal Femoral Deficiency

Proximal focal femoral deficiency (PFFD) is bilateral in only 10% of cases. Varying degrees of agenesis of the

TABLE 5-7 Graf Angles

Type	α Angle (°)	β Angle (°)	Bony Roof	Ossific Rim	Cartilage Roof	Interpretation
Ia	>60	<55	Good	Sharp	Covers femoral head	Mature
Ib	>60	>55	Good	Usually blunt	Covers head	Mature
IIa	50–59	>55	Deficient	Rounded	Covers head	Physiological ossification delay
IIb	50–59	>55	Deficient	Rounded	Covers head	
IIc	43–49	<77	Deficient	Rounded/flat	Covers head	
IId	43–49	>77	Severely deficient	Rounded/flat	Compressed	On point of dislocation
IIIa	<43	>77	Poor	Flat	Displaced up Echo poor	Dislocated
IIIb	<43	>77	Poor	Flat	Displaced up Reflective	Dislocated
IV	<43	>77	Poor	Flat	Interposed	Dislocated

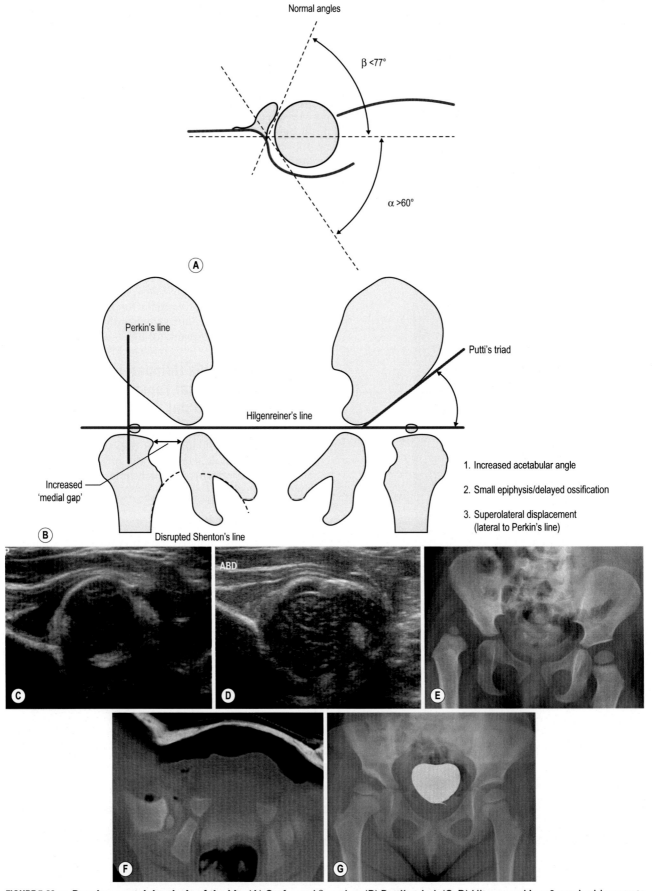

FIGURE 5-30 ■ **Developmental dysplasia of the hip.** (A) Graf α and β angles. (B) Putti's triad. (C, D) Ultrasound in a 2-week-old neonate showing dislocation of the left hip. The dislocated left hip reduces in abduction (D). (E) Dysplastic right acetabulum with dislocated femoral head at 1 year and 5 months. (F) Same patient at 1 year and 7 months. Postoperative axial CT images confirm satisfactory reduction of the femoral head. (G) Same patient at 3 years and 11 months. Shallow right acetabulum with bony fragments beneath the acetabular roof. Flattening of the femoral head. Mild coxa magna.

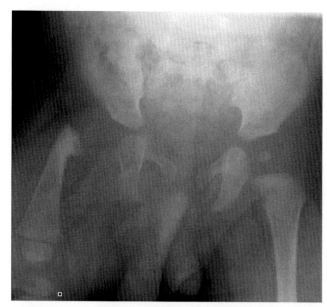

FIGURE 5-31 ■ **Proximal focal femoral deficiency.** Hypoplastic proximal right femur. Absent ossification of the femoral head with a normal acetabulum.

proximal femur occur (Fig. 5-31); there is an association between severity of femoral dysplasia and severity of acetabular dysplasia. Based on the presence or absence of the femoral head and the morphology of the acetabulum and shortened femur, Aitken classified PFFD into four groups of increasing severity from A to D. In addition to the femoral shortening, the lower leg may also be short, and the fibula absent or hypoplastic.

Radiography demonstrates the degree of aplasia and, particularly in younger children, MRI[13] and/or arthrography is useful for the visualisation of unossified cartilage. Because PFFD is associated with absence or deficiency of the cruciate ligaments, MRI also has a role in imaging the knee(s) of affected patients.

Tibia Vara

This refers to unilateral or bilateral bowing of the legs.[14] Bowing may occur at the level of the knee joint or proximal tibia. Causes include physiological bowing (bilateral and self-resolving), rickets, trauma, infection, neurofibromatosis, Ollier's disease, Maffucci syndrome, fibrous dysplasia, focal fibrocartilaginous dysplasia (Fig. 5-32) and Blount's disease (Fig. 5-33).

Focal fibrocartilaginous dysplasia[15] (Fig. 5-32) characteristically affects the proximal tibia, appearing as a linear radiolucency extending inferolaterally from the proximal tibial metadiaphysis. It causes bowing of the affected bone, but is benign and usually self-resolving. Surgery is required in those children with severe bowing or in whom the bowing does not resolve with time.

Blount's disease (Fig. 5-33) affects the medial aspects of the proximal tibial epiphyses. It is unilateral in 40%. There are infantile and adolescent presentations. The infantile form of the disease occurs between the ages of 1 and 3 years. Adolescent Blount's disease has a higher post-surgical recurrence rate than the infantile form.

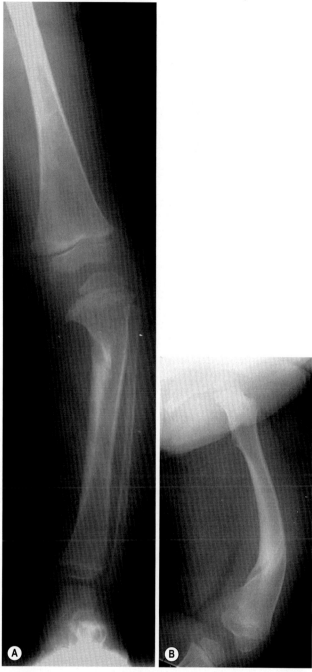

FIGURE 5-32 ■ **Focal fibrocartilaginous dysplasia (FFCD).** (A) Pathognomonic appearance of the proximal tibia with bowing deformity and a cortical radiolucent band. This condition is usually self-resolving and should be managed conservatively. The proximal tibia is the commonest site to be affected. (B) FFCD of the distal femur.

Tibial bowing occurs below the level of the knee. Initial beaking of the medial proximal tibial metaphysis progresses to irregularity, fragmentation and premature fusion of the medial aspect of the proximal tibial growth plate.

Talipes

Talipes equinovarus (congenital clubfoot) consists of varus (inversion) and equinus (fixed plantar flexion) of the

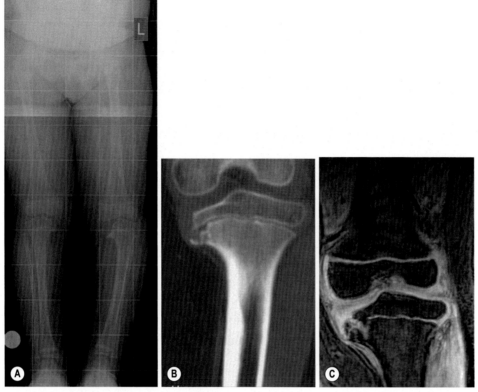

FIGURE 5-33 ■ **Blount's disease.** Fragmentation of the medial half of the left proximal tibial epiphysis. (A) Radiograph showing varus angulation. (B) CT appearance in a different patient with no varus angulation. (C) MRI appearance in the same patient in (B).

TABLE 5-8   Diagnosis of Talipes

Deformity	DP Radiograph	Lateral Radiograph
Hind foot varus	Talocalcaneal angle: <15° Midtalar line lateral to first metatarsal base	Talocalcaneal angle: <25°
Hind foot valgus	Talocalcaneal angle: >50° in newborns; >40° in older children Midtalar angle medial to first metatarsal base	Talocalcaneal angle: >50° in newborns; >45° in older children
Hind foot equines	—	Calcaneotibial angle: >90° plantar flexion of calcaneus
Hind foot calcaneus	—	Calcaneotibial angle: <60° dorsiflexion of calcaneus
Forefoot varus	Narrow with increased overlap of metatarsal bases	Fifth metatarsal most plantar (normal); first metatarsal most dorsal
Forefoot valgus	Broad with reduced overlap of metatarsal bases	First metatarsal most plantar

hindfoot, and varus of the forefoot. It results from abnormal development around the ninth week of gestation. Aetiological considerations include genetic factors and early amniocentesis (before 11 weeks), with recent work providing tentative evidence for aetiologically distinct subtypes.[16] It occurs two to three times more commonly in boys. Useful measurements are summarised in Table 5-8.

Idiopathic Avascular Necrosis of the Femoral Head (Perthes Disease)

Osteonecrosis of the femoral head usually presents with pain or limping between 5 and 8 years of age. It is most often unilateral, but when bilateral (approximately 15%)

is asymmetrical, helping to distinguish it from an epiphyseal dysplasia. There are four stages of disease: devascularisation; collapse and fragmentation; re-ossification; and finally the stage of remodelling.

The earliest radiographic feature is that of a radiolucent subchondral fissure—the crescent sign (Fig. 5-34A). Disease progresses with loss of height, fragmentation and sclerosis of the femoral head (Figs. 5-34B, C). A coxa magna deformity may ensue, with lateral uncovering of the capital femoral epiphysis. There may be associated irregularity of the acetabular margin. The extent of subchondral fracture is said to be a good predictor of the final outcome.[17] Several radiological classification systems have been developed and shown to be reliable when used by an experienced observer.[18]

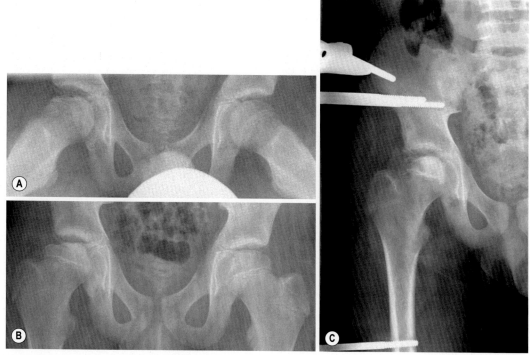

FIGURE 5-34 ■ **Idiopathic avascular necrosis (AVN) of the femoral head (Perthes disease).** (A) Frog lateral on day of presentation showing the characteristic crescent sign of early AVN of the right capital femoral epiphysis. (B) Ten days after (A): rapid progression with irregularity, loss of height and sclerosis of the femoral head. (C) Nine months after (A) and a month following hip distraction.

US may reveal capsular distension from a hip effusion, which if persisting for longer than 6 weeks may be associated with the development of Perthes disease. Additionally, irregularity/fragmentation of the capital femoral epiphysis and poor coverage of the femoral head may be demonstrated.

While skeletal scintigraphy is highly sensitive and specific for detecting AVN, MRI has now largely replaced it (see Fig. 5-41C below). Six patterns of signal abnormality have been described.[19] T1-weighted images show low signal intensity, compared to high signal on T2-weighted, fat-suppressed/inversion recovery (STIR) sequences. In those with normal signal intensity or complete loss of signal on both sequences (dead bone), intravenous enhancement is not necessary. In those with normal/low T1- and high T2-weighted signal, intravenous contrast medium will identify areas of viable bone. Dynamic contrast and DWI MRI have an increasing role in the diagnosis of Perthes disease.[20,21]

Slipped Capital Femoral Epiphysis (SCFE)

This is the commonest hip disorder of adolescence. Anterolateral and rotational forces of the hip muscles on the femoral shaft result in anterosuperior translation of the proximal femoral metaphysis relative to the epiphysis. By definition, a slip occurs through the non-rachitic physis.[22]

It is more common in boys, in Afro-Americans and in the obese. The age range for girls is 11–12 years and for boys 12–14 years. It most commonly occurs at the time of the pubertal growth spurt at Risser grade 0 (see Fig. 5-37 below), and is rarely seen in girls after menarche or in boys after Tanner stage 4. Bilateral slips occur in about 25% of Caucasian and up to 50% of Afro-American children. When unilateral, the left side is more often involved (65%). Endocrine disorders associated with SCFE include hypothyroidism, growth hormone deficiency, hypogonadism and panhypopituitarism.

Clinically, SCFE may be classified based either on duration of symptoms—acute (symptoms for less than 3 weeks); chronic (symptoms for more than 3 weeks); or acute on chronic (symptoms for more than 3 weeks with an acute exacerbation). A second system based on patient mobility classifies SCFE as either stable (patient able to walk with or without crutches) or unstable (patient unable to walk with or without crutches). The condition is most commonly of chronic onset.

Radiography remains the investigation of choice. Klein's line is drawn on the AP projection (Fig. 5-35A) and the slip angle measured on frog lateral radiographs (Fig. 5-35B). Based on the slip angle obtained, SCFE can be classified as mild (≤30°), moderate (31°–50°) or severe (≥51°). It is important to ensure adequate patient positioning if measurements are to be accurate and reliable.[23]

Complications of SCFE include chondrolysis (narrowing of the joint space), AVN and osteoarthritis.

Scoliosis

Scoliosis (a lateral curvature of the spine greater than 10°) may be congenital or idiopathic. In contrast to idiopathic scoliosis, congenital scoliosis is related to a developmental abnormality of the spine. Based on the age of the

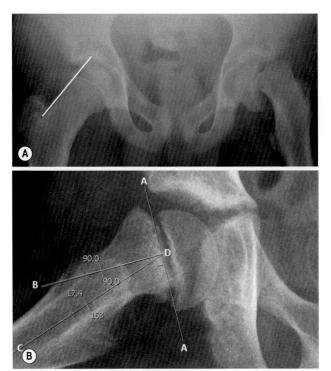

FIGURE 5-35 ■ **Slipped capital femoral epiphysis.** (A) Left slipped capital femoral epiphysis. Klein's line is shown on the right. This line should normally intersect approximately the lateral sixth of the capital femoral epiphysis in the AP projection. (B) The slip angle—between (1) a line [BD] perpendicular to the plane of the growth plate [AA] and (2) a line [CD] parallel to the longitudinal axis of the femoral shaft in the frog lateral projection—is 17.4°.

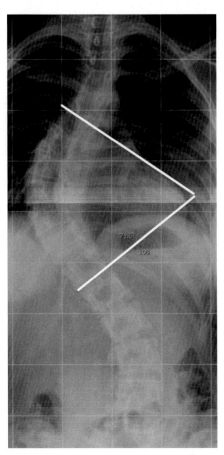

FIGURE 5-36 ■ **Scoliosis concave to the left.** The Cobb angle between the superior end plate of D6 and the inferior end plate of D12 is 71.6°.

patient at diagnosis, idiopathic scoliosis may be further subdivided into infantile (onset before 3 years of age), juvenile (between 3 and 10 years of age) and adolescent (from 10 years to skeletal maturity). The majority of children who present with idiopathic scoliosis do so in the adolescent period.[24] There is a strong hereditary component to idiopathic scoliosis and candidate regions on chromosomes 6, 9, 10 and 16 have been identified.[25,26]

Congenital scoliosis is associated with such vertebral anomalies as hemivertebrae, block vertebrae and butterfly vertebrae. It may be associated with syndromes such as Alagille, spondylocostal and spondylothoracic dysostoses, VACTERL, Goldenhar and Klippel–Feil. Other conditions associated with a scoliosis include connective tissue disorders (Marfan's, Ehlers–Danlos and homocystinuria), neurological conditions (cerebral palsy, tethered cord, neurofibromatosis), and any cause of a leg length discrepancy.

The risk of curve progression depends on the patient's gender (worse in girls), the severity of the curve and the child's growth potential. The latter two may be determined radiographically.

The magnitude of the curve is determined by measuring the Cobb angle (Fig. 5-36). An estimation of growth potential can be made by an assessment of the Tanner stage (clinical) and the Risser grade (radiological; Fig. 5-37). The Risser grade is based on the degree of maturation of the iliac crest apophysis, and gives an estimation

of how much growth remains. It correlates directly with the risk of curve progression.

Cross-sectional imaging (CT and MRI) is useful for the exclusion of underlying vertebral and spinal cord anomalies; indications for cross-sectional imaging include a left thoracic curve, pain, abnormal neurological examination, or other unexpected findings in order to exclude underlying causes such as tumour, syringomyelia or spondylolisthesis.[27]

NEUROCUTANEOUS SYNDROMES

Neurofibromatosis

See Tables 5-1 and 5-6.

Tuberous Sclerosis

Clinical and radiographic features are listed in Table 5-9.

Juvenile Idiopathic Arthritis (JIA)

The 1997 International League of Associations for Rheumatology (ILAR) initial criteria for classification into various JIA subtypes was revised in 2001.[32] JIA is arthritis

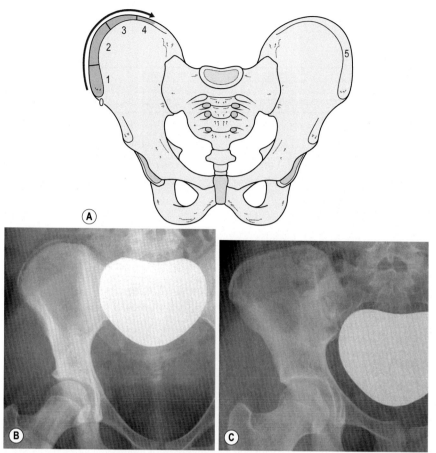

FIGURE 5-37 ■ **Risser grades of maturation of the iliac apophysis.** (A) Grade 0—no ossification. Grades 1 to 4 correspond to sequential 25% increments in ossification. Grade 5 indicates skeletal maturity. (B) Grade 3 in a 12-year-old girl. (C) Grade 4 (very close to complete fusion i.e. grade 5) in a 15-year-old girl.

TABLE 5-9 Clinical and Radiographic Features of Tuberous Sclerosis[30,31]

Clinical Features	Radiographic Features
Adenoma sebaceum	Renal angiomyofibromas[30]
Leukoderma	Cardiac myomas
Shagreen patches	Cyst-like phalangeal lesions
Subungual fibromas	Irregular undulating periosteal reaction along metacarpals and other tubular bones
Café au lait spots	Bone islands in the vertebral bodies and pedicles

of unknown aetiology occurring before the age of 16 years. It is subdivided to include: 'oligoarthritis' (one to four joints affected in the first 6 months of the disease); 'polyarthritis' (more than four joints affected within the first 6 months); 'systemic arthritis' (arthritis accompanied by systemic illness); 'psoriatic arthritis'; 'enthesitis-related arthritis' (often HLA B-27 positive); and 'other arthritis' (disease that does not fall into the listed groups).

The wrist is affected in 61% of patients with polyarticular JIA, being second only to the knee as the most frequently affected joint. The hip and wrist are the most vulnerable joints to radiographically visible destruction.

In some children, isolated involvement of the hips with bilateral protrusio acetabuli has been documented. It has been suggested that this isolated inflammatory coxitis may represent a separate subtype of oligoarthritic JIA.[33]

Joint involvement is characterised by synovial inflammation progressing to synovial hyperplasia and pannus formation. Pannus erodes cartilage and bone and leads to articular destruction and ankylosis. Affected joints are swollen, stiff with reduced motion, painful, erythematous and warm.

The best predictors of poor outcome are severity and extent of joint involvement at onset of disease; early hip and/or wrist involvement; positive rheumatoid factor; and prolonged active disease.[34]

Radiography (Fig. 5-38), dual-energy X-ray absorptiometry (DEXA), ultrasound, CT and MRI are all employed, both for the initial evaluation and diagnosis of patients with JIA and for monitoring response to and complications of therapy.

Radiography allows the assessment of soft-tissue swelling, osteoporosis, erosions, joint destruction and ankylosis. Early in the course of the disease, the presence of effusions causes the joint spaces to appear widened. As disease progresses in severity, the joint spaces are narrowed (seen in the wrist as loss of height of the carpus) until finally there may be bony ankylosis. Inflammation

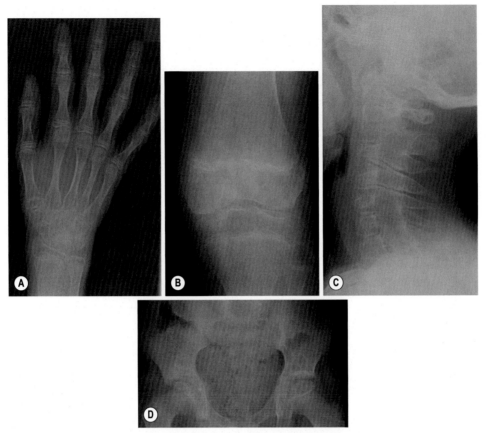

FIGURE 5-38 ■ **Juvenile idiopathic arthritis.** (A) Periarticular osteoporosis, soft-tissue swelling around proximal interphalangeal joints of second to fourth fingers, erosions of carpal bones with loss of joint space of intercarpal and wrist joints. (B) Wide intercondylar notch, reduced bone density, loss of joint space and erosion of the lateral femoral condyle. (C) Ankylosis of the cervical spine. (D) Erosions of both femoral heads, loss of joint spaces and irregular acetabula.

causes hyperaemia with osteopenia, relative overgrowth of the femoral condyles and patella and premature fusion of the epiphyses. The pressure from the hypertrophied synovium causes widening of the intercondylar notch. Evaluation of bone density from digital radiographs has poor sensitivity and interobserver reliability.[35] Other disadvantages of radiography include its low sensitivity for the detection of joint effusions, synovial thickening and differentiation of active from quiescent disease.

MRI has the advantage of not exposing the child to radiation. Furthermore, it allows improved demonstration of articular cartilage, joint effusions, synovial hypertrophy, fibrocartilaginous structures and muscles. Although a recent systematic review concluded that Doppler ultrasound has a higher sensitivity for the identification of synovitis than clinical examination,[36] contrast-enhanced MRI allows assessment of the perfusion of cartilage, synovium and bone and is the most sensitive method for determining whether an arthritic condition is present.[37] Enhancement of thickened synovium suggests active disease and differentiates it from fluid.

AVN is a recognised complication of both JIA and of steroid therapy. The presence of AVN may be determined using either radiography or MRI. Although it is more sensitive than radiography for the detection of early AVN, MRI is said to be less sensitive for the detection of

osteochondral fractures[38]. MRI is also useful for imaging the sacroiliac joints (Fig. 5-39).

Juvenile Dermatomyositis

Juvenile dermatomyositis (JDM) is a multisystem disease defined as affecting those under 18 years of age, although it more commonly affects children aged 2–15 years. It is of unknown aetiology, but both genetic and infectious agents have been implicated. The disease is characterised by a non-suppurative inflammation of skin and skeletal muscle and is associated with a typical (pathognomonic) rash.[39]

Diagnostic criteria include this rash and any three of the following: symmetrical proximal muscle weakness, elevated muscle enzymes, diagnostic histopathology findings and characteristic features on electromyogram (EMG). The latter two are invasive procedures and with the advent of MRI the diagnosis is often based on clinical, laboratory and MRI findings. Indeed, the development of new diagnostic criteria that include MRI findings has been advocated.[40]

Disease activity and response to therapy may be monitored by documenting muscle strength and function, serum muscle enzyme levels, range of joint movement, physician's global assessment and MRI. The Paediatric

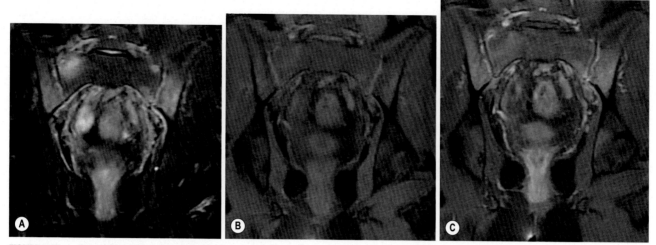

FIGURE 5-39 ■ **Sacroiliitis in a girl with ulcerative colitis.** Coronal fat-saturated T2 (A), coronal T1 (B) and coronal T1 post-gadolinium (C) images show oedema and enhancement of sacroiliac joints and surrounding bones.

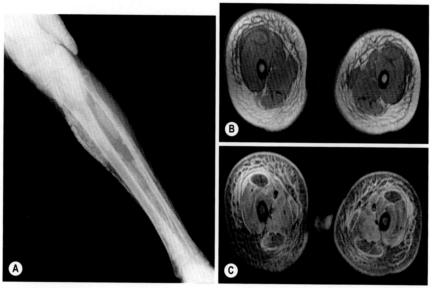

FIGURE 5-40 ■ **Juvenile dermatomyositis.** (A) Significant soft-tissue calcification. (B) T1 axial of both thighs. Marked soft-tissue oedema. (C) Axial STIR image of same patient in (B) more clearly illustrates soft-tissue and muscle oedema and perifascicular fluid.

Rheumatology International Trials Organisation and the Pediatric Rheumatology Collaborative Study Group have recently validated core sets of measures for disease activity and damage assessment in JDM, which bring together several of the tools listed above. However, they include neither ultrasound (because it has not been sufficiently validated), nor MRI (as it is relatively expensive and not universally available).[41]

Abnormal radiographic findings include loss of muscle bulk, disuse osteopenia and soft-tissue calcification (Fig. 5-40A).

Ultrasound will demonstrate oedema of affected muscles, with Doppler highlighting areas of increased vascularity.[42]

The MRI features of active dermatomyositis are best illustrated on axial T1 (Fig. 5-40B) and T2-weighted or inversion recovery (Fig. 5-40C) sequences. Features include increased signal intensity, perimuscular oedema, enhanced chemical-shift artefact and increased signal intensity in subcutaneous fat. More recently it has been shown that the T2 relaxation time can be used as a quantitative measure of muscle inflammation in JDM.[43] Furthermore, a new MRI scoring system has been trialed, is being further developed and may prove useful, particularly as a non-invasive biomarker of response to therapy.[44]

MRI will also demonstrate loss of muscle bulk with relative and absolute increases in subcutaneous fat, fatty infiltration of muscles, and occasionally soft-tissue calcification. The resolution and relapse of signal abnormality during the course of JDM has been documented using serial MRI. However, there have been no controlled studies. Currently there are no recommendations for the timing of MRI in JDM, and it is not known how soon the abnormal signal intensity begins to respond to therapy or when it normalises.

The bisphosphonates are a group of drugs that are pyrophosphate analogues. They act by reducing bone resorption through an inhibitory effect on osteoclast function. Although not yet licensed for children, they are increasingly used in this age group, most commonly to increase bone mass in osteogenesis imperfecta. However, other indications include improvement of bone pain and density in rheumatological conditions such as JIA, JDM and SAPHO (synovitis, acne, palmoplantar pustulosis, hyperostosis and osteitis) syndrome. The radiographic hallmark of bisphosphonate therapy is the presence of dense metaphyseal bands (treatment pulses) alternating with bone of normal density (periods off treatment) (Figs. 5-1 and 5-17F).

NON-INFLAMMATORY DISORDERS

Haemophilia

In this X-linked recessive disorder, a defect in blood coagulation leads to an increased tendency to haemorrhage. Depending on the severity of the disease (and compliance with therapy), bleeding may be spontaneous or occur following relatively mild trauma. Sites of bleeding include the brain, joints, abdomen and retroperitoneal cavity.

Bleeding into the joints is common and usually involves the large joints of the knee (Fig. 5-41A), elbow, ankle (Fig. 5-41B), hip (Fig. 5-41C) and shoulder. Haemarthrosis begins in the first two decades of life, but the number of affected joints stabilises by the age of 20.

Recurrent episodes of intra-articular bleeding cause villous synovial hypertrophy with accumulation of haemosiderin within macrophages. The arthropathy may

progress to cause significant and irreversible cartilage destruction with secondary degenerative disease. Rarely (1–2% of patients), recurrent subperiosteal haemorrhage may become encapsulated and cause bony erosion, giving rise to the so-called haemophilic pseudotumour. This is more common in adult patients.[45]

Based on radiography, five stages of disease may be recognised; however, in any given patient, the chronology may not necessarily follow the stages, nor is progression to the final stages inevitable in all affected joints. The stages are:
- Stage I—soft-tissue swelling and/or joint effusion—normal joint surfaces.
- Stage II—stage I plus periarticular osteoporosis—epiphyseal overgrowth.
- Stage III—erosions, sclerosis and subchondral cysts—joint spaces preserved.
- Stage IV—stage III plus focal/diffuse joint space narrowing.
- Stage V—stiff contracted joint with significant degenerative change.

Although CT and US may be used in the assessment of haemophilic arthropathy, MRI (with its ability to demonstrate early disease, including synovial abnormality, ligamentous tears, periarticular bleeding, cartilaginous and osseous bruising, erosions and joint space narrowing) is the investigation of choice and classification systems based on MRI findings have been developed.[46–48] Intra-articular haemorrhage will usually be evident as a joint effusion; fluid–fluid levels may be demonstrated. Gradient-echo sequences will more readily demonstrate deposits of haemosiderin compared to spin-echo sequences (due to magnetic susceptibility artefact). Three-dimensional spoiled gradient-echo and fast spin-echo sequences allow early identification of focal cartilage defects and thinning.

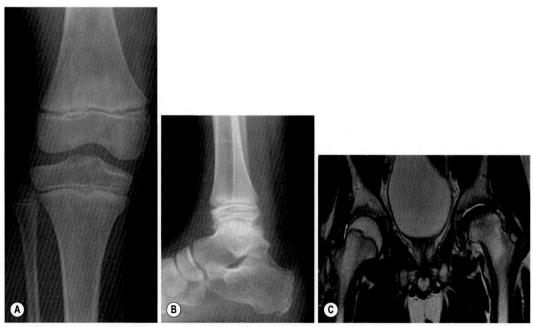

FIGURE 5-41 ■ **Haemophilia.** (A) Wide intercondylar notch. (B) Destructive change secondary to bleeding into the ankle joint. (C) Avascular necrosis of the left capital femoral epiphysis in another patient.

Pigmented Villonodular Synovitis

Pigmented villonodular synovitis (PVNS) refers to benign villous or nodular proliferation of synovium of uncertain aetiology. It most commonly affects a single joint, with the knee being involved in 80%. Although most patients present in the third and fourth decades of life, the disease may also present in childhood. Synovial joints, tendon sheaths, or bursae may be involved.

Presentation is with a slow-growing painless mass that may be tender to palpation. In long-standing cases there may be destruction of cartilage, secondary degenerative change and pain.

Radiographic findings include soft-tissue swelling, joint space narrowing and bony erosion (particularly in the hip where subchondral cysts with sclerotic rims are typical). Calcification is rare.

Non-enhanced CT will show high attenuation due to haemosiderin within the mass. The synovial proliferation enhances following administration of contrast medium.

Diagnostic MRI features include a nodular lesion with areas of haemosiderin (low signal on all sequences) and haemorrhage. Joint effusions and bony erosions are well demonstrated. As with CT, contrast enhancement is typical.

The differential diagnosis includes haemophilia and synovial haemangioma (rare, phleboliths in soft tissue).[49]

Synovial Osteochondromatosis

This benign condition is characterised by synovial membrane proliferation and metaplasia. Fragments of proliferated synovium detach from the synovial surface into the joint, where, nourished by synovial fluid, the fragments may grow, calcify or ossify. The intra-articular fragments may vary in size from a few millimetres to a few centimetres. The extent of calcification seen on radiographs (Fig. 5-42) is variable, and may underestimate the degree of intra-articular bodies. The calcified bodies are well depicted by CT and ultrasound. Although the fragments will appear as foci of reduced signal on MRI (not well seen on gradient-echo sequences),[50] the condition may be confused with PVNS if radiographs or CT is not available. Other features include synovial hypertrophy, joint effusions and changes of osteoarthritis.

METABOLIC AND ENDOCRINE DISORDERS

Metabolic Disorders

Rickets

Rickets is osteomalacia in children. There is an excess of unmineralised osteoid. The serum alkaline phosphatase is elevated, while serum and urinary calcium and phosphate levels are low. Serum levels of calcium and phosphate are controlled in part by vitamin D.

The active form of vitamin D (cholecalciferol) is 1,25-dihydroxy-D_3. Hydroxylation of D_3 occurs first in the liver at the 25-position, and then in the kidney (regulated by parathyroid hormone) at the 1-position. It acts

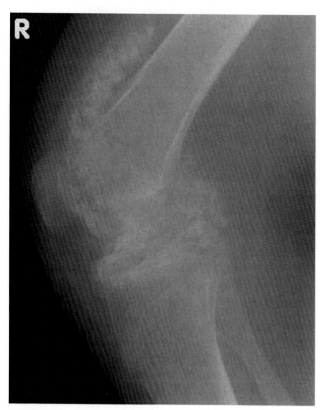

FIGURE 5-42 ■ **Synovial osteochondromatosis.** Multiple calcified intra-articular loose bodies.

(with parathyroid hormone) on bone to stimulate the release of calcium and phosphate from osteoclasts; it stimulates intestinal absorption of calcium and phosphate; it inhibits secretion of parathyroid hormone; and, finally, it stimulates renal tubular re-absorption of phosphate.

The radiographic features of rickets are best seen at sites of rapid growth (metaphyses and epiphyses of the distal radius, ulna and femur and proximal humerus and tibia (Fig. 5-43)). Features include widening and cupping of the metaphyses, which have irregular, frayed margins. There is apparent widening of the physis (due to the unossified zone of provisional calcification). The epiphyses have indistinct margins and are relatively osteopenic. Looser zones may be seen, particularly at the pubic rami, medial margins of the proximal femora, posterior aspects of the proximal ulnae, axillary margins of the scapulae and the ribs. The 'rachitic rosary' occurs as a result of expansion of the costochondral junctions.

Complications include bowing of the long bones (bone softening, especially of the lower limbs), irregular vertebral end plates and fractures. It should be noted that, in a recent study, fractures in children with rickets were only present in those with radiographic evidence of rickets.[51]

Renal Osteodystrophy

Chronic renal failure causes rickets as a result of failure of hydroxylation of inactive 1-hydroxy-D_3 to the active 1,25-dihydroxy-D_3 within the renal glomeruli. In chronic renal failure there is retention of phosphate and hypocalcaemia, which leads to parathyroid hyperplasia and

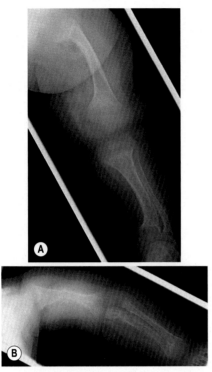

FIGURE 5-43 ▪ **Severe nutritional rickets.** Marked reduction in bone density with bowing deformity. Cupped frayed metaphyses with wide growth plates. Pathological fractures of the humerus and ulna.

secondary hyperparathyroidism. In addition there is reduced gastrointestinal absorption of calcium and end-organ resistance to parathyroid hormone. Serum phosphate and alkaline phosphatase are elevated, while serum calcium is normal or low.

Radiologically, in addition to features of rickets, those of secondary hyperparathyroidism (osteosclerosis, acro-osteolysis and subperiosteal bone resorption) are also present.

Vitamin D-Dependent Rickets

In these autosomal recessive conditions, vitamin D levels are not reduced. Type I is due to a defect in 1-α-hydroxylase, while in Type II vitamin D-dependent rickets there is end-organ resistance to 1,25-dihydroxy-D$_3$. Patients may have alopecia and abnormal dentition.

Vitamin D-Resistant Rickets

In these disorders renal tubular re-absorption of phosphate is defective. Renal excretion of calcium and phosphate is increased. Serum vitamin D levels are normal or even elevated. X-linked hypophosphatasia, vitamin D-resistant rickets with glycosuria (defective glucose and phosphate resorption), Fanconi's syndrome and acquired hypophosphataemic syndrome are the four conditions in which vitamin D-resistant or -refractory rickets may be seen.

Tumour Rickets

Certain tumours are thought to secrete a phosphaturic substance with consequent elevation in urine phosphate

and alkaline phosphatase. Serum calcium is normal. Implicated tumours include haemangiopericytoma, linear sebaceous naevus syndrome, non-ossifying fibroma, giant cell tumour, osteoblastoma, fibrous dysplasia and mixed sclerosing dysplasia. Resection of the tumour leads to resolution of the rickets.

Neonatal Rickets

Radiographic features of neonatal rickets are not usually seen before 6 months of age. Rickets may develop in the neonate because dietary levels of calcium, phosphate and vitamin D cannot meet the needs of a rapidly growing skeleton. Rickets occurring in preterm infants on parenteral nutrition is now relatively uncommon as a result of supplements in feeds.

Scurvy

In this condition there is deficiency (usually dietary) of vitamin C (ascorbic acid). Infants typically present between 6 and 9 months of age. There is defective osteoid production by osteoblasts with reduced endochondral bone ossification.

The bones are osteopenic with relatively dense margins (white lines of scurvy) where mineralisation of osteoid continues. In the epiphyses this pencil outline is termed the 'Wimberger' sign. Other features include metaphyseal (pelcan) spurs, which may fracture, exuberant periosteal reaction (recurrent subperiosteal bleeding), lucent metaphyseal bands and increased density of the end of the metaphyses (white line of Fraenk).

MRI may show broad bands of abnormal metaphyseal signal (low on T1- and high on T2-weighted sequences),[52] or more diffuse marrow signal abnormality. Marrow change may be isolated or coexistent with subperiosteal collections and muscle signal abnormality.

Gaucher's Disease

This autosomal recessive storage disorder occurs most frequently in Ashkenazi Jews. The deficient enzyme is glucocerebrosidase. Glucocerebroside accumulates in the reticuloendothelial system and the bone marrow is infiltrated by lipid-laden Gaucher cells. Infantile and juvenile forms are associated with mental retardation and early death. A milder adolescent form presents in childhood or early adulthood.

Radiological features include osteopenia, bone infarcts, AVN (particularly of the femoral head), flattening of the vertebral bodies, which may be significant (vertebra plana), Erlenmeyer flask deformity of the femora and localised lytic bone lesions (focal deposition of Gaucher cells).

Radiology helps to estimate disease burden, detect skeletal complications and monitor response to treatment. In children, physiological conversion of red to yellow marrow may cause confusion when interpreting MRIs. Radiologists should be aware of the patterns of conversion of low-signal red marrow to high-signal fatty marrow.[53,54]

Endocrine Disorders

Hyperparathyroidism

In hyperthyroidism serum phosphate is decreased, serum calcium and alkaline phosphatase increased, and urine calcium and phosphate increased.

Primary hyperthyroidism is due to a parathyroid adenoma or may occur in multiple endocrine neoplasia and is rare in children. Secondary hyperthyroidism is seen in chronic renal failure and tertiary hyperthyroidism occurs when the parathyroid glands become resistant to the regulatory effects of serum calcium (usually in patients on haemodialysis).

Radiographs reveal features either of bone resorption and/or bone formation. Sites of bone resorption include:
- subperiosteal (radial sides of phalanges)
- subchondral (sacroiliac joints, acromioclavicular joints, with resorption of the acromial ends of the clavicle and symphysis pubis)
- subligamentous (calcaneum at the site of insertion of the Achilles tendon)
- trabecular (diploic space causing a 'salt and pepper' skull)
- intracortical (intracortical tunnelling/striations)
- endosteal.

Additional findings include osteosclerosis (localised or diffuse), rugger-jersey spine, brown tumours, chondrocalcinosis and soft-tissue and vascular calcification.

Neonatal hyperparathyroidism (Fig. 5-44) may occur as a primary disorder or as a result of poorly controlled maternal hypoparathyroidism, pseudohypoparathyroidism, hypocalcaemia, vitamin D deficiency, chronic renal failure and renal tubular acidosis. Radiological features in these infants with failure to thrive include severe osteopenia with an increased tendency to fracture, coarse trabeculae, metaphyseal cupping, metaphyseal spurs and subperiosteal resorption. It may be associated with severe respiratory distress and death. Intrauterine fractures may rarely occur.

Hypoparathyroidism

A reduced level of parathyroid hormone causes hypocalcaemia, hypophosphataemia and neuromuscular malfunction. It may be idiopathic or occur after surgical removal, disease, or trauma.

Radiographs demonstrate osteosclerosis, skull vault thickening, soft-tissue calcification, calcification of the basal ganglia, hypoplastic dentition and thickened lamina dura. Less commonly, osteoporosis, dense metaphyseal bands, dense vertebral end plates, premature fusion of the growth plates, vertebral hyperostosis and enthesopathy may occur.

Pseudohypoparathyroidism and Pseudo-Pseudohypoparathyroidismm

Features in common with hypoparathyroidism include osteosclerosis, dense metaphyseal bands and calcification of the soft tissues and basal ganglia. Secondary hyperparathyroidism may be seen in 10% of patients with

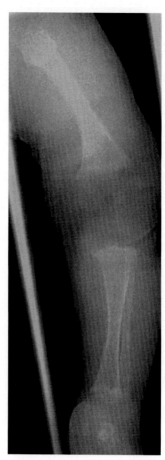

FIGURE 5-44 ■ **Neonatal hyperparathyroidism.** Reduced bone density and metaphyseal spurs.

pseudo-hypoparathyroidism (PHP), but is never seen in pseudo-pseudohypoparathyroidism (PPHP).

Both PHP and PPHP are caused by epigenetic (imprinting) mutations in GNAS.[55]
1. PHP type 1a: Albright's hereditary osteodystrophy (AHO). This is caused by specific loss of function mutations inherited from the mother. There is end-organ resistance to normal or increased serum levels of parathyroid and other hormones. Clinically there is obesity, short stature and a rounded facies. Hypocalcaemia results in muscular tetany. Radiological features include exostoses and brachydactyly (short fourth (and fifth) fingers and toes (Fig. 5-45)) with a positive metacarpal sign (a line joining the heads of the little and middle fingers fails to intersect the head of the fourth metacarpal).
2. Inheritance of the same GNAS mutations from the father gives rise to PPHP. These patients have the skeletal phenotype of PHP; however, serum calcium and phosphate levels are normal. Cone-shaped epiphyses of the tubular bones of the hands and feet fuse prematurely, causing brachydactyly.
3. PHP type 1b is due to a different GNAS mutation, and has no skeletal manifestations. Patients have end-organ resistance to parathyroid hormone.

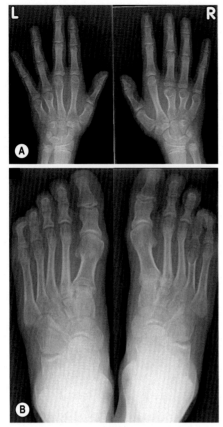

FIGURE 5-45 ■ **Pseudohypoparathyroidism.** (A) Short left fourth and fifth, right third to fifth and both first metacarpals. (B) Short right fourth metatarsal.

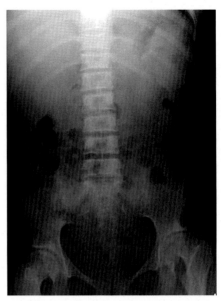

FIGURE 5-46 ■ **Sickle cell anaemia.** Cod fish vertebrae and bilateral avascular necrosis of the femoral heads.

Hypothyroidism

In all types of hypothyroidism (infantile, juvenile and adult) there is either deficiency, or failure, of end-organ response to thyroxine. A mutation in the thyroid hormone receptor alpha gene causing end-organ resistance to thyroxine and presenting with recognised radiographic features of hypothyroidism has recently been identified.[56]

Radiological features in the paediatric age group include delayed bone age, delay in appearance of secondary ossification centres, epiphyseal fragmentation, stippling and short stature. Additional findings include osteoporosis, multiple Wormian bones, delay in closure of the sutures and fontanelles, delayed dentition, dense metaphyseal bands, shortened long bones, increased atlantoaxial distance, kyphosis at the thoracolumbar junction and an increased incidence of slipped capital femoral epiphysis.

TOXIC DISORDERS

Fluorosis

Radiologically, fluorosis manifests as a generalised increase in bone density, particularly of the axial skeleton. There is periosteal proliferation, ligamentous calcification, degenerative enthesopathy and fractures. In children, exposure before the age of 8 years causes patchy opaque areas of the enamel of permanent teeth.

Lead Poisoning

This manifests radiologically as dense metaphyseal bands. Other features include widened sutures (raised intracranial pressure) and radio-opacities on abdominal radiographs (ingested lead).

HAEMOGLOBINOPATHIES

Sickle Cell Disease

Bone pain is the most common reason for hospital admission of patients with sickle cell disease. Thromboembolic infarcts and haemolysis (with chronic anaemia and secondary marrow expansion) is the underlying pathophysiology of the skeletal complications that occur.

Acute bony involvement includes bone infarcts, osteomyelitis, stress fractures, vertebral collapse, bone marrow necrosis, orbital compression (infarction of the orbital bone) and dental complications (caries, mandibular osteomyelitis). Chronic complications include osteoporosis (secondary to marrow hyperplasia), AVN, chronic arthritis and growth failure.[57]

Bone infarcts of the small bones of the hands and feet will lead to dactylitis; of the vertebral end plates to the so-called 'cod fish' or 'H-shaped' vertebrae (Fig. 5-46); of the epiphyses will lead to joint effusions and AVN. Osteomyelitis is common, with *Salmonella* species being isolated in up to 70%. The infection most commonly involves the diaphysis of the humerus, femur and tibia (Fig. 5-47A).

The diagnostic challenge is to differentiate acute osteomyelitis from vaso-occlusive disease. Imaging findings may be very similar. The presence of a collection or

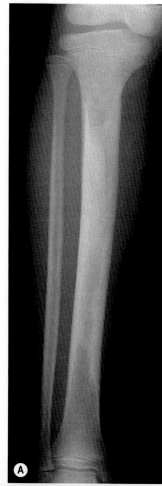

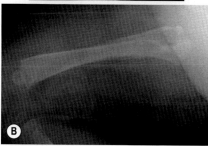

FIGURE 5-47 ■ **Osteomyelitis.** (A) Low-grade infection in a child with sickle cell anaemia showing sclerosis of the tibia. (B) Radiolucency of the proximal femoral metaphysis and periosteal reaction along the proximal femoral shaft in an infant with acute osteomyelitis.

of a break in the cortex makes infection more likely than simple infarction.

Thalassaemia

Skeletal changes in thalassaemia arise from the chronic anaemia associated with the condition.

In the skull, there is widening of the diploic spaces (low signal on all MRI sequences), with thinning of the outer table of the skull vault. The trabecular markings are oriented perpendicular to the inner and outer tables

and on plain radiographs give rise to the 'hair-on-end' appearance. There is frontal bossing and overgrowth of the facial bones with reduced pneumatisation of the paranasal sinuses. The so-called 'rodent facies' arises from marrow hyperplasia in the maxillae, causing lateral displacement of the orbits and ventral displacement of the central incisors.

In the spine there may be marked osteoporosis and cortical thinning, resulting in fractures of the vertebral bodies and platyspondyly. Imaging may reveal paraspinal masses (as a result of extramedullary haematopoiesis). Cord compression can result if these masses extend into the extradural space. MRI findings are secondary to blood transfusion and chelation therapy.

There may be expansion of the head and neck of the ribs and osteoporosis. A rib within a rib appearance may result. Extramedullary haematopoiesis can cause erosions of the inner cortex of the ribs or manifest as a posterior mediastinal soft-tissue mass.

Premature fusion of the growth plates (particularly of the proximal humerus and distal femur) is a recognised feature. Irregular sclerosis at the metaphyses and anterior rib ends is a recognised complication of treatment with desferrioxamine.[58]

INFECTION OF THE BONES AND JOINTS

Osteomyelitis

Infection may reach the bone through the bloodstream (haematogenous), from direct implantation (e.g. penetrating injury, surgery), or from infection elsewhere adjacent to bone (e.g. soft tissues). Because of the rich blood supply, osteomyelitis of the long bones in children most commonly affects the metaphyses. In infants, metaphyseal vessels penetrate the growth plate, and therefore in this age group there is a higher incidence of epiphyseal and joint involvement.

Infection of the bones may be acute, subacute (Brodie's abscess) or chronic.

Acute osteomyelitis is most commonly seen in infants (*Staphylococcus aureus*, *Escherichia coli*) and young children (*S. aureus*, *Streptococcus pyogenes*, *Haemophilus influenzae*). Patients with sickle cell disease are more disposed to *Salmonella* infection. Subacute and chronic osteomyelitis result from incomplete eradication of infection following acute osteomyelitis, or from infection by less virulent organisms. Mycobacterial osteomyelitis occurs from haematogenous spread in a patient with primary tuberculosis. Fungal causes include coccidioidomycosis, blastomycosis and cryptococcosis.

In acute disease there is oedema, vascular congestion and thrombosis of small vessels. Clinical features include fever, irritability, lethargy and local signs including swelling, erythema and warmth (inflammation). If not treated promptly (or aggressively), the vascular compromise leads to areas of dead bone (sequestra), which are the hallmark of chronic infection.[59,60] Periosteal new bone formation is another feature of chronic osteomyelitis. This new bone (involucrum) encases areas of live bone. Pus may track from the medullary cavity through gaps in the involucrum into the soft tissues. These tracks may eventually penetrate the skin surface (sinus tracts).

Radiographic changes (Fig. 5-47B) may not be apparent for up to 2 weeks after the onset of disease, and therefore radiographs may appear entirely normal. More specific signs include soft-tissue swelling, cortical irregularity (bony destruction) and periosteal reaction. A Brodie's abscess may be seen as a well-defined lytic lesion with a sclerotic rim. In chronic infection, sequestra appear as dense foci, and soft-tissue wasting and sinus tracts may be appreciated. Even on appropriate therapy, radiographic signs of improvement may lag behind clinical recovery. Spina ventosa implies tuberculous dactylitis. Radiographically there are cyst-like cavities associated with diaphyseal expansion. It more commonly affects the bones of the hands than the feet.[61]

High-resolution US provides a simple and non-invasive assessment of infants and children with osteomyelitis. US helps to localise the site and extent of disease, and to confirm the presence and degree of the fluid component of the abscess, and provides guidance for interventional procedures. Chau and Griffith provide a useful review of the US appearances of musculoskeletal infection.[62]

Skeletal scintigraphy is useful if multifocal infection is suspected.

CT helps to define the extent of cortical destruction and to exclude the presence of sequestra.

MRI has the highest sensitivity and specificity for detecting osteomyelitis in children. In subacute infection a characteristic penumbra sign may be recognised.[63] This consists of a peripheral relatively high-signal ring (granulation tissue) surrounding a low-signal central zone (abscess cavity). Enhanced fat-suppressed sequences show avid enhancement of the granulation tissue. Contrast medium also helps to identify soft-tissue abscesses. On T2-weighted sequences the high signal of reactive oedema may exaggerate the extent of infection.

Complications include joint destruction, damage to growth plates and resorption of bone (Fig. 5-48), resulting in limb-length discrepancies, angular deformity and premature osteoarthritis.

Chronic Recurrent Multifocal Osteomyelitis

This is a condition of unknown aetiology characterised by a fluctuating clinical course of relapses and remissions. It affects multiple sites (synchronous or metachronous) and most commonly involves the long bones, clavicle, spine and pelvis. The ribs and sternum may also be affected. No causative agent is found. When associated with acne and palmoplanter pustulosis it is termed SAPHO syndrome.

Radiographic features (Fig. 5-49) suggest subacute or chronic osteomyelitis; however, abscess formation, involucra and sinus tracts are not a feature. In the tubular bones lytic metaphyseal lesions sometimes extending to the diaphysis are typical. Quiescent periods are characterised by bony expansion and sclerosis. In the clavicle, lytic medullary lesions are a feature of active disease, with expansion and sclerosis again being features of a

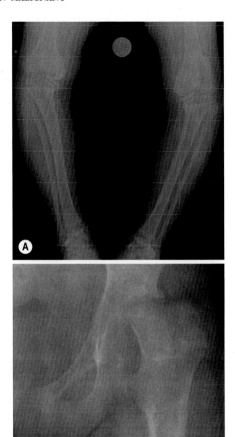

FIGURE 5-48 ■ **Complications of infection.** (A) Premature fusion of the distal femoral and proximal tibial growth plates with genu varum following meningococcal septicaemia (bilateral knee and ankle arthrograms were performed prior to obtaining this image). (B) Almost complete resorption of the femoral head following infective arthritis.

quiescent phase. Chronic recurrent multifocal osteomyelitis (CRMO) manifests in the spine as loss of height of the affected vertebral bodies and is a differential diagnosis of vertebra plana.

Bone scintigraphy is useful for the detection of asymptomatic lesions. MRI, by failing to demonstrate abscesses and sinus tracts, excludes chronic osteomyelitis. Active disease is confirmed by the presence of high signal marrow on T2/STIR sequences.

Infective Arthritis

As with osteomyelitis, infection may spread to joints via the bloodstream, direct inoculation, or spread from a contiguous site. The most common organism is *S. aureus*. Imaging features (Fig. 5-50) include soft-tissue swelling, oedema and joint effusion. In infants, effusions may lead to dislocation (particularly in the hip joint). Other findings include metaphyseal irregularity, destruction and avascular necrosis. Septic arthritis in children is a clinical emergency, and early drainage is required to prevent severe bony destruction with resultant shortening and deformity. In this regard US is helpful, both to exclude

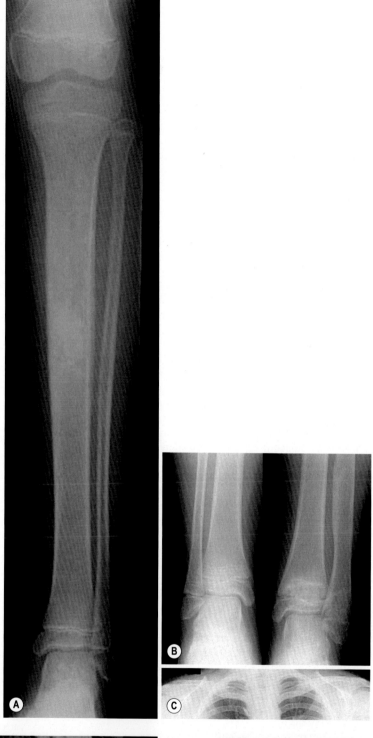

FIGURE 5-49 ■ **Chronic recurrent multifocal osteomyelitis.** (A) Periosteal reaction with sclerosis of the mid-tibial shaft. (B) Lucent lesions with a permeative appearance adjacent to the growth plates of the left distal tibia and fibula. Broad left distal fibula with cortical thickening. (C) Broad medial ends of the clavicles (right more than left).

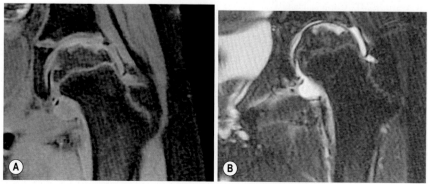

FIGURE 5-50 ■ **Infective arthritis in a child with thalassaemia.** Coronal fat-saturated T1 (A) and T2 (B) images show a joint effusion and avascular necrosis of the femoral head.

the presence of an effusion (a difference of 1–2 mm between the two sides is suggestive) and to assist in its drainage.

Infection of the Spine (Discitis and Osteomyelitis)

Discitis refers to infection of the intervertebral disc space, whereas osteomyelitis of the spine implies pyogenic destruction of the vertebral body, which may then spread to involve the disc. Differentiation of the two is important, as management may differ. Discitis can involve any spinal level, but most commonly affects the lumbar region in children younger than 5 years of age.[64] Generally children with discitis are younger, and clinically less toxic than those with osteomyelitis.[64] Children with either condition will present with back pain, refusal to mobilise, or irritability depending on age at presentation. Although there is much debate as to the aetiology of discitis, a low-grade infection has been postulated. In 70% of cases, the causative organism is not identified. When an organism is cultured, it is most commonly *S. aureus*. In discitis, radiological changes are confined to the disc and adjacent vertebral end plates, in comparison to osteomyelitis, in which the disease begins in and destroys the vertebral body. Infection may then spread to an adjacent vertebral body either via the intervertebral disc or via the subligamentous spread of pus (e.g. in spinal tuberculosis).

In discitis, radiographs/CT of the spine show characteristic features, including loss of disc height and irregularity of the adjacent vertebral end plates. Vertebral body height is preserved. It has been suggested that in the clinical context of suspected discitis, further imaging is not required if the radiographs demonstrate characteristic findings. However, if radiographs are normal or equivocal, or the child is toxic (suggesting spinal osteomyelitis), then further imaging is indicated.[65]

MRI can exclude intraspinal or other soft-tissue (e.g. psoas) collections. T1 sagittal and axial and T2 sagittal views are often sufficient. In equivocal cases, intravenous administration of contrast medium may be helpful. The pattern of enhancement may aid in differentiating tuberculous spondylitis (avid, heterogeneous rim enhancement, involving several vertebral bodies) from vertebral osteomyelitis. However, regardless of the pattern of enhancement, tissue should be obtained for microbiological examination, usually by CT-guided biopsy.

REFERENCES

1. Warman ML, Cormier-Daire V, Hall C, et al. Nosology and classification of genetic skeletal disorders: 2010 revision. Am J Med Genet A 2011;155A:943–68.
2. Offiah AC, Hall CM. Radiological diagnosis of the constitutional disorders of bone. As easy as A, B, C? Pediatr Radiol 2003;33:153–61.
3. Winter Baraitser Dysmorphology Database (WBDD). Available from London Medical Databases <http://www.lmdatabases.com>. Accessed April 2012.
4. European Skeletal Dysplasia Network (ESDN). Available from <http://www.esdn.org>. Accessed April 2012.
5. Digital radiological electronic atlas for malformation syndromes (dREAMS). Available from <http://www.d-reams.org>. Accessed April 2012.
6. Victoria T, Epelman M, Bebbington M, et al. Low-dose fetal CT for evaluation of severe congenital skeletal anomalies: preliminary experience. Pediatr Radiol 2012;42(Suppl. 1):S142–9.
7. Applegate KE. Can MR imaging be used to characterize fetal musculoskeletal development? Radiology 2004;233:305–6.
8. Cannie MM, Jani JC, Van Kerkhove F, et al. Fetal body volume at MR imaging to quantify total fetal lung volume: normal ranges. Radiology 2008;247:197–203.
9. Laker SR, Concannon LG. Radiologic evaluation of the neck: a review of radiography, ultrasonography, computed tomography, magnetic resonance imaging, and other imaging modalities for neck pain. Phys Med Rehabil Clin N Am 2011;22:411–28.
10. Dilli A, Ayaz UY, Damar C, et al. Sprengel deformity: magnetic resonance imaging findings in two pediatric cases. J Clin Imaging Sci 2011;1:13.
11. Shorter D, Hong T, Osborn DA. Screening programmes for developmental dysplasia of the hip in newborn infants. Cochrane Database Syst Rev 2011;CD004595.
12. Roposch A, Liu LQ, Offiah AC, et al. Functional outcomes in children with osteonecrosis secondary to treatment of developmental dysplasia of the hip. J Bone Joint Surg Am 2011;93:e145.
13. Biko DM, Davidson R, Pena A, Jaramillo D. Proximal focal femoral deficiency: evaluation by MR imaging. Pediatr Radiol 2012;42:50–6.
14. Cheema JI, Grissom LE, Harcke HT. Radiographic characteristics of lower-extremity bowing in children. Radiographics 2003;23:871–80.
15. Jouve JL, Kohler R, Mubarak SJ, et al. Focal fibrocartilaginous dysplasia ('fibrous periosteal inclusion'): an additional series of eleven cases and literature review. J Pediatr Orthop 2007;27:75–84.
16. Cardy AH, Sharp L, Torrance N, et al. Is there evidence for aetiologically distinct subgroups of idiopathic congenital talipes equinovarus? A case-only study and pedigree analysis. PLoS One 2011;6:e17895.
17. Wiig O, Svenningsen S, Terjesen T. Evaluation of the subchondral fracture in predicting the extent of femoral head necrosis in Perthes disease: a prospective study of 92 patients. J Pediatr Orthop B 2004;13:293–8.
18. Wiig O, Terjesen T, Svenningsen S. Interobserver reliability of radiographic classifications and measurements in the assessment of Perthes disease. Acta Orthop Scand 2002;73:523–30.
19. Mahnken AH, Staatz G, Ihme N, Gunther RW. MR signal intensity characteristics in Legg–Calve–Perthés disease. Value of fat-suppressed (STIR) images and contrast-enhanced T1-weighted images. Acta Radiol 2002;43:329–35.
20. Lamer S, Dorgeret S, Khairouni A, et al. Femoral head vascularisation in Legg–Calve–Perthés disease: comparison of dynamic gadolinium-enhanced subtraction MRI with bone scintigraphy. Pediatr Radiol 2002;32:580–5.
21. Merlini L, Combescure C, De Rosa V, et al. Diffusion-weighted imaging findings in Perthes disease with dynamic gadolinium-enhanced subtracted (DGS) MR correlation: a preliminary study. Pediatr Radiol 2010;40:318–25.
22. Loder RT. Unstable slipped capital femoral epiphyses. J Pediatr Orthop 2001;21:694–9.
23. Richolt JA, Hata N, Kikinis R, et al. Quantitative evaluation of angular measurements on plain radiographs in patients with slipped capital femoral epiphysis: a 3-dimensional analysis of computed tomography-based computer models of 46 femora. J Pediatr Orthop 2008;28:291–6.
24. Reamy BV, Slakey JB. Adolescent idiopathic scoliosis: Review and current concepts. Am Fam Physician 2001;64:111–16.
25. Miller NH, Justice CM, Marosy B, et al. Identification of candidate regions for familial idiopathic scoliosis. Spine 2005;30:1181–7.
26. Marosy B, Justice CM, Vu C, et al. Identification of susceptibility loci for scoliosis in FIS families with triple curves. Am J Med Genet 2010;152A:846–55.
27. Thomsen M, Abel R. Imaging in scoliosis from the orthopaedic surgeon's point of view. Eur J Radiol 2006;58:41–7.
28. Vitale MG, Guha A, Skaggs DL. Orthopaedic manifestations of neurofibromatosis in children: an update. Clin Orthop Relat Res 2002;402:107–18.
29. Jacquemin C, Bosley TM, Liu D, et al. Reassessment of sphenoid dysplasia associated with neurofibromatosis type 1. Am J Neuroradiol 2002;23:644–8.

30. Casper KA, Donnelly LF, Chan B, et al. Tuberous sclerosis complex: renal imaging findings. Radiology 2002;225:451–6.

31. Morris BS, Garg A, Jadhav PJ. Tuberous sclerosis: a presentation of less commonly encountered stigmata. Australas Radiol 2002;46: 426–30.

32. Petty RE, Southwood TR, Manners P, et al; (International League of Associations for Rheumatology). International League of Associations for Rheumatology classification of juvenile idiopathic arthritis: second revision, Edmonton, 2001. J Rheumatol 2004;31: 390–2.

33. Adib N, Owers KL, Witt JD, et al. Isolated inflammatory coxitis with protrusio acetabuli: a new form of juvenile idiopathic arthritis? Rheumatology 2005;44:219–26.

34. Ravelli A, Martini A. Early predictors of outcome in juvenile idiopathic arthritis. Clin Exp Rheumatol 2003;21:S89–93.

35. Mulugeta PG, Jordanov M, Hernanz-Schulman M, et al. Determination of osteopenia in children on digital radiography compared with a DEXA reference standard. Acad Radiol 2011;18:722–5.

36. Collado P, Jousse-Joulin S, Alcalde M, et al. Is ultrasound a validated imaging tool for the diagnosis and management of synovitis in juvenile idiopathic arthritis? A systematic literature review. Arthritis Care Res 2012;64(7):1011–19.

37. Lamer S, Sebag GH. MRI and ultrasound in children with juvenile chronic arthritis. Eur J Radiol 2000;33:85–93.

38. Stevens K, Tao C, Lee S-U, et al. Subchondral fractures in osteonecrosis of the femoral head: comparison of radiography, CT and MR imaging. Am J Roentgenol 2003;180:363–8.

39. Martin N, Krol P, Smith S, et al; Juvenile Dermatomyositis Research Group. A national registry for juvenile dermatomyositis and other paediatric idiopathic inflammatory myopathies: 10 years' experience; the Juvenile Dermatomyositis National (UK and Ireland) Cohort Biomarker Study and Repository for Idiopathic Inflammatory Myopathies. Rheumatology 2011;50:137–45.

40. McCann LJ, Juggins AD, Maillard SM, et al; Juvenile Dermatomyositis Research Group. The Juvenile Dermatomyositis National Registry and Repository (UK and Ireland)–clinical characteristics of children recruited within the first 5 yr. Rheumatology 2006;45: 1255–60.

41. Ruperto N, Ravelli A, Pistorio A, et al; Paediatric Rheumatology International Trials Organisation (PRINTO); Pediatric Rheumatology Collaborative Study Group (PRCSG). The provisional Paediatric Rheumatology International Trials Organisation/American College of Rheumatology/European League Against Rheumatism Disease activity core set for the evaluation of response to therapy in juvenile dermatomyositis: a prospective validation study. Arthritis Rheum 2008;59:4–13.

42. Walker UA. Imaging tools for the clinical assessment of idiopathic inflammatory myositis. Curr Opin Rheumatol 2008;20:656–61.

43. Maillard SM, Jones R, Owens C, et al. Quantitative assessment of MRI T2 relaxation time of thigh muscles in juvenile dermatomyositis. Rheumatology 2004;43:603–8.

44. Davis WR, Halls JE, Offiah AC, et al. Assessment of active inflammation in juvenile dermatomyositis: a novel magnetic resonance imaging-based scoring system. Rheumatology 2011;50: 2237–44.

45. Kerr R. Imaging of the musculoskeletal complications of hemophilia. Semin Musculoskelet Radiol 2003;7:127–36.

46. Kilcoyne RF, Nuss R. Radiological assessment of haemophilic arthropathy with emphasis on MRI findings. Haemophilia 2003; 9(Suppl. 1):57–63.

47. Lundin B, Babyn P, Doria AS, et al. Compatible scales for progressive and additive MRI assessments of haemophilic arthropathy. Haemophilia 2005;11:109–15.

48. Doria AS, Lundin B, Kilcoyne RF, et al. Reliability of progressive and additive MRI scoring systems for evaluation of haemophilic arthropathy in children: expert MRI Working Group of the International Prophylaxis Study Group. Haemophilia 2005;11:245–53.

49. Masih S, Antebi A. Imaging of pigmented villonodular synovitis. Semin Musculoskelet Radiol 2003;7:205–16.

50. Kim HK, Zbojniewicz AM, Merrow AC, et al. MR findings of synovial disease in children and young adults: Part 1. Pediatr Radiol 2011;41:495–511.

51. Chapman T, Sugar N, Done S, et al. Fractures in infants and toddlers with rickets. Pediatr Radiol 2010;40:1184–9.

52. Brennan CM, Atkins KA, Druzgal CH, et al. Magnetic resonance imaging appearance of scurvy with gelatinous bone marrow transformation. Skeletal Radiol 2012;41:357–60.

53. Maas M, Poll WL, Terk MR. Imaging and quantifying skeletal involvement in Gaucher disease. Br J Radiol 2002;75(Suppl. 1): A13–24.

54. Bembi B, Ciana G, Mengel E, et al. Bone complications in children with Gaucher disease. Br J Radiol 2002;75(Suppl. 1):A37–44.

55. Mantovani G, de Sanctis L, Barbieri AM, et al. Pseudohypoparathyroidism and GNAS epigenetic defects: clinical evaluation of Albright hereditary osteodystrophy and molecular analysis in 40 patients. J Clin Endocrinol Metab 2010;95:651–8.

56. Bochukova E, Schoenmakers N, Agostini M, et al. Growth retardation and severe constipation due to a dominant negative mutation in the thyroid hormone receptor alpha gene. N Engl J Med 2012;366:243–9.

57. Almeida A, Roberts I. Bone involvement in sickle cell disease. Br J Haematol 2005;129:482–90.

58. Chan Y-L, Pang L-M, Chik K-W, et al. Patterns of bone disease in transfusion-dependent homozygous thalassaemia major: predominance of osteoporosis and desferrioxamine-induced bone dysplasia. Pediatr Radiol 2002;32:492–7.

59. Lazzarini L, Mader JT, Calhoun JH. Osteomyelitis in long bones. J Bone Joint Surg (Am) 2004;86:2305–18.

60. Offiah AC. Acute osteomyelitis, septic arthritis and discitis: differences between neonates and older children. Eur J Radiol 2006;60: 221–32.

61. Andronikou S, Smith B. Spina ventosa—tuberculous dactylitis. Arch Dis Child 2002;86:206.

62. Chau CLF, Griffith JF. Musculoskeletal infections: ultrasound appearances. Clin Radiol 2005;60:149–59.

63. Davies AM, Grimer R. The penumbra sign in subacute osteomyelitis. Eur Radiol 2005;15:1268–70.

64. Early SD, Kay RM, Tolo VT. Childhood diskitis. J Am Acad Orthop Surg 2003;11:413–20.

65. Fernandez M, Carrol CL, Baker CJ. Discitis and vertebral osteomyelitis in children: An 18-year review. Pediatrics 2000;105: 1299–304.

CHAPTER 6

Paediatric Musculoskeletal Trauma and the Radiology of Non-accidental Injury and Paediatric Fractures

Karen Rosendahl • Jean-François Chateil • Karl Johnson

Fractures account for up to 25% of all injuries in children, being commoner in boys.[1] The type and distribution of injuries varies between different age groups in children and adults because of the physiology of the developing skeleton. A child's bones are more elastic than those of an adult. When a force is applied to a bone, it will generate stresses within that bone, which may be compressive, tensile or shearing. These stresses will result in deformity of the bone, which will progress as the stress increases. When the force is removed, the bone may eventually return to normal. However, at some point, namely the yield stress, the bone enters a phase of plastic deformity, resulting in microscopic fractures on the tensile side of the bone.[2] This bone may initially be radiographically normal, but follow-up radiographs may show evidence of a healing periosteal reaction in response to these microfractures. With further increases in the deforming force, the bone's ultimate stress point will be reached and the bone then fractures.

In adults, the yield point and ultimate stress points are very close together, so plastic deformity is rare. In the younger child, the greater degree of elasticity of the bone means that there can be a significant difference between the yield point and ultimate point, with a greater propensity for plastic deformity. Cortical bone will tolerate compressive stresses better than tensile or shearing forces. Consequently, childhood fractures may be complete or partial (incomplete). A complete fracture occurs when there is complete discontinuity between two or more bone fragments. An incomplete fracture involves trauma and damage to the bone, but a portion of the cortex remains intact due to the increased elasticity of the bone.

Greenstick, buckle and plastic bowing fall into the category of incomplete fractures (Fig. 6-1). Stress injuries can occur due to repeated forces acting upon the bone, which are less than the force needed to fracture the bone (Fig. 6-2). Fractures may also be classified with regards to the fracture line; a simple fracture is where there is only a single fracture line. These fractures can be further described as transverse, oblique or spiral, depending on the appearances of the fracture line with respect to the bone's long axis. A comminuted fracture is where there are several fracture lines and these include segmental fractures and those with butterfly fragments (Fig. 6-3). Open or compound fractures occur when a wound extends from the skin surface to the fracture. Displacement refers to when there is a space and altered alignment between the fracture fragments.

For the majority of injuries, a good-quality anteroposterior and lateral radiograph is the only imaging which will be required. From these projections, the fracture pattern, along with any shortening or angulation, can be determined. Rotation is best assessed from the relative position of the joints above and below the fracture, which should be included on the radiograph as standard practice. Careful inspection of a fracture may allow the mechanism of injury to be determined, which may have implications as to the stability and hence help determine management.

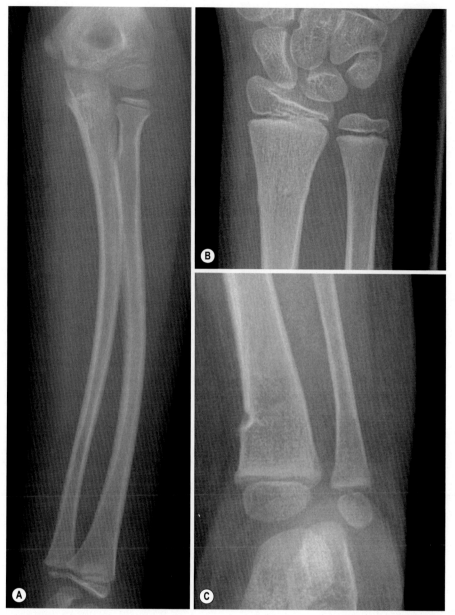

FIGURE 6-1 ■ (A) Fracture of the left radius and ulna. (B) Torus fracture of the distal right radius. (C) Greenstick fracture of the distal left tibia.

PHYSEAL INJURIES

A cartilaginous physis (growth plate) occurs between a bone and its epiphysis or apophysis. An epiphysis contributes to longitudinal growth while an apophysis does not. In early childhood, not all the epiphysis or apophysis will be ossified and so will not be visible on a radiograph. The transitional zone between the physeal cartilage and the metaphyseal portion of the bone, 'the zone of provisional calcification', is the weakest point in the growing skeleton. The physeal cartilage is weaker than bone, which, in turn, is weaker than the surrounding ligaments.

Injuries which may result in a ligamental tear or joint dislocation in an adult are more likely to cause a physeal

injury in a child.[3] Up to 15% of fractures of the tubular bones in children affect the growth plate and the majority of physeal fractures are due to shearing or avulsion stresses. The classification of physeal injuries typically uses the system of Salter and Harris, which separates fractures into five main types (Figs. 6-4 and 6-5).[4] Other fracture types and other categories of injury have been proposed since the original classification.[5,6] The importance of the classification system is that for higher grades of injuries, there is an increased likelihood that the growth plate will be damaged, which will result in long-term complications such as malunion, premature fusion (resulting in growth impairment) and avascular necrosis (Fig. 6-6). The latter is most likely to occur in fractures of the femoral or radial neck. Whilst

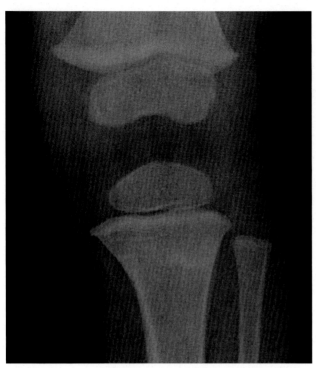

FIGURE 6-2 ■ Healing stress fracture of the proximal tibia.

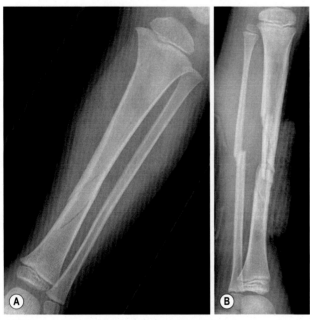

FIGURE 6-3 ■ (A) Spiral fracture of the left tibia. (B) Comminuted fracture of the right tibia with associated fracture of the fibula.

the majority of injuries are clearly shown on standard radiographs, magnetic resonance imaging (MRI) can be used to better visualise the physeal cartilage and the non-ossified portion of the epiphysis (Fig. 6-7).[7]

The other site of potential physeal damage is at the musculotendinous insertion into an apophysis,

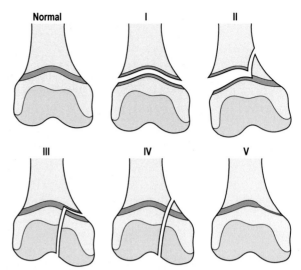

FIGURE 6-4 ■ **Illustration of the Salter–Harris classification of fractures.** (Type I) The fracture is isolated to the growth plate and causes epiphyseal separation, without adjacent bone fracture. The fracture line passes through the hypertrophic layer of the physis. (Type II) This is the most common growth plate fracture and is usually seen in children between the ages of 10 and 16. As a result of shearing or avulsive force, the fracture splits the growth plate and then passes into the metaphysis, separating a small fragment of bone. (Type III) The fracture line passes through the epiphysis, and then horizontally across the growth plate. This is most commonly seen at the distal tibia in children aged 10–15. (Type IV) This is a vertically orientated fracture, involving both the epiphysis and metaphysis, and crossing the growth plate. This is most commonly seen in the distal humerus and tibia. (Type V) This fracture, results from a compressive force, crushing the growth plate. Damage to the growth plate can cause subsequent deformity. The diagnosis is often made retrospectively when growth arrest is discovered at a later date.

particularly following an avulsion injury. In children, the apophyseal physis is the weakest point of the bone, tendon and muscle interface and, consequently, severe traction on the muscle will result in avulsion of a bone or cartilaginous fragment. Avulsion injuries are common sports injuries and most usually seen around the pelvis and elbow (Figs. 6-8 and 6-9).

Low-energy repetitive traction forces can result in microtrauma, causing a chronic apophysitis. Around the medial epicondyle of the humerus, this is eponymously called 'little leaguer's elbow'. Radiographs are usually sufficient to diagnose acute avulsion injuries, providing the avulsed fragment is ossified. MR imaging or ultrasound can be helpful in demonstrating soft-tissue swelling, effusion and marrow oedema in the more chronic presentations.

THE UPPER LIMB

Shoulder/Humerus

Fractures of the clavicle can occur from either a direct blow or a fall onto the shoulder or outstretched arm. Typically, they occur in the middle third and there is a

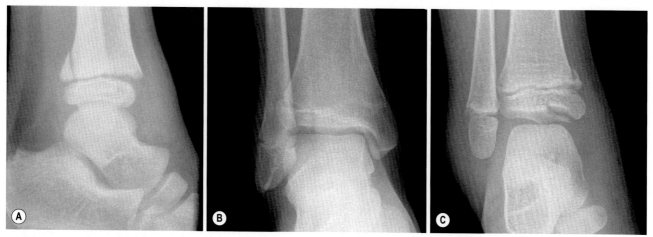

FIGURE 6-5 ■ **Various Salter–Harris fractures.** (A) Salter–Harris II fracture of the distal left tibia. (B) Salter–Harris III fracture of the distal right tibia. (C) Salter–Harris fracture of the distal left tibia.

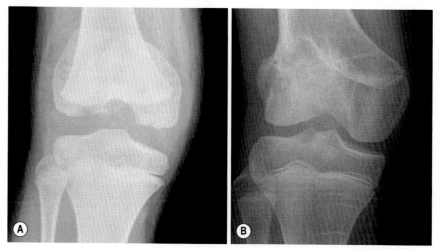

FIGURE 6-6 ■ (A) Fracture through the growth plate of the distal right femur with significant displacement and distortion of the epiphysis. (B) Follow-up radiographs after surgical correction show premature fusion of the lateral aspect of the distal femoral physis, resulting in abnormal remodelling and development.

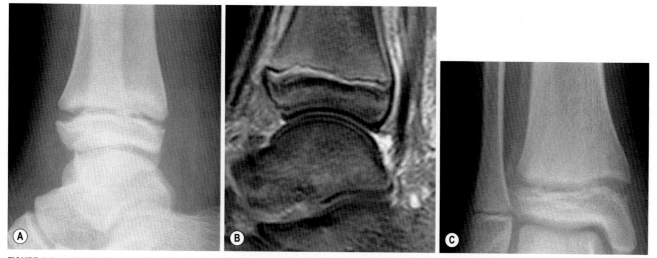

FIGURE 6-7 ■ (A) Salter–Harris I fracture of the distal right tibia. Note widening of the growth plate. (B) MRI of the same patient showing abnormal increased signal on the T2-weighted sequences through the growth plate. (C) Follow-up films in the same patient as (A) show subperiosteal new bone formation around the fracture site confirming the injury.

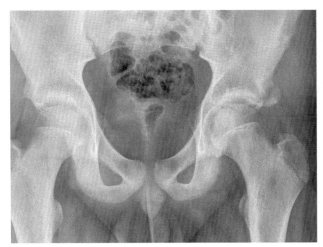

FIGURE 6-8 ■ Avulsion fracture of the left anterior inferior iliac spine.

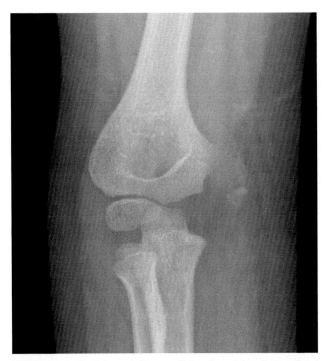

FIGURE 6-9 ■ Avulsion of the medial epicondyle of the distal humerus.

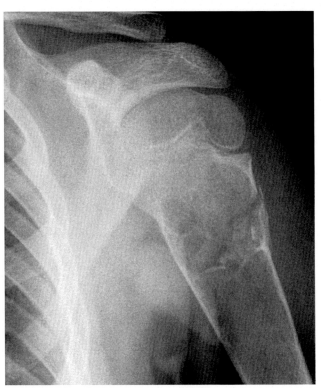

FIGURE 6-10 ■ **Pathological fracture of the proximal left humerus through a simple bone cyst.** There is a small bony fragment within the cystic cavity.

high propensity for greenstick injuries due to the plastic nature of the periosteum.[8] The clavicle is the commonest site of birth-related fracture and is associated with shoulder dystocia and obstetric brachial plexus palsy. This may cause the neonate to present with reduced arm movement, the differential diagnosis of which includes septic arthritis, osteomyelitis, shoulder dislocation and non-accidental injury (NAI).[9]

Shoulder dislocation is uncommon under 10 years of age, the presence of the humeral physis appearing to be in some way protective. Displacement is typically anteriorly and the humeral head lies under the coracoid process on the AP radiograph. On the axial view, the humeral head is displaced anteriorly and no longer covers the glenoid.

Proximal humeral fractures are uncommon, with those involving the physis representing just 3% of such injuries. However, the consequences of fractures here may be significant as the physis accounts for 80% of longitudinal growth of the humerus. Care must be taken in reviewing the proximal humerus, as the normal growth plate has an irregular contour which should not be mistaken for a fracture.[10]

Under 10 years of age, the fractures are typically metaphyseal, whilst in adolescents, they are usually a Salter–Harris type II fracture. Conversely, the proximal humerus is a relatively common site for pathological fractures, typically through a simple bone cyst, creating the 'fallen fragment sign', due to a piece of cortical bone lying within the fluid-filled cavity (Fig. 6-10).[11]

Elbow

There are six separate ossification centres around the elbow joint which appear and fuse in a relatively predictable temporal sequence. These are shown in Table 6-1. Recognition of this sequence is important in determining the presence and type of any injury. While some variation in the appearances can be seen, the internal apophysis should always appear before that of the trochlea, and any deviation from this, with a history of trauma, is suspicious for an avulsed or malpositioned internal apophysis (Fig. 6-11).[12]

TABLE 6-1	The Ossification Centres around the Elbow Joint	
	Age Range at Which The Ossification Centre Becomes Visible Radiographically (Years)	Age Range at Which They Fuse (Years)
Capitellum	0–2	13–16
Radial head	3–6	13–17
Internal (medial) epicondyle	3–9	Up to 20
Trochlea	7–13	13–16
Olecranon	8–10	13–16
Lateral (external) epicondyle	8–12	13–16

The age at which they appear and then subsequently fuse. In general it occurs earlier in girls than in boys.

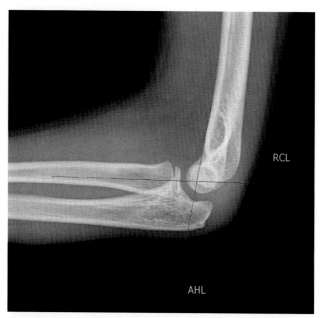

FIGURE 6-12 ■ **Normal lateral film of the elbow.** The two lines drawn on the radiograph are used to assess the elbow joint. Anterior humeral line (AHL): one-third of the capitellum should lie anterior to this line. In the young child where there is only partial ossification of the capitellum, this measurement is less valid. RCL—on a lateral film, a line drawn along the shaft of the proximal radius should pass through the capitellum.

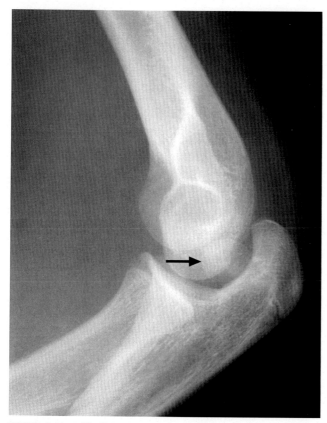

FIGURE 6-11 ■ **Medial epicondyle epiphysis (arrow) trapped within the elbow joint following avulsion.**

A good-quality AP and lateral radiograph is essential for evaluating the elbow joint following trauma, for the important assessment of crucial anatomical landmarks (Figs. 6-12 and 6-13). Fracture, haematoma or effusion into the elbow joint will cause capsular distension and elevation of the fat pads overlying it. A visible posterior fat pad should be regarded as abnormal due to a potential occult injury, particularly a fracture/dislocation of the radial head or undisplaced supracondylar fracture.

A visible anterior fat pad may be a normal finding. The absence of any visible fat pad does not exclude the presence of a fracture. The medial and lateral epicondyles are extracapsular and so are not associated with capsular distension.

Supracondylar fractures are the commonest fractures under the age of 7 years. The majority are the extension type, with posterior displacement of the distal fracture fragment, typically due to a fall on an outstretched arm. Flexion-type fractures with anterior displacement are due to a direct blow on a flexed elbow and are often unstable (Fig. 6-14).[13]

Complications include nerve entrapment, malunion (leading to either cubitus valgus or varus) and vascular compromise. The absence of the radial pulse may be an indication for arteriography prior to surgical exploration.

Lateral condylar fractures are due to a varus force on an extended elbow. It is important to realise that this fracture may extend through the unossified portion of the capitellum into the joint space (Salter–Harris type IV).[14]

Forearm/Wrist/Hand

Radial and ulnar fractures can occur together or in isolation, the radius being the commoner single injury site. Forearm fractures may also occur with dislocation at either the elbow or wrist joint, the so-called Monteggia and Galeazzi fractures. To avoid missing a dislocation, it is vital the joints above and below a forearm fracture are visualised properly (Fig. 6-15).

Incomplete fractures of the distal forearm metadiaphysis are common, the mechanism of injury typically being a fall on an outstretched hand. The peak incidence

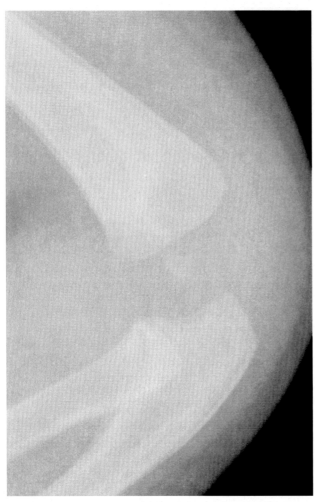

FIGURE 6-13 ■ **Dislocated radial head.** Note a line along the proximal radius does not pass through the capitellum.

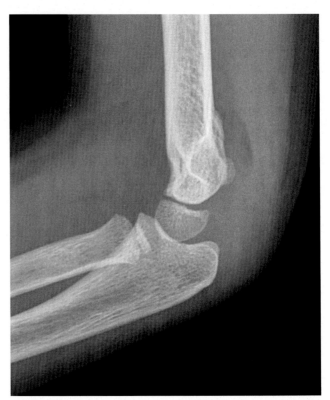

FIGURE 6-14 ■ **Left supracondylar fracture with posterior displacement and a large elbow effusion.**

in boys is between 12 and 14 and in girls 10 and 12 years.[15] This corresponds to the adolescent growth spurt and relative weakness of the metadiaphysis (Fig. 6-1).

Carpal injuries in childhood are infrequent, the commonest being the scaphoid, which more typically occurs in adolescence. The site of injury is more likely to be the distal third of the scaphoid, compared with the waist in adults, and so the risk of vascular compromise is lower in children. Scaphoid fractures may be radiographically occult, and MR imaging is useful in confirming the diagnosis and expediting appropriate management (Fig. 6-16).[16]

Metacarpal fractures have an increased incidence in older schoolchildren where the mechanism is usually punching or contact sports. The metacarpal of the little finger is most often injured, with the commonest type of fracture being a Salter–Harris type II.[17]

The phalanges may fracture from direct trauma or as a result of avulsion forces. Crush injuries of the phalanges are typically seen in the preschool child. It is important that all the ossified phalangeal epiphyses are reviewed, as any avulsed fragments may travel a significant distance proximally.

THE LOWER LIMB

Pelvis

A number of classifications of pelvic fractures have been proposed, with the general aim being to predict the degree of morbidity associated with the injury and to try to assess the mechanism and force vectors involved in the causation. An improved understanding of causation helps plan treatment. In principle, the classification systems all detail the type of fracture and the anatomical sites within the pelvis. Unsurprisingly, the more severe injuries which result in significant disruption of the pelvis are associated with greater long-term morbidity. They are generally associated with high-velocity impacts and often occur with injuries in other anatomical areas, particularly the brain.[18–21]

The least severe fractures are avulsion injuries, which are common in adolescence and are typically the result of athletic activity. These can occur at a number of sites related to muscle attachments.

Standard AP radiographs are usually the initial investigation and are useful in assessing for avulsion injuries. For higher-grade injuries, CT is a more sensitive investigation and in most circumstances is part of a more general screening of a child following high energy/impact trauma.

Acetabular, Hip and Femur

Acetabular fractures are an uncommon, but significant, injury in childhood, because if the triradiate cartilage is

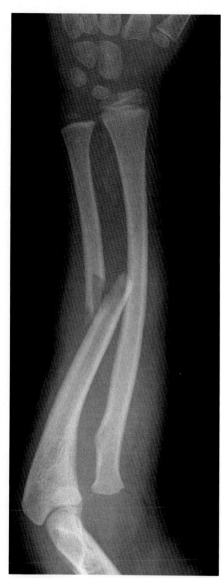

FIGURE 6-15 ■ Monteggia fracture of the left radius and ulna (fractured ulna dislocated radial head).

involved, growth and acetabular development may be affected.

Posterior dislocation of the hip is commoner than anterior, and while dislocation in children is less likely to result in acetabular injury, avascular necrosis of the femoral capital epiphysis is a serious potential complication if the femur remains unreduced for over 24 hours. With dislocations, proper assessment of the acetabular margins is vital to exclude occult fractures and this will be improved with CT or MR imaging (Fig. 6-17).[22,23]

Femoral head and neck fractures are relatively uncommon and may be associated with femoral head dislocation. They are classified with reference to their location along the femoral neck: namely, transepiphyseal, transcervical, cervicotrochanteric and intratrochanteric. Complications include osteonecrosis (the occurrence of which is increased the more significant the fracture displacement), premature physeal fusion, varus deformity and non-union.[24]

Femoral diaphyseal fractures may be associated with significant displacement if the fracture line means that there is unopposed muscle traction of the bone fragment. It is vital to check for rotation, as this will not be corrected without manipulation.

Knee

Acute knee trauma is a common childhood symptom. Studies which have been validated in paediatrics have devised rules to determine the need for radiographs within this cohort of patients. Radiographs are only indicated when there is isolated tenderness of the patella and head of the fibula, an inability to flex the knee to 90° or if the patient cannot weight bear. AP and lateral radiographs are standard and the use of the skyline view is arbitrary.[25]

An effusion within the knee joint will outline the suprapatellar region and obliterate fat planes. A horizontal beam lateral film will show a lipohaemarthrosis due to the different densities of fat and blood within the joint. The presence of a lipohaemarthrosis is suspicious of an intra-articular injury.

Outside of acute trauma, MR imaging is the modality of choice when assessing for pathological conditions of the knee, as it will obviously provide an assessment of ligaments, menisci and cartilage. CT is valuable for detecting intra-articular fracture displacement and detached bony fragments.

In contrast to adults, anterior tibial spine fractures are more likely to occur in childhood compared with anterior cruciate ligament (ACL) ruptures. This occurs when there is forced hyperextension and rotation of the knee. In children, the tensile strength of the ACL is greater than that of the bone, causing avulsion of the tibial spine. The detached bony fragment may be seen on radiographs within the knee joint. Both CT and MRI are more sensitive in assessing the degree of displacement and rotation (Fig. 6-18).

Osteochondral fractures are associated with traumatic lateral dislocation of the patella or axial compressive loading on the femur. Typical sites for injury are the lateral femoral condyle or patella. The fracture is through the subchondral bone and there may be a small bony (loose) fragment within the knee joint.

Osteochondritis dissecans is a defect within the subchondral region of the distal femur, typically occurring on the posterolateral aspect of the medial femoral condyle. Other anatomical sites are the talar dome and capitellum. The full aetiology is unknown, but there is necrosis of the subchondral bone which may be the result of repetitive overloading. On radiographs, there is an oval lucency adjacent to the articular margin.[26]

The patella is infrequently fractured in children, the commonest types being the comminuted and transverse. Sleeve fractures are avulsion injuries of the inferior pole of the patella with a small amount of detached ossified periosteum, but a large amount of unossified cartilage and retinaculum. This may be difficult to detect on standard radiographs as there is only a small of flake of detached bone, but it is well shown on MR imaging.

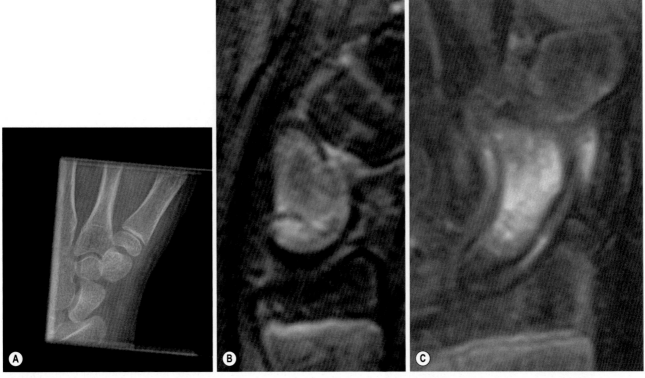

FIGURE 6-16 ■ (A) Normal radiographs of the left scaphoid. (B, C) MR images in the same patient demonstrate extensive marrow oedema within the scaphoid and a fracture line.

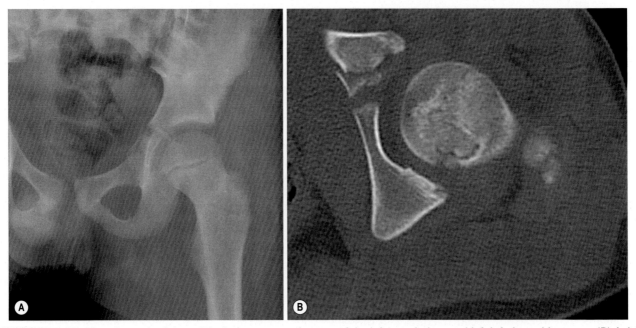

FIGURE 6-17 ■ (A) AP radiograph of the pelvis demonstrates a fracture of the left acetabulum and left inferior pubic ramus. (B) Axial CT confirms the presence of the acetabular fracture and demonstrates involvement of the triradiate cartilage.

Tibia/Ankle/Foot

Tibia

The classical toddler's fracture is an undisplaced fracture of the middle/distal tibial diaphysis, which may not be initially visible on the convential AP and lateral radiograph (being more discernible on oblique views). The toddler's fracture is a cause for a child to be non-weight bearing. If there are no other clinical concerns, follow-up imaging is not routinely indicated, due to radiation dose considerations. However, if repeat imaging

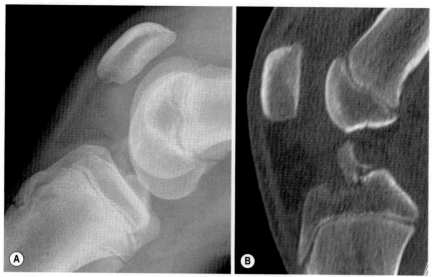

FIGURE 6-18 ■ (A) Lateral radiograph of the right knee demonstrates a bony fragment within the knee joint due to an avulsed tibial spine. (B) Avulsed tibial fragment clearly shown on sagittal reformatted CT image.

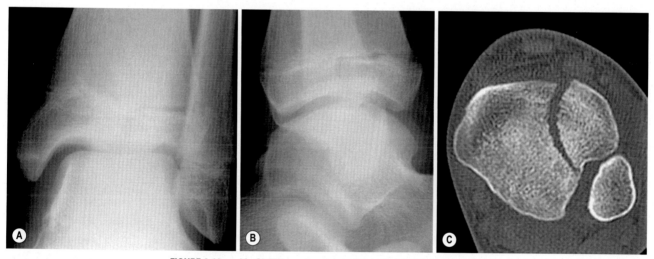

FIGURE 6-19 ■ (A–C) Tillaux fracture of the distal tibial epiphysis.

is performed, periosteal reaction and sclerosis along the fracture line may become visible after about a week (Fig. 6-3).

Stress fractures of the tibia are generally located in the upper third in children aged around 10–15 years and are associated with excessive or continuous physical exercise (Fig. 6-2). Approximately 70% of tibial shaft fractures are isolated, with the remainder also involving the fibula. The tibia shows a reduced tendency to remodel and there may be a risk of varus angulation due to the pull of the long flexors and an intact fibula. Isolated fibular fractures are rare and usually occur from a direct blow.[27]

Ankle

Most ankle fractures are adequately assessed with standard radiographs (i.e. AP, lateral ± mortice view). Some confusion can occur from the numerous accessory ossification centres which may be visible, particularly adjacent to the malleoli.

Epiphyseal, avulsion and Salter–Harris type I and II fractures of the distal tibia account for the majority of injuries. Injuries are usually caused by indirect trauma with the foot being fixed and forced either into dorsiflexion, plantar flexion, eversion, inversion or rotation (external or internal). The physes of the distal tibia and fibula fuse at the same time, initially centrally followed by medially and then laterally. If only one physis is visible, the suspicion of an epiphyseal injury is raised.

Transitional fractures (triplane and juvenile tillaux) occur in adolescence, as the name implies, as the skeleton becomes more mature (Figs. 6-19 and 6-20). Triplane injuries are fractures caused by external rotation which causes the fracture to extend in the axial, sagittal and

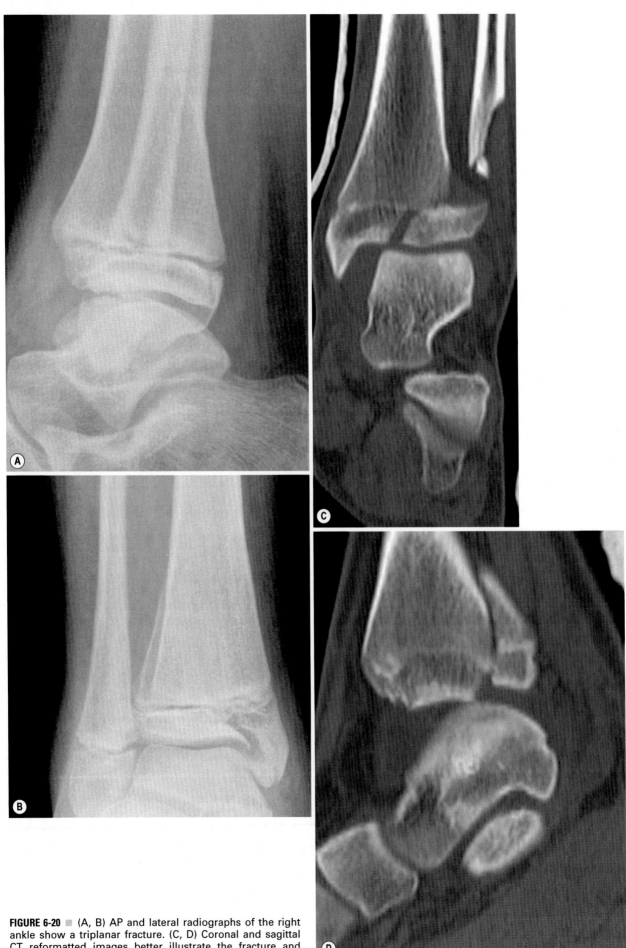

FIGURE 6-20 ■ (A, B) AP and lateral radiographs of the right ankle show a triplanar fracture. (C, D) Coronal and sagittal CT reformatted images better illustrate the fracture and degree of displacement.

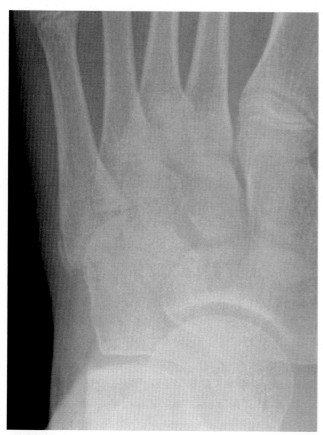

FIGURE 6-21 ■ **The normal apophysis of the fifth metatarsal, which runs in a longitudinal direction parallel to the metatarsal.** Fractures are typically transverse.

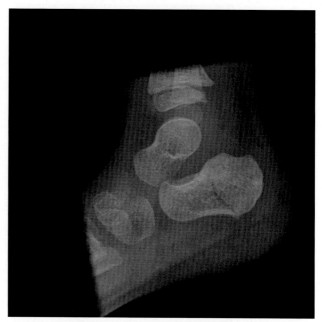

FIGURE 6-22 ■ **Fracture of the calcaneum.**

coronal planes. If the fibula is also fractured, it suggests a more severe rotational force. The lateral radiograph may suggest a Salter–Harris type II fracture while the AP view demonstrates a type II injury.[28]

Tillaux fractures are Salter–Harris type III fractures of the epiphysis and the unfused anterolateral portion of the distal tibial physis, due to avulsion of the anterior tibiofibular ligament. The lack of a fracture component in the coronal plane distinguishes it from a triplane fracture.[29,30]

In all Salter–Harris type III and IV fractures, there will be intra-articular extension of the fracture line and any degree of displacement should be properly evaluated with CT. Displacement greater than 2 mm often requires precise surgical reduction and fixation.

Foot

Foot fractures account for less than 10% of paediatric fractures,[31] the majority of which occur in the metatarsals and phalanges, particularly the fifth metatarsal. However, children under 5 years have a higher proportion of first metatarsal fractures, of which greenstick and torus are the commonest types. It is important not to confuse the apophysis of the fifth metatarsal with a fracture (Fig. 6-21).

The calcaneum is the commonest tarsal bone to be fractured, classically as a result of a fall from a height

(Fig. 6-22). An extra-articular fracture which involves the tuberosity and avoids the posterior facet is commoner in the immature skeleton. There is an association with other injuries to the limb. Bohler's angle is unreliable under the age of 10 years and a normal Bohler's angle does not exclude a fracture.[32] CT is the imaging modality of choice for all suspected tarsal injuries.

Talar fractures are uncommon, as it is believed that the high cartilage to bone ratio in the young child is protective. Displaced fractures of the talar neck carry the risk of avascular necrosis. Isolated fractures of the cuboid, navicular and cuneiforms are rare and tend to be simple avulsions.

Stress fractures in the athletic child may occur in any tarsal bone.

CERVICAL SPINAL INJURIES

Paediatric spinal trauma is uncommon, with childhood injuries accounting for less than 10% of reported spinal injuries. Spinal fractures account for no more than 2% of all paediatric fractures,[33] the majority of which are the result of road traffic accidents.

Due to the disproportionate size of a young child's head and underdeveloped neck musculature, injuries under the age of 12 typically affect the first and second cervical bodies. Younger children are more likely to suffer distraction and subluxation injuries compared with the adult pattern of fractures which occur in the older child.

In children, the spinal column has significantly more flexibility than the spinal cord. Consequently, severe flexion extension injuries may not result in a fracture or ligamental disruption, but will cause significant spinal cord injury. The term 'spinal cord injury without radiographic abnormality' (SCIWORA) was described.[34] The increased use of MR imaging has been able to demonstrate abnormal cord findings in these patients. However,

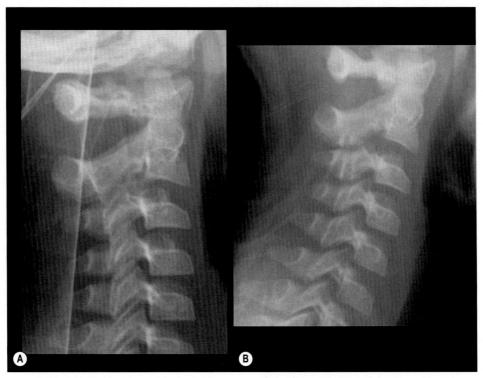

FIGURE 6-23 ■ **(A, B) A Pseudosubluxation of C2 upon C3.** In the same patient, extension view shows normal anterior alignment.

there is a small group of patients where even the MR imaging is normal despite clinical evidence of cord injury and damage.

It is important that normal anatomical variations are not misinterpreted as possible injuries. The commonest variant is pseudosubluxation at the C2/3 and C3/4 levels. Pseudosubluxation of up to 4 mm is acceptable. A line connecting the anterior aspects of the spinous processes (spinolaminar junction) of C1–C3 should pass within 2 mm of the spinolaminar junction of C2 (Fig. 6-23).

When the C2 spinolaminar junction lies 2 mm or more behind this line then the possibility of a fracture or true subluxation is raised. On an open mouth view, a pseudo-Jefferson fracture may be observed due to ossification of the lateral mass of C1 exceeding that of C2, so that they appear to overhang the axis by up to 6 mm. Pseudo anterior wedging of the vertebral bodies of up to 3 mm can be a normal variation and is particularly common at the C3 level.

Unfused apophyses and ossification centres may cause some confusion with fractures.

Atlantoaxial rotatory fixation (AARF) may or may not follow trauma in children and is a commoner occurrence than in adults.

Four types have been described and CT is the imaging modality of choice. An axial CT is performed in a neutral position, followed by repeat imaging in voluntary, maximal, ipsilateral and contralateral head rotation. In patients with fixation, no rotation of the atlas on the axis is observed while with transient torticollis, a reverse or reduction of rotation occurs.

Thoracic and lumbar injuries are typically the result of hyperflexion, which will result in stable anterior wedge compression fractures, and are commoner in children more than 8 years of age.

Flexion distraction forces causing bone and ligament disruption to the lumbar spine can occur with lap seat-belt restraint. Multilevel injuries are common and warrant imaging evaluation of the entire spinal column. The prognosis for neurological recovery is related to the initial severity of the injury. Some children with significant spinal cord injuries can recover substantial neurological function. Associated injuries within the thorax and abdomen are not uncommon.

NON-ACCIDENTAL INJURY

The incidence of physical abuse, a subset of child abuse, varies according to age, ethnicity and the specific definition used, and is both under-reported and under-recorded. Common to all definitions is the presence of an injury that the child sustains at the hands of his (or her) caregiver(s) (<http://www.yesican.org/definitions/CAPTA.html>, <http://www.yesican.org/definitions/WHO.html>, <http://www.yesican.org/articles.html>). These injuries are also referred to as inflicted or non-accidental injuries, battered child syndrome[35] or shaken baby syndrome.[36] When first described in 1946, the shaken baby syndrome included subdural and retinal haemorrhages in conjunction with fractures; however, during the past decade this term has been more and more linked to the abusive head injuries sustained by shaking.

During the past decades, efforts have been made to systematically register the occurrence and nature of child abuse. In the USA, the National Child Abuse and Neglect

Data System (NCANDS) has reported annually since 1990 (<http://www.acf.hhs.gov>). For 2010, the unique victim rate was 9.2 per 1000 children in the total population, increasing to around 20 per 1000 for those below 1 year of age. Victimisation was split between the sexes, with boys accounting for 48.5%. As in prior years, the greatest percentage of children was neglected while 17.6% suffered physical abuse. The overall rate of child fatalities was 2.1 deaths per 100,000 children, with nearly 80% being younger than 4 years old. Boys had a higher child fatality rate than girls; 2.5 versus 1.7 per 100,000. Around one-third of child fatalities were attributed exclusively to neglect, while around 40% were caused by multiple maltreatment types, i.e. neglect, physical abuse, psychological maltreatment and/or sexual abuse. More than 80% of duplicate perpetrators of child maltreatment were parents, and another 6% were other relatives of the victim. Of the perpetrators who were parents, more than 80% were the biological parent of the victim. In the USA, child abuse is responsible for approximately 1400 deaths per year[37] (<http://www.childwelfare.gov/pubs/factsheets/fatality.cfm>).

The UK does not publish statistics on the number of substantiated child abuse cases recorded every year; however, as at March 2010, there were 46,700 children on child protection registers or the subject of child protection plans, i.e. at risk of abuse (National Society for the Prevention of Cruelty to Children, NSPCC, <http://www.nspcc.org.uk/Inform/research/statistics/statistics_wda48748.html>). A UK-wide study of child maltreatment carried out by the NSPCC in 2009 suggested that one in 14 children (6.9%) aged 11–17 have experienced severe physical violence at the hands of an adult.[38]

Further, in England, the Department for Education and the Office for National Statistics have collected and reported statistics on children being looked after every year since 1989 (<http://www.education.gov.uk/rsgateway/DB/SFR>). At 31 March 2011, there were 65,520 looked after children in England, an increase of 9% since 2007. Overall, the main reason why social services first engaged with these looked after children was because of abuse or neglect (54%).

In Australia, the 13th annual comprehensive child protection report (*Child Protection Australia 2008–09*) showed that the number of children subject to a notification of child abuse or neglect increased by 47% from 4.8 to 7.0 per 1000 children over the past 5 years.[39]

Taken together, the rate of physical child abuse is fairly high in industrialised countries. Infants and young children are at greatest risk, with up to 80% of cases being younger than 5 years and up to half being infants (< 1 year of age).

CLINICAL PRESENTATION AND THE ROLE OF THE RADIOLOGIST

The clinical presentation takes many forms, but the physically abused child typically presents with an obvious injury such as soft-tissue swelling, haematomas, bruises, burns and/or fractures. Fractures are seen in a high proportion of physically abused children and more often in

infants.[40,41] It is not uncommon, however, for the abused child to present with symptoms of occult injury, particularly in cases of head and abdominal trauma.

Infants with head injuries may present with non-specific symptoms, such as lethargy, irritability, persistent, unexplained vomiting, apnoea, coma or seizures. Abusive head injury is the most common cause of NAI-related death.[42] Similar to head injury, severe abdominal trauma may present without visible external signs or history to suggest such an injury.

As radiologists, we have important medical and legal roles in the diagnosis of cases of child abuse. We may be the first to raise a question of abuse, if characteristic or unexplained findings are encountered during imaging. The possibility of physical abuse when the parent or another adult caregiver offers conflicting, unconvincing, or indeed no explanation for the child's injury, should always be considered. Immediate and direct communication with the referring physician and also a named and designated child protection colleague (if available) is imperative in all such cases. If there is any doubt as to the presence or significance of a lesion, a second opinion should be sought from a paediatric radiologist experienced in NAI cases, as both a missed, and also an incorrect, diagnosis may be devastating for the child and the family.

INJURY PATTERNS

Our current understanding of injuries and injury patterns in physical abuse is the result of early observations by neurosurgeons, identifying an association between trauma-induced subdural haemorrhages (SDHs) and retinal haemorrhages.[43] Subsequently, in the 1940s, radiologists noticed SDHs in conjunction with skeletal injuries.[36] Physicians' recognition of abuse as the cause of these injuries emerged in the 1950s.[35,44] Observational studies of accidental versus non-accidental injuries are summarised in a recent review,[45] large epidemiological series on fractures in children,[46,47] cadaver and animal studies,[48] and more recently, biomechanical studies.[49]

Physical abuse can produce various injuries and injury patterns in children, of which none are pathognomonic for non-accidental injury.[45] In various clinical series, fractures are observed in approximately 30% of the children and more often in infants,[44] burns are observed in 10%, bruises are common and are present in approximately 40% of maltreated children, and inflicted CNS injury is observed in around a quarter of children treated for head injury.[50] Abdominal trauma is rare, with a reported incidence of 1% of abused children, and is more predominantly seen after the child is able to move around freely.[51]

Shaken Baby Syndrome

The description of findings referred to as the 'shaken baby syndrome' (SBS) has been widely ascribed to the paediatric radiologist John Caffey, who, in 1946, observed and published case reports on six infants suffering chronic subdural haematoma.[36] These six patients also had fractures of long bones, without evidence of an underlying, predisposing skeletal disorder or a history of trauma. During subsequent years he continued to collect data, and in 1974, he published his sentinel paper in which he linked violent manual shaking of an infant to brain damage, retinal haemorrhage and residual mental retardation.[52,53]

Since then our understanding of this syndrome has been modified as a result of new medical research and multiple legal challenges. Biomechanical studies have repeatedly failed to show that shaking alone can generate the triad of subdural haemorrhage, retinal haemorrhage and encephalopathy, in the absence of significant neck injury.[49] Moreover, the importance of a concomitant impact has been recognised, i.e. 'shaken baby—impact syndrome'. More recently, an even wider term, namely 'abusive head trauma', has been introduced to cover the whole spectrum of CNS pathology sustained by violent shaking.[54] Controversy still exists, however, as to the cause and mechanisms of the observed head and spinal injuries. The majority of all cases of abusive head injury are limited to children under 2–3 years of age, and most often seen in infants younger than 6 months.[55] Small children and infants are at a high risk due to their small size in comparison to their adult perpetrators.

GENERAL IMAGING STRATEGIES

The appropriate imaging of children being evaluated for suspected physical child abuse depends on the age of the child and the presence of neurological, thoracic or abdominal signs and symptoms. Several referral and imaging guidelines exist, of which the American College of Radiology (ACR) Appropriateness Criteria,[56] recommendations by the Royal College of Radiologists/the Royal College of Paediatrics and Child Health (RCR-RCPCH)[57] and referral guidelines from the Royal College of Radiologists (RCR)[58] have been widely adopted.

Both the ACR and the RCR recommend a skeletal survey in all children younger than 2 years of age in whom there is suspicion of abuse. As for the use of additional imaging, there are minor differences between the two, and the radiologist should be familiar with the local policy.

The RCR referral guidelines include:
- Skeletal survey, including skull radiographs, as these are essential to demonstrate skull fractures even when CT of the brain is performed.
- Brain CT, indicated for:
  - any infant (< 1 year) where there is evidence of physical abuse[57]
  - any child who presents with evidence of physical abuse with encephalopathic features, focal and neurological signs or haemorrhagic retinopathy.
- Brain MRI is helpful if CT shows evidence of subdural haemorrhage or brain injury, or if there is neurological deficit.
- Consider including the cervical spine.[59]
- Bone scintigraphy, of value if the skeletal survey is equivocal or if there are ongoing clinical concerns despite a normal survey. It should, however, only be performed in departments which have expertise in bone scanning in infants.

For the older children, 2–5 years of age, a skeletal survey is of less value, but should be considered for each specific case, individually. Alternatively, the radiographs may be tailored to the area(s) of suspected injury.[56]

Furthermore, all children with suspected injury to the chest or abdomen should have an enhanced CT scan, following per-oral contrast if possible. Children suffering sudden infant death should have a skeletal survey before an autopsy is undertaken.

SKELETAL INJURY

The role of skeletal imaging in cases of suspected child abuse is to accurately detect, and possibly date, any injuries, to exclude normal variants of growth (which may mimic injuries or fractures) and possibly to diagnose any underlying metabolic or genetic disorders of bone, which may predispose a child to pathological fractures.[60]

The Skeletal Survey

The skeletal survey should be performed by experienced radiographers, under the supervision of a consultant radiologist. High-quality images of each anatomical site, and not a whole-body radiograph ('babygram'), should be performed, and all images should be appropriately labelled and stored. The following views are advised:[57]
- Skull (anteroposterior (AP) and lateral; additional Townes view if there is a suspected occipital fracture).
- Spine (lateral views of cervical, thoracic and lumbar spine); if the whole of the spine is not included on the chest and abdominal radiographs then additional views will be required.
- Chest (AP, including the clavicles, and oblique views of both sets of ribs).
- Abdomen, including pelvis and hips (AP).
- Long bones (AP views of both humeri, both forearms, both femora and both tibiae and fibulae).
- Hands (PA).
- Feet (DP).

When an abnormality is suspected, these views should be supplemented with:
- Lateral views of any suspected shaft fracture.
- AP and lateral coned views of the elbows, wrist, knees and ankles, when a fracture is suspected at these sites—as directed by the supervising consultant radiologist. These may demonstrate metaphyseal injuries in greater detail than AP views of the limb alone.[57]

Follow-up radiographs have been shown to be of value in improving the detection of rib and metaphyseal fractures.[61,62] Repeat radiographs after 11–14 days should be considered if there are questionable areas or areas of persistent clinical concern, particularly to rule out rib fractures. This is pertinent as up to two-thirds of acute fractures may be missed.[63] In cases of suspected metaphyseal injury, a repeat radiograph after 2 weeks may show ongoing healing, while a repeat radiograph after 5–6 weeks may clarify whether a metaphyseal irregularity represents a normal variant, as most fractures will have healed at this stage.

Bone Scintigraphy

The role of bone scintigraphy in diagnosing child abuse is controversial, and the technique is not routinely used in large parts of Europe.[64] According to the guidelines (as published by the ACR and RCR-RCPCH), bone scintigraphy may be considered in cases with a normal radiographic skeletal survey, but with a high clinical index of suspicion of child abuse. To increase sensitivity, the bone scan should include the use of pinhole collimators and differential counts of the metaphysis. A bone scan is especially good for detecting periosteal trauma, and rib, scapular, spinal, diaphyseal, pelvic and acromial fractures, whilst the sensitivity is lower for fractures of flat bones, old healed fractures and metaphyseal injuries.[65] Scintigraphy becomes positive within hours of an injury.[66] Familiarity with the normal scintigraphic appearances in children is crucial, in particular the normal high metaphyseal uptake, which should not be mistaken for a metaphyseal injury.

Magnetic Resonance Imaging (MRI)

MRI is not routinely used for the assessment of bony injury in infants with suspected NAI, and the literature is sparse as to its validation. One study demonstrated a low sensitivity for both metaphyseal and rib fractures.[67] Others have shown that more than half of healthy children aged 5–15 years have findings consistent with bone oedema in at least one of the carpal bones, reflecting a wide normal variation of the MRI appearances within paediatric bones.[68,69]

Ultrasound

Ultrasound may be a useful supplementary technique in selected cases of bony injury; however, its use in NAI has not been validated, and it cannot be advocated as a primary tool for the investigation of bone injury. Of note is the mild periosteal 'elevation' close to the growth plate, which can be seen as a normal feature, and thus should not be mistaken for injury (Fig. 6-24).

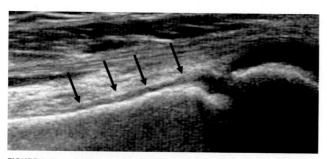

FIGURE 6-24 ■ Ultrasound of the distal femur in a 6-month-old female, showing a normal, diaphyseal elevated periosteum, not to be mistaken for an injury.

Fracture Patterns in Accidental vs Non-Accidental Injury

Fractures are a common problem in childhood, with approximately one-third of girls and boys sustaining at least one fracture before 16–17 years of age.[46,70] Rates are higher among boys than girls, with peak incidences at 14 and 10–11 years of age, respectively.[70,71] The most common site affected in both sexes is the radius/ulna, although the type and location varies considerably at different stages of the child's age and development.[46,72] In toddlers, fractures to the tibia and fibula predominate (Fig. 6-25), while fractures of the clavicle and skull are more common in infants.[71] Multiple fractures are uncommon, and seen in only 16% of non-abused versus 74% of abused children.[41]

In various clinical series of non-accidental injury, skeletal fractures are diagnosed in up to a third of the children, and more often in those under the age of 2.[41,50] Any bone can be involved, but some locations are more frequent than others.

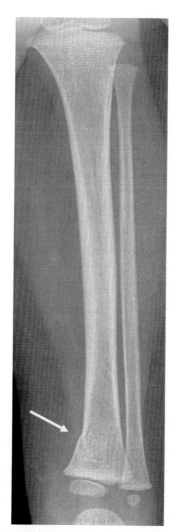

FIGURE 6-25 ■ Buckle fracture (arrow) of the distal metaphysis in a toddler.

TABLE 6-2   **Specificity of Skeletal Injuries in Child Abuse; Highest Specificity Applies in Infants[75]**

Specificity	Type of Fracture/Skeletal Lesion
High specificity	Classic metaphyseal lesion
	Rib fractures, especially posterior
	Scapular fractures
	Spinous process fractures
	Sternal fractures
Moderate specificity	Multiple fractures, specifically bilateral
	Fractures of different ages
	Epiphyseal separation
	Vertebral body fractures and subluxations
	Digital fractures
	Complex skull fractures
Common but low specificity	Subperiosteal ne-bone formation
	Clavicular fractures
	Long bone shaft fractures
	Linear skull fractures

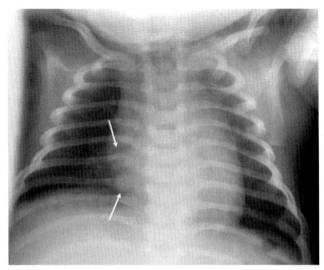

FIGURE 6-26 ■ **Healing fractures to the posterior right seventh and eighth ribs (arrows).** Also note a healing fracture to the left clavicle.

Overall, long tubular bones are affected in about one-third of cases, metaphyses in a quarter, ribs in a quarter and skull fractures in approximately 15%.[73] No fracture is considered pathognomonic for physical abuse on its own, although fractures to the ribs, particularly to the posterior aspects and to the long bone metaphysis, should raise particular concern.[45] In a recent systematic review on fracture patterns in child abuse, the authors conclude that physical abuse should be considered in the differential diagnosis when a child (under 18 months of age) presents with a fracture, in the absence of an overt history of important trauma or a known medical condition that predisposes to bone fragility. The authors present several features associated with possible child abuse[45] such as multiple fractures, rib fractures—(regardless of type), for example femoral fractures—in particular in children who are not yet walking and humeral fractures (in particular affecting the mid-shaft) and skull fractures.

Additional features found to be associated with abuse are metaphyseal injuries,[74] uncommon fractures for example at the scapula, especially at the spinous process, the sternum, and any fracture with a delayed presentation (Table 6-2).[41,75]

Careful correlation of the observed radiological findings with the proposed mechanism of injury, with the child's age and clinical status, is crucial in the evaluation, knowing that a missed diagnosis could lead to a second and potentially fatal abusive injury.

Rib Fractures

Because of the relative elasticity of the thoracic cage, rib fractures in otherwise healthy infants and young children are rare. Any such injury should be regarded with suspicion if no plausible explanation, such as an underlying diseases leading to bone fragility, a motor vehicle accident or violent trauma, is offered.[45,76]

A child with rib fractures has a 7 in 10 chance of having been abused.[45] Most rib fractures are clinically occult, in contrast to around 60% of extremity fractures, and are discovered incidentally during imaging.[77] They are not usually associated with bruising of the chest wall, although finger marks may be an accompanying clinical sign. Abusive rib fractures can occur at any point along the rib, from the costovertebral articulations to the costochondral junctions, but fractures to the posterior rib arches are believed to be particularly associated with NAI[78–80] (Figs. 6-26–6-29). A recent literature review has, however, challenged this assumption, as findings of posterior rib fractures were variable.[45] While Barsness and colleagues found that posterior rib fractures were significantly more common in abuse than in non-abuse,[80] their findings were not supported by others.[81,82]

Abusive rib fractures are typically multiple, positioned immediately above each other in a line, are unilateral in up to 50%, but may also be solitary.[76] In up to 29% of cases, one or more rib fractures are the only skeletal finding in an abused child, underscoring the importance of high-quality radiographs and a keen eye for detail.[80]

The mechanism of rib fractures is believed to be thoracic compression by adult hands, causing fractures along the rib arches, including the posterior aspects, when the posterior end of the rib is levered over the transverse process[48] (Fig. 6-30). Most posterior rib fractures occur near the costovertebral articulations, but can also involve the rib head and neck.[76] Mid-posterior fractures are typically seen in conjunction with fractures to the rib neck in adjacent ribs, whilst lateral and anterior fractures can have the appearances of greenstick or buckle fractures. Injuries to the costochondral junction mirror the classic metaphyseal lesion (CML) due to similar anatomy, with a growth plate present between the osseous anterior rib end and the costal cartilage (Fig. 6-31). As opposed to the others, and similar to the CMLs, these fractures appear to heal by a process of consolidation without callus formation. They can also be associated with abdominal visceral injury.

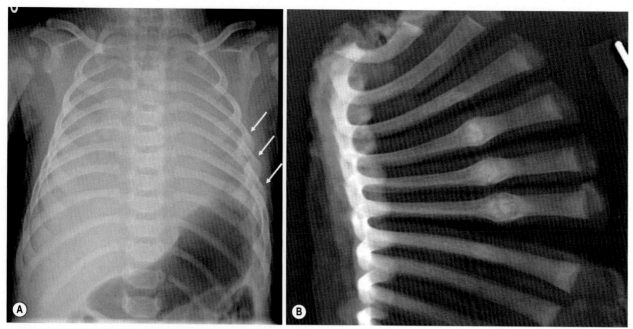

FIGURE 6-27 ■ Healing fractures to the lateral left fourth through sixth ribs (arrows) in a 3-month-old infant. (A) Pre- and (B) postautopsy.

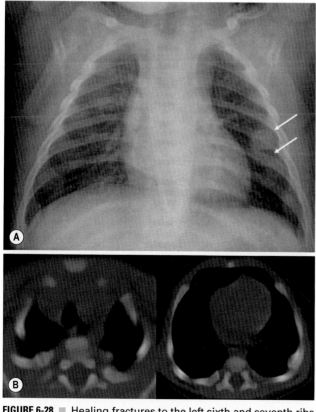

FIGURE 6-28 ■ Healing fractures to the left sixth and seventh ribs as shown on a chest radiograph (A) (arrows). A CT performed 4 days later also demonstrated healing fractures to the second through fifth right ribs, and to the second left rib, all of which had been missed on the initial, slightly suboptimal radiograph (B).

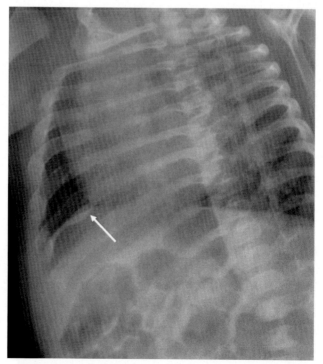

FIGURE 6-29 ■ Old fracture to the right seventh rib (arrow).

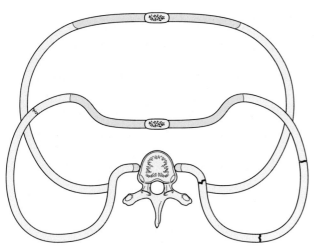

FIGURE 6-30 ■ **During violent shaking, the perpetrator's hands wrap around the child's chest, exerting a bidirectional force.** The vertebrae act as a fulcrum, resulting in posterior rib fractures. Lateral and anterior fractures may also occur. (Illustration courtesy of E M Hoff, Department of Photo and Drawing, University of Bergen.)

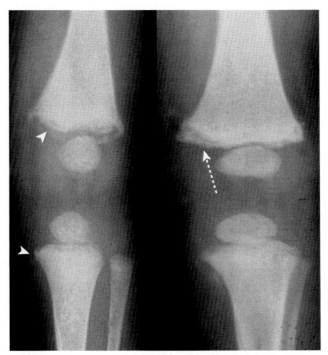

FIGURE 6-32 ■ **Classic metaphyseal lesions with different appearances.** 'Corner fracture' (a thick rim only, arrowhead), 'bucket handle' (a thick rim projected away from the shaft, arrow) and a thin disk with a thick rim (stippled arrow).

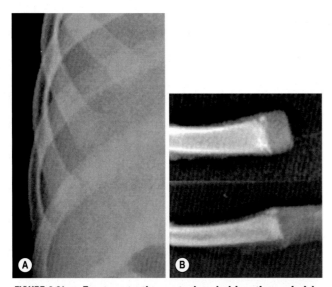

FIGURE 6-31 ■ **Fracture to the costochondral junction, mimicking a classic metaphyseal lesion.** (A) Pre- and (B) postautopsy.

Rib fractures can also be seen after blunt trauma to the chest wall. Unlike in the adult skeleton, rib fractures due to cardiopulmonary resuscitation are uncommon, and if present, involve the lateral or anterior arches of the ribs.[83,84] Recently, however, there have been some reports on rib fractures, posterior, anterior and lateral, after two-handed CPR delivered by trained medical personnel.[85] Similarly, fractures caused by physiotherapy in children treated for bronchiolitis have been reported.[86] However, fractures to the first rib are rare.

Metaphyseal Injury

Metaphyseal injury, or classic metaphyseal lesions (CMLs), are seen in a high proportion of physically abused infants, most commonly in non-mobile infants under the age of 12 months.[87] CMLs have been perceived as strong predictors of abuse,[76] although the literature is inconclusive.[45,74] Histologically, the CML is a series of microfractures across the entire width of, or part thereof the metaphysis, through the immature portion of the primary spongiosa.[88] The injury is a result of 'shearing forces' sustained during violent shaking or handling of the infant, outside those forces associated with daily care. The CMLs are usually asymptomatic and not evident clinically. They are most frequently seen in the distal femur, the tibia and the proximal humerus, but also occur in the elbow and wrist. They may be uni- or bilateral.

Radiographically, the CML appears as:
1. a thin wafer of bone separated from the metaphysis, thicker at the periphery ('bucket handle fracture');
2. a thick rim only ('corner fracture'); or
3. a thin disk with a thick rim (Fig. 6-32).

Small CMLs tend to heal without callus formation, by gradual bone consolidation, within 4–8 weeks.[76] When the adjacent periosteum is injured, or stripped by the shearing forces, a subperiosteal haemorrhage occurs, which, during the healing process, is evident as a periosteal reaction. Occasionally the fracture heals with a local disturbance of growth.

CMLs must be differentiated from normal growth variations, which may take the form of subtle irregularities, 'step-off' (also termed a metaphyseal collar) (Fig. 6-33) or even mimic a bucket handle fracture (Fig. 6-34). In children over the age of 15 months, metaphyseal fragmentation can be seen in bow-legs due to abnormal stresses associated with early weight bearing.[89]

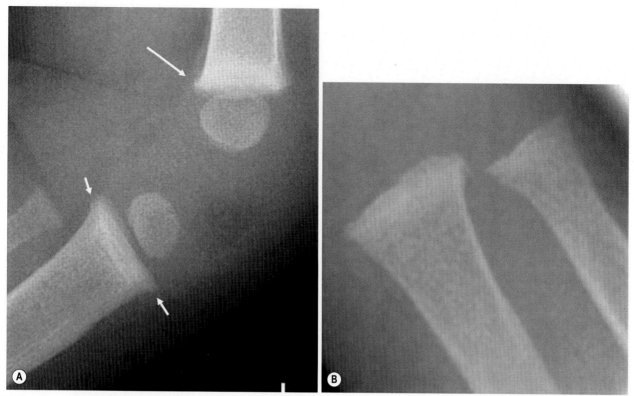

FIGURE 6-33 ■ Normal metaphyseal irregularities in the distal femur (A) and in the distal radius (B) in an 8-month-old boy who had a skeletal survey after presenting with a head injury suspect of abuse.

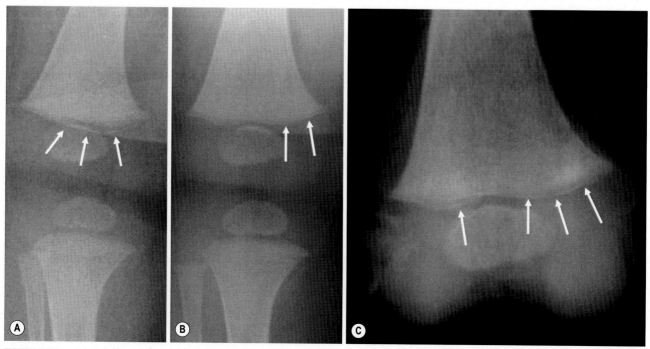

FIGURE 6-34 ■ Lucent line through the distal right femur metaphysis (arrows), mimicking a CML (bucket handle fracture) in a 3-month-old boy who died from abusive head injury. (A, B) Initial radiographs and (C) post-mortem specimen. No fracture was found at autopsy.

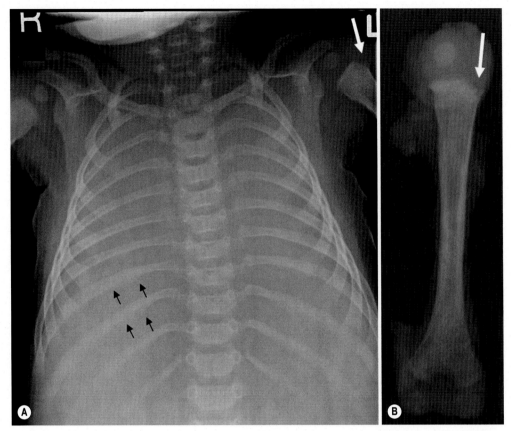

FIGURE 6-35 ■ **Avulsion fracture to the proximal left humerus (white arrows) in a 3-month-old boy who died from abusive head trauma.** (A) Initial radiograph and (B) radiograph of the specimen at autopsy. Note the normal, flanged appearances of the postero-lateral ribs, not to be mistaken for periosteal reaction (short, black arrows).

Long Bone Fractures

Fractures to the long tubular bones are seen in about one-third of physically abused children, most commonly involving the femur, humerus and tibia (Fig. 6-35).

There is no specific fracture pattern or type specific to NAI.[45] The type of fracture may suggest a possible mechanism that, again, can assist the clinician in attempting to assess the truthfulness of the explanation given by the carers.

In general, a spiral fracture indicates a twisting force; an oblique fracture may result from levering, for instance by lifting a child by a limb; and a transverse fracture may be the result of a direct impact. A greenstick or buckle fracture, commonly seen in toddlers, will be caused by compression in relation to a fall.

Overall, a child with a femoral fracture has approximately a 1 in 3 chance of having being abused, and femoral fractures resulting from abuse are more commonly seen in children who are not yet walking.[45] Similarly, a child under the age of 3 years with a humeral fracture has a 1 in 2 chance of having been abused. Midshaft diaphyseal fractures are more common in abuse than non-abuse, whereas supracondylar fractures are more likely to have non-abusive causes.[45]

The significance of long bone fractures increases when they are multiple (Fig. 6-36), particularly when of different ages, when bilateral, and when associated with clinical findings suggestive of physical abuse.

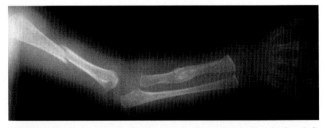

FIGURE 6-36 ■ **A recent fracture to the midshaft of the left humerus, and an old, healing fracture to the mid-radius in a 6-week-old girl, highly suggestive of abuse.**

Periosteal new bone formation along the shaft of the long bones is a normal feature in up to 35% of infants between the ages of 1 and 3–4 months of age, and should be differentiated from subperiosteal new bone formation (SPNBF) as a result of an occult fracture, or a gripping injury (Fig. 6-37).[90] SPNBF is usually bilateral but can also be unilateral, and most commonly involves the femur or tibia, and less commonly the humerus or forearm.[76] It is confined to the diaphysis and never extends to the metaphysis.

Unusual Fractures

Fractures to the spine, scapula (most commonly the acromion), sternum, pelvis, fingers and toes, in a

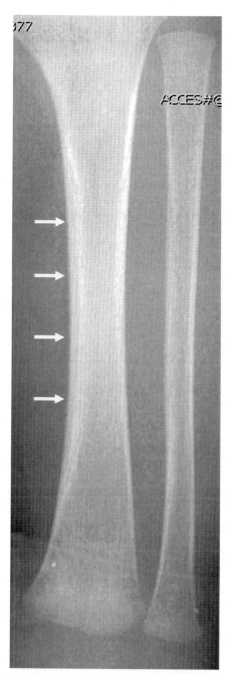

FIGURE 6-37 ■ A smooth band of mineralised density separate from the underlying cortex, not exceeding 2-mm thickness, along the tibial shaft in a 4-week-old, healthy boy, consistent with physiological SPNBF.

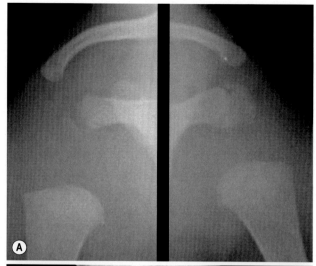

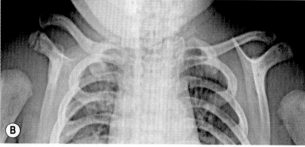

FIGURE 6-38 ■ Lucent, irregular lines with surrounding sclerosis through both acromions in a 3-month-old boy having a skeletal survey for suspected abuse. (A) Initial radiographs and (B) follow-up radiograph after 6 weeks, showing healing of the left, but not the right, suggestive of a healing, left-sided fracture from unrecognised trauma.

non-ambulant child are rare, and should raise concern when no plausible explanation can be provided.

Acromial fractures, which tend to be clinically overt, must be differentiated from normal variations in acromial ossification[76,91] (Fig. 6-38). In acromial fractures, the radiolucent defect appears to be initially smooth or slightly irregular but then, probably within a month, the margins become quite irregular and sclerotic, indicating early healing.[88] More advanced or complete healing of the fracture is usual thereafter. In the developmental anomaly, the margins of the defect remain smooth and corticated for more than a year, becoming thickened and slightly irregular thereafter. The defect becomes progressively narrow and remains visible for 3 years or more. Both injury and ossification defects can be bilateral, but can also be unilateral. Fractures are thought to be the result of indirect forces, and have also been observed in severe neonatal tetanus.

Vertebral compression fractures, particularly to the thoracolumbar region, very occasionally occur during violent shaking.

Fracture Healing

Radiological dating of fractures is of medicolegal importance, but unfortunately the evidence base for current methods of dating is sparse.

Most radiologists date fractures based on their own clinical experience, and guidance offered by textbooks (Table 6-3).[76,92,93] The radiological features of bone healing are a continuum with considerable overlap,[94] and depend on age of the child, fracture site and mobility. A systematic review of the international, scientific literature from 2005 concluded that:[94]

• Radiologists can clearly differentiate recent from old fractures.

TABLE 6-3 **Chronology (in Days) of Radiographic Changes during Fracture Healing**[75]

	Early	Peak	Late
Appearance of SPBNF	4–10	10–14	14–21
Loss of fracture line definition owing to formation of soft callus	10–14	14–21	
Appearance of hard callus (formation of lamellar bone)	14–21	21–42	42–90

- Periosteal reaction is seen as early as 4 days and is present in at least 50% of the cases by 2 weeks after the injury.
- Remodelling peaks 8 weeks after the injury and, moreover, bone scintigraphy has no place in fracture dating, as fractures show increased uptake for as long as a year.

A recent study, addressing the timetable for the radiographic features of fracture healing, concluded that fractures in young children may be dated as acute (< 1 week), recent (8–35 days), or old (≥ 36 days) on the basis of six key radiological features; soft-tissue swelling, periosteal reaction, soft callus, hard callus, bridging and remodelling.[95]

Differential Diagnosis

The differential diagnoses include accidental injury, including birth trauma, and generalised bone disease.

Birth Trauma

Birth trauma most commonly involves the clavicle, femur or humerus, but classical metaphyseal lesions have also been reported.[96] Clavicular fractures typically affect the middle third, and when left sided, must be differentiated from congenital pseudarthrosis. The fracture may be noted during birth, or later when a carer palpates the forming callus. The absence of callus 11 days or more after birth excludes a birth-related injury.

Accidental Injury

The most common explanation offered for a fracture and its plausibility will rest on relating the fracture morphology to the mechanism of injury, radiological age to temporal history of events, and personal and published data on common injuries at different ages. Numerous registries on paediatric injuries and fractures have been established worldwide during the 20 years.

Generalised Bone Disease

Differential considerations for bone injury include metabolic disorders such as rickets; copper deficiency, particularly Menkes syndrome; metaphyseal chondrodysplasia of the Schmid type; spondylometaphyseal dysplasia; corner fractures; and the occasional fragmentation occurring in osteogenesis imperfecta.

BRAIN INJURIES

Brain injuries are a major cause of morbidity and mortality in abused children under 2 years of age.[97] The clinical presentation may be hyperacute (respiratory failure, cerebral oedema), acute or subacute. Again, lack of a plausible explanation to the child's symptoms and clinical findings should raise concern. The clinical signs may be non-specific, such as changes in the mental status, vomiting, pallor, apathy, cyanosis, seizures, and even shock or severe respiratory distress. Children with hypoxic-ischaemic injury often present with apnoea and loss of consciousness. Notably, an interval of several hours to days may exist between the initial trauma and the first neurological manifestations, underscoring the importance of a meticulous medical history.

Differentiation between accidental and non-accidental head injury (NAHI) is of major legal importance, but remains difficult.[98] In one retrospective study, cases in which a perpetrator confessed to violence toward the child were compared with cases in which there was no confession. There was no significant difference between the two groups for any of the variables studied: gender, mortality, fractures, retinal haemorrhage, ecchymosis, symptoms and SDH pattern. In cases with confession, shaking was described as extremely violent (100%) and was repeated (55%) from 2 to 30 times (mean, 10) because it stopped the infant's crying (62.5%). Impact was reported in around a quarter of the cases. No correlation was found between repeated shaking and SDH densities on CT.[99] There is reason to believe that some of the NAHI cases remain undiagnosed, and the converse that is some 'unexplained sudden infant deaths' may represent NAHI.[100]

Pathophysiology of Skull, Brain and Spinal Canal Lesions

From a pathophysiological point of view, NAHI, or abusive head trauma,[54] may be caused by direct trauma with skull fractures and underlying brain damage, repeated trauma, shaking, or even strangulation. These mechanisms could lead to subdural/subarachnoid haemorrhage, contusion and intraparenchymal haemorrhage as well as other injuries such as diffuse axonal (shear) injuries and hypoxic-ischaemic damage.[101-103] The overall prognosis of intracranial lesions in this context is generally relatively pejorative compared to isolated head injuries.

Shaking injuries to the head and neck usually occur in infants younger than 1 year of age, but can be seen up to 2 years. Infants this age have relatively large heads compared to body size, and their neck muscles are weak, providing little head support.[99] Thus, repeat whiplash movements can result in ruptured cortical veins at their influx to the fixed sagittal sinus, with subarachnoid and/or subdural haemorrhage, often bilateral.[55,104,105] Further, axonal injuries can occur in the brain parenchyma due to differences in density between white and grey matter, and also in the midbrain, due to the limited mobility of the upper brainstem (set by the tentorium).

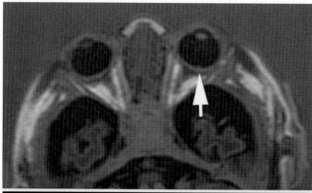

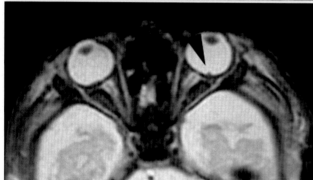

FIGURE 6-39 ■ **Axial T1- and T2*-weighted images showing left retinal haemorrhages in a 3-month-old girl with a subdural haematoma.** The findings were also demonstrated on fundoscopy.

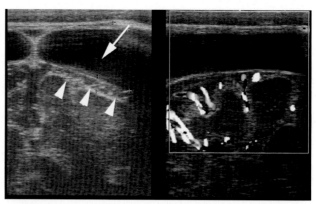

FIGURE 6-40 ■ **A 9-month-old boy presenting with hypotonia and macrocrania.** Cranial ultrasound demonstrates a bilateral subdural chronic haematoma (arrow) with compressed subarachnoid space (arrowhead) containing vessels between subdural spaces and brain.

Shaking also causes retinal haemorrhages, which must be systematically searched for ophthalmoscopically, and described in detail as to location, severity, extent and bilaterality.[106,107] Notably, both retinal and vitreous haemorrhages can also be seen on MRI (Fig. 6-39).[108,109]

Spinal injuries can be associated with NAHI. Parenchymal cord injury, meningeal haemorrhage (epidural/subdural), nerve root avulsion or ganglion haemorrhages have been reported in post-mortem examinations. They usually occur without evidence of muscular or ligamentous damage, or of bone dislocation or fracture.[110] A recent study demonstrated that 60% of children with abusive head trauma also suffered spinal canal subdural bleeding. The two proposed mechanisms regarding the origin of spinal subdural hemorrhage are mainly tracking of intracranial subdural haemorrhage[104] or, more uncommonly as a consequence of, direct injury to vessels in or around the spinal cord, but within the dural compartment.[111]

Imaging in NAHI

Skull radiographs, including AP and lateral views, are mandatory to demonstrate skull vault fractures. An additional Townes view may help diagnose occipital fractures, as well as the presence and number of Wormian bones, which may be of value for the differential diagnoses, such as osteogenesis imperfecta and Menkes' disease.

The value of head ultrasound is limited in the diagnosis of NAHI; however, it may add useful information when the initial presentation is misleading (macrocrania, stupor).[112] Pericerebral spaces are well seen with high-frequency probes. A subdural haematoma is visible outside the subarachnoid space, as a peripheral anechoic collection limited by a deep echoic thin line separating the two spaces, causing a compression more or less marked on the adjacent cortical sulci (Fig. 6-40). Parenchymal contusions, when located in an area accessible to the probe, at the convexity, can be found with hypoechoic, hypoechoic or cystic lesions, particularly at the junction of grey matter and white matter.

CT is the initial examination in suspected head trauma,[113] and should include thin, contiguous slices of the entire skull and of the craniocervical junction. Parenchymal algorithm reconstructions should be completed by specific bony reconstruction with VRT projections.

MRI is indicated when CT is equivocal or discordant with clinical signs, or to give more details about pericerebral spaces or parenchymal lesions.[114] In most cases sedation or general anaesthesia is required. The examination should include T1-weighted images (two orthogonal planes), T2-weighted (axial or coronal) or gradient-echo T2* to better detect degradation products of haemoglobin; susceptibility-weighted imaging (SWI) is more sensitive for small haemorrhages and is considered as the best tool to depict a bleed. FLAIR can be difficult to analyse during the first months of life, but is also useful for demonstrating an extra-axial, acute bleed.[59]

Diffusion-weighted imaging (DWI) is now mandatory, especially in the initial phase of trauma, to look for hypoxic-ischaemic changes and axonal injuries.[112]

Additional, alternative sequences include MR angiography and MR spectroscopy. Sagittal T1- and T2-weighted images of the spine are useful to detect intraspinal haemorrhage, and should be supplemented with axial scans in cases of equivocal or positive findings.

In most cases, the use of contrast medium, both in CT and MRI, is unnecessary;[112] it may in some cases be useful to confirm the presence of a subdural haematoma.[53,73,115]

Skull Fractures

Most skull fractures, both accidental and abusive, are linear. The presence of bilateral, stellar or depressed fractures or fractures through the midline, increase the clinical suspicion of abuse, in particular when there is a history of a mild trauma or no trauma (fall from a couch).[116] Dating is difficult, as skull fractures heal without any callus formation, within 6 months.

Loss of fracture-line definition can be seen after around 2 weeks' interval. A growing fracture with leptomeningeal cyst formation is more commonly seen in NAHI than in accidental injury. With CT, some parallel linear fractures in the plane of slices may be missed, highlighting the need for conventional radiographs. CT with thin sections and 3D volume reconstruction and VRT views are useful to demonstrate these fractures[53] (Fig. 6-41). Bone scintigraphy, on the other hand, may fail to visualise skull fractures due to low osteoblastic activity during fracture repair.

Extra-Axial Haemorrhages

Acute extradural haemorrhage is rare, and can be found in both abusive and accidental head injury.[113]

Subarachnoid haemorrhage (SAH) is better seen in the initial phase with CT than with conventional T1 and T2 WSE MRI,[117] but FLAIR (hyperintensity) and SWI (hypointensity) are still sensitive. In young infants, the diagnosis may be overdiagnosed on CT since the difference in density between the dura and parenchyma is higher than in the older child.

Subdural haematoma (SDH) is the most frequent haemorrhage encountered in NAHI. It is caused by the primary trauma, and not secondary hypoxia or brain swelling.[101,118] At the time of presentation, SDHs can be acute, subacute or chronic and seen as a hyper-, iso- or hypodense collection, respectively, on CT.[109]

In the context of abuse, SDHs are frequently bilateral, closely related to the falx, layering over the tentorium and then highly suggestive of abuse, especially if they are accompanied by cerebral oedema[116] (Figs. 6-42A-C). Haemorrhages can also occur within the falx itself.[119,120] In accidental trauma, SDHs are mainly localised over the cerebral convexities, while involvement of the posterior fossa is more common in abusive trauma.

MRI is more sensitive than CT for detecting small collections, and is also useful in the differentiation between CSF in the subarachnoidal space and chronic SDHs in cases where the CT scan shows low-attenuation extra-axial fluid[116] (Figs. 6-42B, 6-43A, B and 6-44A, B). Dating of haemorrhages is inaccurate on both CT and MRI.[101,121] After the acute phase, several concentric compartments can be seen within the SDH, with different signal regarding the weighted sequences. Is appears very difficult to affirm that they correspond to repetitive trauma, or to give a specific calendar of these bleedings, because in case of SDH, new spontaneous bleedings can occur within the first one.

Moreover, in terms of differential diagnosis, it should be remembered that a subdural collection is not necessarily related to abuse, but may also occur in children

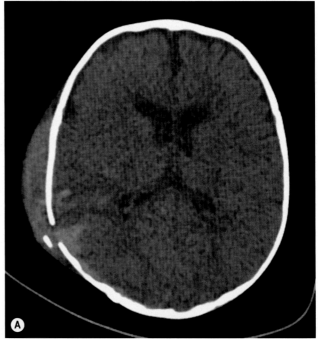

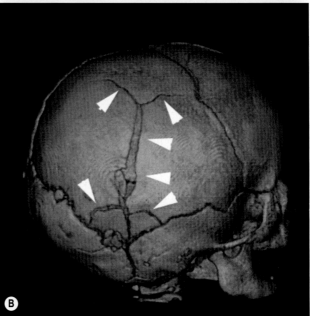

FIGURE 6-41 ■ (A) Cerebral CT in a 6-month-old boy, showing a soft-tissue swelling in the right parietal region with an underlying skull fracture and haemorrhagic brain contusions. The baby had been thrown to the floor. (B) A 3D reconstruction of the skull, demonstrating a stellar parietal fracture.

with 'benign macrocrania', with enlarged transitional subarachnoid spaces and tensioning of the cortical veins. Searching for an association between a sudden increase in head circumference and intraparenchymal lesions is therefore important in order to avoid overdiagnosis of NAHI.[104,109,122,123]

It remains difficult, without previous imaging studies demonstrating a 'benign' enlargement of subarachnoid spaces, to affirm that an acute or subacute SDH is present only in relation to this pre-existent situation.[53,124] Other

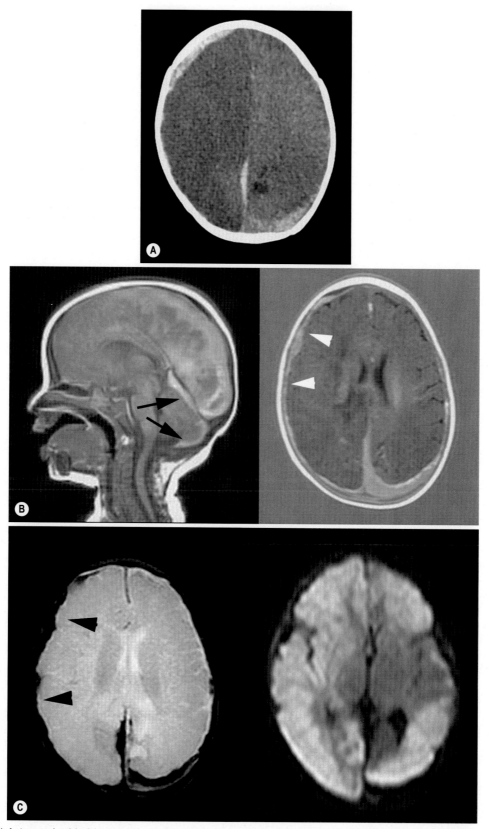

FIGURE 6-42 ■ (A) A 4-month-old girl presenting with apnoea and loss of consciousness. The initial CT demonstrated acute, subdural haematomas in the right frontal and left parietal regions, a haemorrhage within the posterior part of the falx and oedema of the right hemisphere with loss of grey–white matter differentiation. (B) Continuing, sagittal and axial T1-weighted MR images confirmed the hemispheric subdural acute haematoma (arrowheads). Note also a subdural bleeding within the posterior fossa (arrows). (C) Continuing, an axial T2*-weighted MR image shows hypointensity in relation to blood. Diffusion-weighted image confirms restriction of water diffusion within the right hemisphere, but also in the left frontal and parietal lobes.

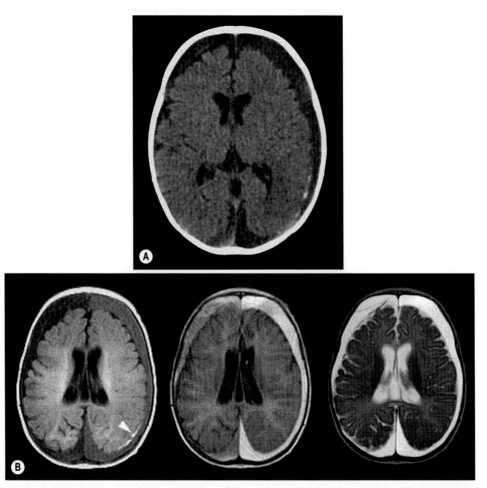

FIGURE 6-43 ■ (A) A 4-month-old boy, somnolent, presenting with a right periorbital haematoma. CT demonstrated subacute, sub-dural collections bilaterally, with recent bleeding on the left side. (B) Continuing, MRI performed 3 days later. Axial T1, flair and T2-weighted images. Right and left subdural collections exhibit different signal intensities, maybe in relation to different bleeding but also to blood concentration in each collection. Note also subarachnoid bleeding on the left side, better seen on T1 (arrowhead). Skeletal survey revealed multiple rib fractures.

options to be considered would be coagulopathies, sub-dural collections after acute dehydratation or meningitis, or in relation to congenital metabolic diseases, such as glutaric aciduria type I or Menke's disease.

Intraventricular haemorrhage may occur in the 'shaken baby' in connection with a subependymal venous injury, and is easily detected on CT in the acute phase. On MRI, changes on T2*-weighted or SWI sequences will remain for a while. Secondary, obstructive hydro-cephalus may be seen.

Parenchymal Brain Injuries

Focal or generalised brain injury can be related to the severity of the trauma itself, or to hypoxic-ischaemic change. CT is useful for detecting focal haemorrhages in the acute phase, while MRI is more sensitive for their recognition at any stage.

Intraparenchymal haemorrhagic contusions, visible at the white matter and cortex junction, are spontane-ously hyperdense on CT in the acute phase and become hypodense after a few days. They are also secondarily better seen with MRI, due to the presence of degradation products of haemoglobin, with increased signal intensity

on T1, at the intermediate phase, then a low signal on T2*, SWI in the late phase (Fig. 6-44C). It may, however, be difficult, once again, to precisely date the haemor-rhage.[73] Non-haemorrhagic lesions are well depicted by MRI. Multiple subcortical lesions affect the neurodevel-opmental outcome and prognosis.[125]

Shearing lesions (diffuse axonal lesions) are sought in the subcortical region, but also at the centrum ovale, in the corpus callosum and the cerebral peduncles. They can be haemorrhagic, and then initially visible on CT, or in most of cases non-haemorrhagic: MRI (FLAIR, T2 and DWI) is then essential to demonstrate them.[126] DWI is useful to look for changes in regional brain anisotropy and fibre tracking helps to characterise axonal lesions, although this is not routine clinical practice.

Diffuse Hypoxic-Ischaemic Lesions

The association of focal ischaemic lesions, in multiple locations, either in the MCA territory, with a subarach-noid haemorrhage is highly suggestive of abuse. Ischae-mic lesions preferentially involve the basal ganglia. Moreover, the lesions are more diffuse, preserving only the posterior fossa (especially in lesions resulting from

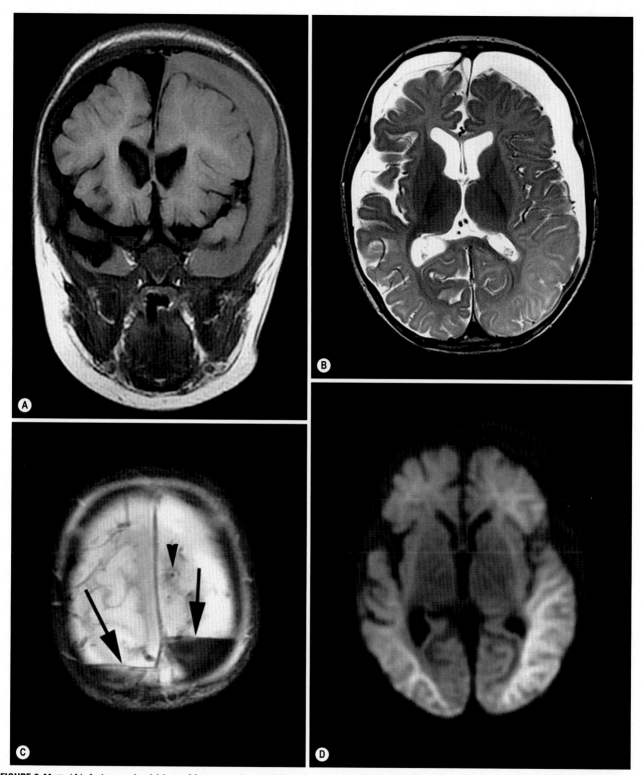

FIGURE 6-44 ■ (A) A 4-month-old boy. Macrocrania, malaise. Coronal FLAIR image demonstrates circumferential bilateral subdural collections. (B) Continuing, T2 axial slice confirms subdural collections, with hyperintensity of the posterior regions of the brain. (C) Continuing, susceptibity-weighted image shows punctiform parenchyma bleeding (arrowhead) and fluid–fluid levels within the surrounding subdural collections. (D) Continuing, diffusion-weighted image better demonstrates bilateral cortico-subcortical ischaemic lesions.

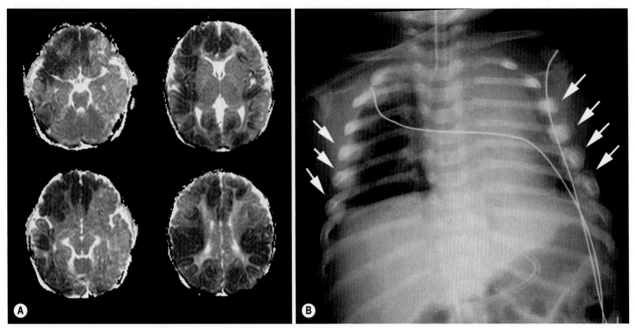

FIGURE 6-45 ■ (A) A 3-month-old girl. Sudden pallor, loss of consciousness, then seizures; blood found with lumbar puncture. DWI with ADC maps reveals multiple ischaemic lesions. (B) Continuing, chest radiographs after resuscitation in the intensive care unit: multiple rib fractures with callus (arrows). Shaken baby.

strangulation), sometimes associated with specific signs of shock.

CT may show parenchymal hypoattenuation or loss of grey–white matter differentiation, and the 'reversal sign', where the cerebellum is of higher attenuation than the cerebral hemispheres. MRI with DWI is very sensitive in demonstrating early hypoxic-ischaemic changes, by demonstrating cytotoxic oedema with restriction of water diffusion (Figs. 6-42C, 6-42D and 6-45). MR spectroscopy adds some prognostic information when a high relative concentration of lactate, compared to creatine and *N*-acetylaspartate (NAA), is obvious[53,109] (Fig. 6-46). CT or MRI will secondarily depict late outcome with brain atrophy or multicystic encephalomalacia.[127]

Intraspinal Lesions

Spinal injuries in NAHI are believed to be underdiagnosed,[110,128] and additional MRI series covering the whole spine are therefore recommended by some authors.[111] Signal abnormality of the cord may suggest contusion or infarction. Haemorrhage in the epidural or subdural spaces is suspected when there is a nodular or smooth dural thickening, a mass effect upon the cord and/or effacement of the subarachnoid space. Recognition of the normal epidural fat allows for distinction between epidural or subdural location.[111] Spinal ultrasound represents a valuable alternative to demonstrate a spinal subdural haematoma.[129]

Strategy and Prognosis

In summary, the initial work-up of children having sustained a head injury should include skull radiographs, an unenhanced head CT and an ophthalmic examination.

In the majority of cases, MRI is indicated to better depict the parenchymal lesions and is particularly useful for follow-up. The MRI should include T1-weighted series, T2, T2* or SWI and DWI. The assessment and report should preferably be done by a neuroradiologist or a paediatric radiologist with experience in NAHI cases, and should include a thorough description of the nature and the extent of the lesions, possible mechanisms and possible differential diagnoses. Dating intracranial lesions should be performed with caution.[113] The evaluation of head injuries in infants requires a high level of awareness and thorough and systematic examination by a trained multidisciplinary team.[57,98]

Overall, prognosis is worse in NAHI than in accidental trauma. Parenchymal haemorrhages and cerebral contusions, better seen on MRI with SWI and DWI, correlate with poor clinical outcome.[130] Preventative efforts must be focused within the child welfare system, assisting parents and caregivers as well as child welfare professionals to facilitate early identification of abusive head injury.[54,131,132]

ABDOMINAL AND CHEST INJURIES

Non-accidental skeletal and cerebral trauma are features of the non ambulant child, whilst visceral injuries are common after the child is mobile, with an average age of 2 years.[51] The incidence of these injuries is lower than that reported for skeletal and head injury, but the mortality rate is as high as 50%.

This could be related to the vague clinical history at presentation and consequent delayed diagnosis.[76] The clinical presentation can be acute, with symptoms

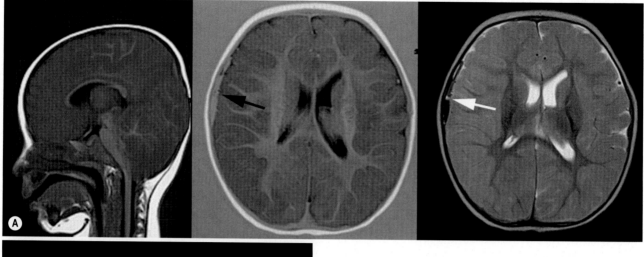

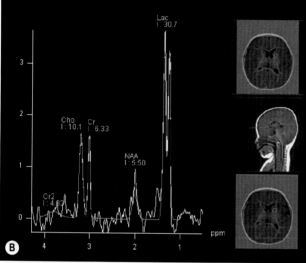

FIGURE 6-46 ■ (A) A 4-month-old boy. Acute respiratory distress, admitted for near-miss syndrome. Sagittal and axial T1-weighted images, axial T2-weighted slice demonstrate massive brain oedema without visibility of cerebral cisterns. Note also subdural bleeding on the right side (arrows). (B) Continiuing, MR spectroscopy demonstrates a low N-acetylaspartate (NAA) peak and a very high concentration of lactate. Post-mortem pathological confirmation of an acute subdural haematoma with rupture of bridging veins.

suggestive of perforation, obstruction or bleeding, such as vomiting, severe pain, tenderness, shock or sepsis.

Others may present with more ill-defined, chronic symptoms like weight loss, malaise or non-specific abdominal pain. The radiologist should be familiar with the different scenarios, and also be aware that incidental findings, e.g. rib fractures on an abdominal radiograph, may represent markers for abuse. The most common abdominal injuries involve the duodenum, pancreas and mesentery, but injuries to the liver, kidney and spleen also occur. Injuries to the chest are rare, and include pneumothorax/pneumomediastinum, haemothorax, chylothorax, contusions to the lung and heart, as well as injuries to the oesophagus.

Imaging

In unstable patients, a focused assessment with sonography (FAST) ultrasound, which has now become an extension of the physical examination of the trauma patient, should be considered. Performed in the trauma room by properly trained and credentialed staff, it allows the timely diagnosis of potentially life-threatening haemorrhage and is a decision-making tool to help determine the need for transfer to the operating room, CT scanner or angiography suite.

CT scans of the chest, abdomen and/or the pelvis are indicated if there are signs and symptoms of abuse or if abnormal findings are seen on conventional radiography, particularly if there is a discrepancy with clinical history.[56]

The chest scan should generally be performed with intravenous contrast to detect vascular injuries, while CT scans for suspected intra-abdominal injury should include contrast-enhanced images of both the abdomen and pelvis, as well as oral contrast where possible.

REFERENCES

1. Landin LA. Epidemiology of children's fractures. J Pediatr Orthop B 1997;6(2):79–83.
2. Rang M, editor. Children's Fractures. Phildelphia: Lippencott; 2005.
3. Rogers LF. The radiography of epiphyseal injuries. Radiology 1970;96(2):289–99.
4. Salter RB, Harris WR. Injuries involving the epiphyseal plate. J Bone Joint Surg Am 1963;45:587–622.
5. Ogden JA. Injury to the growth mechanisms of the immature skeleton. Skeletal Radiol 1981;6(4):237–53.
6. Peterson HA. Physeal fractures: Part 3. Classification. J Pediatr Orthop 1994;14(4):439–48.

7. Stevens MA, El-Khoury GY, Kathol MH, et al. Imaging features of avulsion injuries. Radiographics 1999;19(3):655–72.

8. Allman FL Jr. Fractures and ligamentous injuries of the clavicle and its articulation. J Bone Joint Surg Am 1967;49(4):774–84.

9. Lam MH, Wong GY, Lao TT. Reappraisal of neonatal clavicular fracture. Relationship between infant size and risk factors. J Reprod Med 2002;47(11):903–8.

10. Schwendenwein E, Hajdu S, Gaebler C, et al. Displaced fractures of the proximal humerus in children require open/closed reduction and internal fixation. Eur J Pediatr Surg 2004;14(1):51–5.

11. Killeen KL. The fallen fragment sign. Radiology 1998;207(1):261–2.

12. Ouellette H, Bredella M, Labis J, et al. MR imaging of the elbow in baseball pitchers. Skeletal Radiol 2008;37(2):115–21.

13. Adirim TA, Cheng TL. Overview of injuries in the young athlete. Sports Med 2003;33(1):75–81.

14. Fick DS, Lyons TA. Interpreting elbow radiographs in children. Am Fam Physician 1997;55(4):1278–82.

15. Kramhøft M, Bødtker S. Epidemiology of distal forearm fractures in Danish children. Acta Orthop Scand 1988;59(5):557–9.

16. Johnson KJ, Haigh SF, Symonds KE. MRI in the management of scaphoid fractures in skeletally immature patients. Pediatr Radiol 2000;30(10):685–8.

17. Rajesh A, Basu AK, Vaidhyanath R, Finlay D. Hand fractures: a study of their site and type in childhood. Clin Radiol 2001;56(8):667–9.

18. Burgess AR, Eastridge BJ, Young JW, et al. Pelvic ring disruptions: effective classification system and treatment protocols. J Trauma 1990;30(7):848–56.

19. Manson T, O'Toole RV, Whitney A, et al. Young–Burgess classification of pelvic ring fractures: does it predict mortality, transfusion requirements, and non-orthopaedic injuries? J Orthop Trauma 2010;24(10):603–9.

20. Tile M. Acute pelvic fractures: I. Causation and classification. J Am Acad Orthop Surg 1996;4(3):143–51.

21. Shore BJ, Palmer CS, Bevin C, et al. Pediatric pelvic fracture: a modification of a preexisting classification. J Pediatr Orthop 2012;32(2):162–8.

22. Heeg M, de Ridder VA, Tornetta P 3rd, et al. Acetabular fractures in children and adolescents. Clin Orthop Relat Res 2000;(376):80–6.

23. Harris JH, Coupe KJ, Lee JS, Trotscher T. Acetabular fractures revisited: a new CT-based classification. Semin Musculoskelet Radiol 2005;9(2):150–60.

24. Salisbury RD, Eastwood DM. Traumatic dislocation of the hip in children. Clin Orthop Relat Res 2000;(377):106–11.

25. Moore BR, Hampers LC, Clark KD. Performance of a decision rule for radiographs of pediatric knee injuries. J Emerg Med 2005;28(3):257–61.

26. Pill SG, Ganley TJ, Milam RA, et al. Role of magnetic resonance imaging and clinical criteria in predicting successful nonoperative treatment of osteochondritis dissecans in children. J Pediatr Orthop 2003;23(1):102–8.

27. Shannak AO. Tibial fractures in children: follow-up study. J Pediatr Orthop 1988;8(3):306–10.

28. Brown SD, Kasser JR, Zurakowski D, Jaramillo D. Analysis of 51 tibial triplane fractures using CT with multiplanar reconstruction. Am J Roentgenol 2004;183(5):1489–95.

29. Spiegel PG, Cooperman DR, Laros GS. Epiphyseal fractures of the distal ends of the tibia and fibula. A retrospective study of two hundred and thirty-seven cases in children. J Bone Joint Surg Am 1978;60(8):1046–50.

30. Berson L, Davidson RS, Dormans JP, et al. Growth disturbances after distal tibial physeal fractures. Foot Ankle Int 2000;21(1):54–8.

31. Kay RM, Tang CW. Pediatric foot fractures: evaluation and treatment. J Am Acad Orthop Surg 2001;9(5):308–19.

32. Ogden J, editor Foot. In: Skeletal Injury in the Child. Heidelberg: Springer Verlag; 2000. pp. 1091–158.

33. Kokoska ER, Keller MS, Rallo MC, Weber TR. Characteristics of pediatric cervical spine injuries. J Pediatr Surg 2001;36(1):100–5.

34. Pang D, Wilberger JE Jr. Spinal cord injury without radiographic abnormalities in children. J Neurosurg 1982;57(1):114–29.

35. Kempe CH, Silverman FN, Steele B, et al. The battered-child syndrome. JAMA 1962;181:17–24.

36. Caffey J. Multiple fractures in the long bones of infants suffering from chronic subdural hematoma. Am J Roentgenol Radium Ther 1946;56(2):163–73.

37. Child Welfare Information Gateway 2006 Child Abuse and Neglect Fatalities: Statistics and Interventions, 2004. Updated July 24, 2006.

38. Radford L, Corral S, Bradley C, et al. Child abuse and neglect in the UK today. London: NSPCC; 2009.

39. AIHW. Child Protection Australia 2008-09. Child Welfare Series 47, Cat. CWS 35. Canberra: AIHW; 2010.

40. King J, Diefendorf D, Apthorp J, et al. Analysis of 429 fractures in 189 battered children. J Pediatr Orthop 1988;8(5):585–9.

41. Worlock P, Stower M, Barbor P. Patterns of fractures in accidental and non-accidental injury in children: a comparative study. Br Med J (Clin Res Ed) 1986;293(6539):100–2.

42. Kellogg ND. Evaluation of suspected child physical abuse. Pediatrics 2007;119(6):1232–41.

43. Al-Holou WN, O'Hara EA, Cohen-Gadol AA, Maher CO. Non-accidental head injury in children. Historical vignette. J Neurosurg Pediatr 2009;3(6):474–83.

44. Woolley PV Jr, Evans WA Jr. Significance of skeletal lesions in infants resembling those of traumatic origin. J Am Med Assoc 1955;158(7):539–43.

45. Kemp AM, Dunstan F, Harrison S, et al. Patterns of skeletal fractures in child abuse: systematic review. BMJ 2008;337:a1518.

46. Landin LA. Epidemiology of children's fractures. J Pediatr Orthop B 1997;6(2):79–83.

47. Brudvik C, Hove LM. Childhood fractures in Bergen, Norway: identifying high-risk groups and activities. J Pediatr Orthop 2003;23(5):629–34.

48. Kleinman PK, Schlesinger AE. Mechanical factors associated with posterior rib fractures: laboratory and case studies. Pediatr Radiol 1997;27(1):87–91.

49. Squier W. Shaken baby syndrome: the quest for evidence. Dev Med Child Neurol 2008;50(1):10–14.

50. Loder RT, Bookout C. Fracture patterns in battered children. J Orthop Trauma 1991;5(4):428–33.

51. Cooper A, Floyd T, Barlow B, et al. Major blunt abdominal trauma due to child abuse. J Trauma 1988;28(10):1483–7.

52. Caffey J. The whiplash shaken infant syndrome: manual shaking by the extremities with whiplash-induced intracranial and intraocular bleedings, linked with residual permanent brain damage and mental retardation. Pediatrics 1974;54(4):396–403.

53. Hedlund GL, Frasier LD. Neuroimaging of abusive head trauma. Forensic Sci Med Pathol 2009;5(4):280–90.

54. Christian CW, Block R. Abusive head trauma in infants and children. Pediatrics 2009;123(5):1409–11.

55. Duhaime AC, Christian CW, Rorke LB, Zimmerman RA. Nonaccidental head injury in infants—the 'shaken-baby syndrome'. N Engl J Med 1998;338(25):1822–9.

56. American College of Radiology. ACR Appropriateness Criteria Suspected Physical Abuse—Child. 2009. Available at <http://www.acr.org/>.

57. Intercollegiate report from the Royal College of Radiologists and the Royal College of Paediatrics and Child Health. Standards for radiological investigations of suspected non-accidental injury. RCR and RCPCH; 2008.

58. Royal College of Radiologists. RCR Referral Guidelines. 2012. Available at <http://www.rcr.ac.uk/>.

59. Kemp AM. Abusive head trauma: recognition and the essential investigation. Arch Dis Child Educ Pract Ed 2011;96(6):202–8.

60. Johnson K. Skeletal aspects of non-accidental injury. Endocr Dev 2009;16:233–45.

61. Zimmerman S, Makoroff K, Care M, et al. Utility of follow-up skeletal surveys in suspected child physical abuse evaluations. Child Abuse Negl 2005;29(10):1075–83.

62. Kleinman PK, Nimkin K, Spevak MR, et al. Follow-up skeletal surveys in suspected child abuse. Am J Roentgenol 1996;167(4):893–6.

63. Weber MA, Risdon RA, Offiah AC, et al. Rib fractures identified at post-mortem examination in sudden unexpected deaths in infancy (SUDI). Forensic Sci Int 2009;189(1–3):75–81.

64. Bilo R, Robben S, van Rijn R. Forensic Aspects of Paediatric Fractures. Berlin-Heidelberg: Springer; 2010.

65. Conway JJ, Collins M, Tanz RR, et al. The role of bone scintigraphy in detecting child abuse. Semin Nucl Med 1993;23(4): 321–33.

66. Sty JR, Starshak RJ, Hubbard AM. Radionuclide evaluation in childhood injuries. Semin Nucl Med 1983;13(3):258–81.

67. Perez-Rossello JM, Connolly SA, Newton AW, et al. Whole-body MRI in suspected infant abuse. Am J Roentgenol 2010;195(3): 744–50.

68. Muller LS, Avenarius D, Damasio B, et al. The paediatric wrist revisited: redefining MR findings in healthy children. Ann Rheum Dis 2011;70(4):605–10.

69. Ording Muller LS, Avenarius D, Olsen OE. High signal in bone marrow at diffusion-weighted imaging with body background suppression (DWIBS) in healthy children. Pediatr Radiol 2011; 41(2):221–6.

70. Cooper C, Dennison EM, Leufkens HG, et al. Epidemiology of childhood fractures in Britain: a study using the general practice research database. J Bone Miner Res 2004;19(12):1976–81.

71. Mayranpaa MK, Makitie O, Kallio PE. Decreasing incidence and changing pattern of childhood fractures: A population-based study. J Bone Miner Res 2010;25(12):2752–9.

72. Brudvik C, Hove LM. Childhood fractures in Bergen, Norway: identifying high-risk groups and activities. J Pediatr Orthop 2003;23(5):629–34.

73. Carty H, Pierce A. Non-accidental injury: a retrospective analysis of a large cohort. Eur Radiol 2002;12(12):2919–25.

74. Kleinman PK, Perez-Rossello JM, Newton AW, et al. Prevalence of the classic metaphyseal lesion in infants at low versus high risk for abuse. Am J Roentgenol 2011;197(4):1005–8.

75. Saperia J, Lakhanpaul M, Kemp A, Glaser D. When to suspect child maltreatment: summary of NICE guidance. BMJ 2009; 339:b2689.

76. Kleinman PK. Diagnostic Imaging of Child Abuse. 2nd ed. London: Mosby; 1998.

77. Merten DF, Radkowski MA, Leonidas JC. The abused child: a radiological reappraisal. Radiology 1983;146(2):377–81.

78. Kleinman PK, Marks SC Jr, Nimkin K, et al. Rib fractures in 31 abused infants: postmortem radiologic-histopathologic study. Radiology 1996;200(3):807–10.

79. Kleinman PK, Marks SC, Adams VI, Blackbourne BD. Factors affecting visualization of posterior rib fractures in abused infants. Am J Roentgenol 1988;150(3):635–8.

80. Barsness KA, Cha ES, Bensard DD, et al. The positive predictive value of rib fractures as an indicator of nonaccidental trauma in children. J Trauma 2003;54(6):1107–10.

81. Cadzow SP, Armstrong KL. Rib fractures in infants: red alert! The clinical features, investigations and child protection outcomes. J Paediatr Child Health 2000;36(4):322–6.

82. Bulloch B, Schubert CJ, Brophy PD, et al. Cause and clinical characteristics of rib fractures in infants. Pediatrics 2000;105(4): E48.

83. Maguire S, Mann M, John N, et al. Does cardiopulmonary resuscitation cause rib fractures in children? A systematic review. Child Abuse Negl 2006;30(7):739–51.

84. Spevak MR, Kleinman PK, Belanger PL, et al. Cardiopulmonary resuscitation and rib fractures in infants. A postmortem radiologic-pathologic study. JAMA 1994;272(8):617–18.

85. Matshes EW, Lew EO. Two-handed cardiopulmonary resuscitation can cause rib fractures in infants. Am J Forensic Med Pathol 2010;31(4):303–7.

86. Gorincour G, Dubus JC, Petit P, et al. Rib periosteal reaction: did you think about chest physical therapy? Arch Dis Child 2004; 89(11):1078–9.

87. Kleinman PK, Sarwar ZU, Newton AW, et al. Metaphyseal fragmentation with physiologic bowing: a finding not to be confused with the classic metaphyseal lesion. Am J Roentgenol 2009; 192(5):1266–8.

88. Kleinman PK, Marks SC, Blackbourne B. The metaphyseal lesion in abused infants: a radiologic-histopathologic study. Am J Roentgenol 1986;146(5):895–905.

89. Kleinman PK, Marks SC Jr. A regional approach to the classic metaphyseal lesion in abused infants: the distal femur. Am J Roentgenol 1998;170(1):43–7.

90. Kwon DS, Spevak MR, Fletcher K, Kleinman PK. Physiologic subperiosteal new bone formation: prevalence, distribution, and thickness in neonates and infants. Am J Roentgenol 2002;179(4): 985–8.

91. Kleinman PK, Spevak MR. Variations in acromial ossification simulating infant abuse in victims of sudden infant death syndrome. Radiology 1991;180(1):185–7.

92. Currarino G, Prescott P. Fractures of the acromion in young children and a description of a variant in acromial ossification which may mimic a fracture. Pediatr Radiol 1994;24(4):251–5.

93. Offiah A, Hall C. Radiological Atlas of Child Abuse. 1st ed. New York: Radcliffe Medical; 2009.

94. Prosser I, Maguire S, Harrison SK, et al. How old is this fracture? Radiologic dating of fractures in children: a systematic review. Am J Roentgenol 2005;184(4):1282–6.

95. Prosser I, Lawson Z, Evans A, et al. A timetable for the radiologic features of fracture healing in young children. Am J Roentgenol 2012;198(5):1014–20.

96. O'Connell A, Donoghue VB. Can classic metaphyseal lesions follow uncomplicated caesarean section? Pediatr Radiol 2007; 37(5):488–91.

97. Sieswerda-Hoogendoorn T, Boos S, Spivack B, et al. Educational paper: Abusive Head Trauma part I. Clinical aspects. Eur J Pediatr 2012;171(3):415–23.

98. Vinchon M, De Foort-Dhellemmes S, Desurmont M, Delestret I. Confessed abuse versus witnessed accidents in infants: comparison of clinical, radiological, and ophthalmological data in corroborated cases. Childs Nerv Syst 2010;26(5):637–45.

99. Adamsbaum C, Grabar S, Mejean N, Rey-Salmon C. Abusive head trauma: judicial admissions highlight violent and repetitive shaking. Pediatrics 2010;126(3):546–55.

100. Reece RM. Fatal child abuse and sudden infant death syndrome: a critical diagnostic decision. Pediatrics 1993;91(2):423–9.

101. Jaspan T. Current controversies in the interpretation of non-accidental head injury. Pediatr Radiol 2008;38(Suppl. 3): S378–87.

102. Case ME. Inflicted traumatic brain injury in infants and young children. Brain Pathol 2008;18(4):571–82.

103. Gerber P, Coffman K. Nonaccidental head trauma in infants. Childs Nerv Syst 2007;23(5):499–507.

104. Squier W. The 'shaken baby' syndrome: pathology and mechanisms. Acta Neuropathol 2011;122(5):519–42.

105. Squier W, Mack J. The neuropathology of infant subdural haemorrhage. Forensic Sci Int 2009;187(1–3):6–13.

106. Levin AV, Christian CW. The eye examination in the evaluation of child abuse. Pediatrics 2010;126(2):376–80.

107. Togioka BM, Arnold MA, Bathurst MA, et al. Retinal hemorrhages and shaken baby syndrome: an evidence-based review. J Emerg Med 2009;37(1):98–106.

108. Altinok D, Saleem S, Zhang Z, et al. MR imaging findings of retinal hemorrhage in a case of nonaccidental trauma. Pediatr Radiol 2009;39(3):290–2.

109. Fernando S, Obaldo RE, Walsh IR, Lowe LH. Neuroimaging of nonaccidental head trauma: pitfalls and controversies. Pediatr Radiol 2008;38(8):827–38.

110. Brennan LK, Rubin D, Christian CW, et al. Neck injuries in young pediatric homicide victims. J Neurosurg Pediatr 2009;3(3): 232–9.

111. Choudhary AK, Bradford RK, Dias MS, et al. Spinal subdural hemorrhage in abusive head trauma: a retrospective study. Radiology 2012;262(1):216–23.

112. Sieswerda-Hoogendoorn T, Boos S, Spivack B, et al. Abusive head trauma. Part II: radiological aspects. Eur J Pediatr 2012;171(4): 617–23.

113. van Rijn RR, Spevak MR. Imaging of neonatal child abuse with an emphasis on abusive head trauma. Magn Reson Imaging Clin N Am 2011;19(4):791–812.

114. Foerster BR, Petrou M, Lin D, et al. Neuroimaging evaluation of non-accidental head trauma with correlation to clinical outcomes: a review of 57 cases. J Pediatr 2009;154(4):573–7.

115. Kleinman PK, Ragland RL. Gadopentetate dimeglumine-enhanced MR imaging of subdural hematoma in an abused infant. Am J Roentgenol 1996;166(6):1456–8.

116. Stoodley N. Neuroimaging in non-accidental head injury: if, when, why and how. Clin Radiol 2005;60(1):22–30.

117. Zimmerman RA, Bilaniuk LT. Pediatric head trauma. Neuroimaging Clin N Am 1994;4(2):349–66.
118. Matschke J, Voss J, Obi N, et al. Nonaccidental head injury is the most common cause of subdural bleeding in infants <1 year of age. Pediatrics 2009;124(6):1587–94.
119. Harwood-Nash DC. Abuse to the pediatric central nervous system. Am J Neuroradiol 1992;13(2):569–75.
120. Kemp AM, Jaspan T, Griffiths J, et al. Neuroimaging: what neuroradiological features distinguish abusive from non-abusive head trauma? A systematic review. Arch Dis Child 2011;96(12): 1103–12.
121. Vezina G. Assessment of the nature and age of subdural collections in nonaccidental head injury with CT and MRI. Pediatr Radiol 2009;39(6):586–90.
122. Zahl SM, Egge A, Helseth E, Wester K. Benign external hydrocephalus: a review, with emphasis on management. Neurosurg Rev 2011;34(4):417–32.
123. Ghosh PS, Ghosh D. Subdural hematoma in infants without accidental or nonaccidental injury: benign external hydrocephalus, a risk factor. Clin Pediatr (Phila) 2011;50(10):897–903.
124. Vinchon M, Delestret I, DeFoort-Dhellemmes S, et al. Subdural hematoma in infants: can it occur spontaneously? Data from a prospective series and critical review of the literature. Childs Nerv Syst 2010;26(9):1195–205.
125. Bonnier C, Marique P, Van HA, Potelle D. Neurodevelopmental outcome after severe traumatic brain injury in very young children: role for subcortical lesions. J Child Neurol 2007;22(5): 519–29.
126. Gentleman SM, Roberts GW, Gennarelli TA, et al. Axonal injury: a universal consequence of fatal closed head injury? Acta Neuropathol 1995;89(6):537–43.
127. Matlung SE, Bilo RA, Kubat B, van Rijn RR. Multicystic encephalomalacia as an end-stage finding in abusive head trauma. Forensic Sci Med Pathol 2011;7(4):355–63.
128. Koumellis P, McConachie NS, Jaspan T. Spinal subdural haematomas in children with non-accidental head injury. Arch Dis Child 2009;94(3):216–19.
129. Edelbauer M, Maurer K, Gassner I. Spinal subdural effusion—an additional sonographic sign of child abuse. Ultraschall Med 2012;33(7):E339–43.
130. Colbert CA, Holshouser BA, Aaen GS, et al. Value of cerebral microhemorrhages detected with susceptibility-weighted MR imaging for prediction of long-term outcome in children with nonaccidental trauma. Radiology 2010;256(3):898–905.
131. Bennett S, Ward M, Moreau K, et al. Head injury secondary to suspected child maltreatment: results of a prospective Canadian national surveillance program. Child Abuse Negl 2011;35(11): 930–6.
132. Russell BS. Revisiting the measurement of Shaken Baby Syndrome Awareness. Child Abuse Negl 2010;34(9):671–6.

CHAPTER 7

BONE TUMOURS AND NEUROBLASTOMA IN CHILDREN

Paul Humphries • Claudio Granata

BONE TUMOURS

The most common presenting symptom of bone neoplasms is skeletal pain. Plain radiography remains the first diagnostic step. Lesion location, appearance and patient age may help suggest a diagnosis. Magnetic resonance imaging (MRI) defines soft tissue, intramedullary extent, joint involvement and relationship to muscular compartments and neurovascular structures. If a malignant lesion is suspected, computed tomography (CT) of the chest and bone scintigraphy are used to evaluate distant metastatic disease.

In the paediatric population, unusual clinical presentation, suspected metastatic spread from an unknown primary, adult-type neoplasms, chemo- and radiotherapy-induced malignancies and tumours associated with genetic syndromes may lead to diagnostic dilemmas. Imaging must be closely coordinated with clinical assessment and histology. It is essential that all potentially malignant lesions in children be referred to an expert centre with an appropriate multidisciplinary team so that discussion about potential biopsy is discussed with the surgeon and oncologists who will be responsible for future care. A biopsy should be obtained through tissue planes related to subsequent surgery to avoid the risk of tumour seeding, and this may avoid contamination of uninvolved muscle compartments.[1]

The aim of initial tumour assessment is to differentiate aggressive from chronic disease and to distinguish benign from malignant lesions (Table 7-1).[2]

MALIGNANT BONE TUMOURS

Primary bone tumours have a peak incidence between 10 and 20 years, with Ewing's sarcoma family of tumours most commonly occurring before 9 years and osteosarcoma most common between 10 and 29 years.[3]

Osteosarcoma

Osteogenic sarcoma (OS) is the most common primary malignant tumour of bone in children and accounts for 55% of all bone tumours seen in adolescence. The aetiology is unknown but there are recognised associations with previous retinoblastoma, prior alkylating agent treatment, prior radiotherapy and some genetic syndromes, such as Rothmund–Thomson syndrome. Often, patients have a history of trauma, which brings the problem to clinical attention.

Radiographically, OS is variable but most frequently appears as a destructive metaphyseal long bone lesion, with poorly demarcated margins, osteoid production, aggressive periosteal reaction and a soft-tissue mass (Fig. 7-1). The lesion may cross the growth plate. Locoregional staging is performed using MRI and pulmonary metastatic disease using CT. Distant bony metastases are usually assessed using scintigraphy.

MRI staging should include wide field-of-view T1-weighted sequences to assess the entire bone involved,

TABLE 7-1   **Types of Bone Tumours Seen in Children**

Type of Tumour	Benign	Malignant
Bone forming	Osteoid osteoma, osteoblastoma, enostosis	Osteosarcoma
Fibro-osseous	Non-ossifying fibroma, fibrous dysplasia, osteofibrous dysplasia	Fibrosarcoma, malignant fibrous histiocytoma
Cartilage forming	Enchondroma, chondroblastoma, chondromyxoid fibroma, osteochondroma	Chondrosarcoma
Vascular/connective tissue	Haemangioma, lymphangioma, myofibrosis, Gorham's disease	Haemangiopericytoma
Cystic	Simple bone cyst, aneurysmal bone cyst	
Small round cells		Ewing's sarcoma family of tumours, lymphoma
Other	Langerhans cell histiocytosis	

Modified from Wootton-Gorges S L 2009 MR imaging of primary bone tumors and tumor-like conditions in children. Magn Reson Imaging Clin N Am 17(3):469–487.[2]

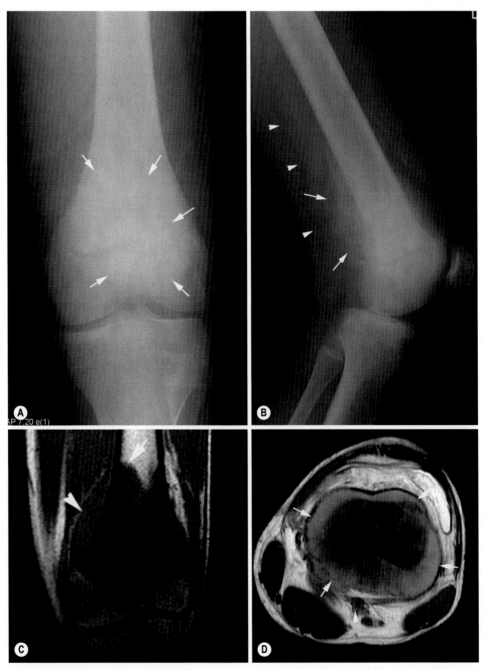

FIGURE 7-1 ■ **Osteosarcoma.** AP radiograph (A) showing a poorly defined dense lesion within the distal left femoral metaphysis, crossing the growth plate into the epiphysis (short arrows). Lateral radiograph (B) demonstrating new bone formation (short arrows) and displacement of surrounding fat planes by an extraosseous mass. Coronal T1-weighted MRI (C) showing both the intramedullary tumour (arrow) and extraosseous soft-tissue mass (arrowhead). Axial PD-weighted MRI (D) demonstrating the circumferential nature of the extraosseous soft-tissue mass (arrows) and the relationship to the popliteal neurovascular bundle (arrowhead).

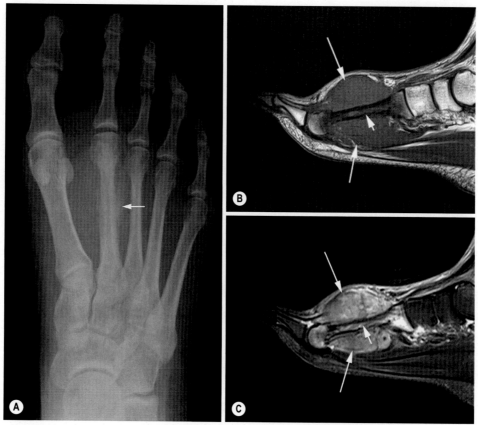

FIGURE 7-2 ■ **Ewing's sarcoma.** DP radiograph (A) demonstrating a periosteal reaction of the second metatarsal. Sagittal T1- (B) and STIR-weighted MRI (C) showing a surrounding soft-tissue mass (long arrows) and bone marrow replacement (short arrows).

and the contralateral side to look for skip and synchronous contralateral lesions.

Paediatric OS variants include telangiectatic OS characterised by dilated blood-filled cavities, periosteal OS arising from the deep periosteal layer and high-grade surface OS involving the bone surface.

Treatment with chemotherapy may lead to a decrease in tumour volume, haemorrhagic signal change and organisation of periosteal reaction. Diffusion-weighted imaging, dynamic MRI contrast imaging and positron emission tomography are all said to assess tumour response and necrosis fraction, an important prognostic indicator, but these are currently research tools.[4-6]

Ewing's Sarcoma Family of Tumours (ESFTs)

ESFTs are the second most common bone tumour in adolescents and children. The pathogenesis of ESFT is unknown. ESFT occurs more commonly in adolescents but a peak of incidence in very young children is well recognised. Classically, flat bone involvement (such as ribs or iliac crest) is seen in ESFT, but any bone may be involved, with 50% arising in the femur or pelvis.

The clinical presentation is non-specific: local pain, fever and swelling can mimic an acute osteomyelitis, delaying the diagnosis. Children with a chest wall tumour usually present with pain. The destructive rib lesion is often initially overlooked and by the time of diagnosis, a pleural effusion is usually present. Metastatic spread is haematogenous, and metastases occur to the lungs, bones and bone marrow. Lymph node, liver and skip metastases are rare. Radiographic features include a permeative appearance, with an 'onion skin' periosteal reaction. There is often a large associated soft-tissue mass (Fig. 7-2), which in the case of pelvic origin tumours may not be clinically apparent and radiographically may be difficult to interpret, possibly delaying diagnosis. ESFT staging is as for OS; however, PET may have some advantages over scintigraphy in evaluating bone metastases in ESFT.[7]

Bone Metastases

Bone metastases are not as common in children when compared to adults. Metastases as the first manifestation of a primary tumour are unusual, as the primary tumour is usually evident initially. Metastatic bone disease in children is most frequently due to leukaemia and neuroblastoma, but lymphoma, ESFT, rhabdomyosarcoma and medulloblastoma may metastasise to bone (Figs. 7-3 and 7-4).

Lytic appearances ± periosteal reaction are the most common radiographic characteristics in metastatic locations, but sclerotic lesions are also reported, particularly in medulloblastoma and leukaemia. Metaphyseal radiolucent lines are typically described in leukaemia and, less commonly, neuroblastoma. Bone scintigraphy, MRI or

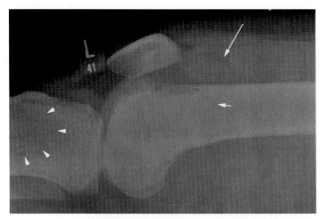

FIGURE 7-3 ■ **Leukaemic infiltration.** Lateral knee radiograph showing an ill-defined permeative osteolytic lesion within the tibia (arrowheads), further permeative lesion within the distal femur (short arrow) and an associated joint effusion (long arrow).

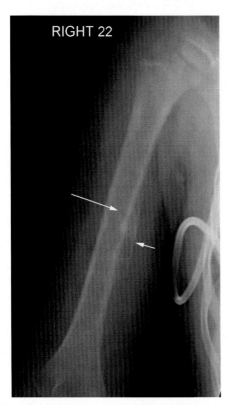

RIGHT 22

FIGURE 7-4 ■ **Neuroblastoma metastases.** AP humeral radiograph demonstrating an ill-defined permeative appearance of the right humerus (long arrow), with an associated periosteal reaction (short arrow). Note the similarity to the lesions in Fig. 7-3.

metaiodobenzylguanidine (mIBG) studies may be utilised, depending on the clinical scenario.

Rare Malignant Bone Tumours in Children

- Chondrosarcoma
- Primary malignant lymphoma of bone
- Haemangiosarcoma of bone.

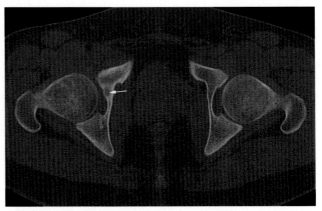

FIGURE 7-5 ■ **Pelvic osteoid osteoma.** Axial CT section depicting a central nidus within the right iliac bone (arrow), with surrounding bony sclerosis.

BENIGN BONE TUMOURS

Bone-Forming Tumours

- Enostosis (bone island)
- Osteoid osteoma
- Osteoblastoma.

Osteoid Osteoma

This painful lesion composed of woven bone and osteiod occurs in children and adolescents but more than 80% of cases occur in the second decade of life.[8] The pain is typically worse at night, relieved by aspirin. Classically, lesions occur in tubular bones but they may also affect the vertebral appendages, presenting clinically with painful scoliosis, seen as a dense pedicle, or are identified following positive scintigraphy. Osteoid osteoma may be polyostotic.

Plain radiographs, supplemented by CT with direct visualisation of a central nidus and surrounding sclerotic reaction, provide the diagnosis (Fig. 7-5). Sometimes, the nidus may contain calcification. On MRI, cortical thickening returns low signal on all sequences. The nidus has a variable appearance depending on the site and relative amounts of osteoid and matrix.[9] There may be prominent soft-tissue or bone marrow oedema, which may lead to diagnostic confusion (Fig. 7-6).

A typical tumour pattern on three-phase skeletal scintigrams is described, characterised by focal hypervascularity and high uptake.[10] A negative scintigram excludes the presence of osteoid osteoma. Scintigraphy can confirm recurrence or incomplete removal if pain persists following surgery. Historically, surgical treatment has been the mainstay; however, image-guided ablation therapy, for example using radiofrequency, is now possible.[11]

Osteoblastoma

Osteoblastoma is rare and difficult to differentiate histologically from osteoid osteoma, whilst, radiographically, it is distinct, with a nidus measuring greater than 1.5–2 cm in diameter.[12] The main site is the posterior elements of the spine. Radiographically, osteoblastoma is expansile, and may be either lucent or sclerotic, with a sclerotic rim (Figs. 7-7 and 7-8). The cortex may occasionally be broken. There is usually surrounding oedema (Fig. 7-9).

Tumours of Fibrous Tissue Origin

- Non-ossifying fibroma (NOF)
- Metaphyseal fibrous cortical defects
- Fibrous bone dysplasia (Jaffe–Lichtenstein) (FBD)
- Osteofibrous bone dysplasia (Campanacci) (OBD)

Non-Ossifying Fibroma and Metaphyseal Fibrous Cortical Defects (Synonyms: Fibroxanthoma, Benign Fibrous Histiocytoma)

Although histologically different, these two lesions appear radiologically similar, NOF being greater than 2 cm in

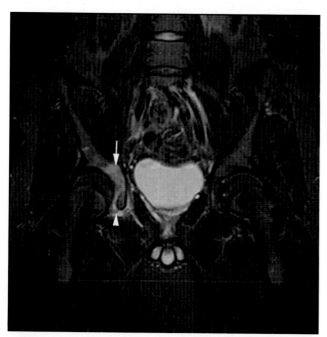

FIGURE 7-6 ■ **Pelvic osteoid osteoma.** Coronal STIR MRI demonstrating marked bone marrow oedema (arrow) and adjacent soft-tissue oedema (arrowhead).

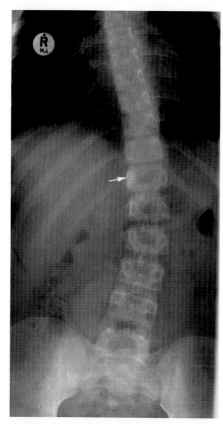

FIGURE 7-7 ■ **Spinal osteoblastoma.** AP spinal radiograph demonstrating a left convex thoracolumbar scoliosis, with a sclerotic right T12 pedicle at the apex of the curve.

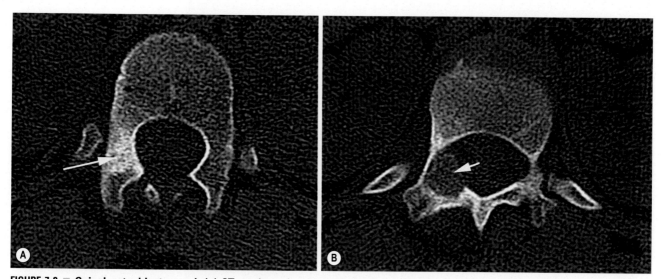

FIGURE 7-8 ■ **Spinal osteoblastoma.** Axial CT sections demonstrating a sclerotic right vertebral pedicle (arrow, panel A), with an adjacent expansile, lytic lesion (short arrow, panel B). The cortex is thinned but intact.

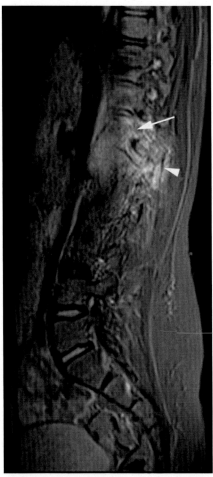

FIGURE 7-9 ■ **Spinal osteoblastoma.** Sagittal STIR MRI depicting both extensive bone marrow (arrow) and adjacent soft-tissue oedema (arrowhead).

size. NOF is the most common benign tumour in children and is typically incidentally encountered during childhood and adolescence, appearing as a well-defined multilocular osteolytic defect in the metaphysis of a long bone, with marginal sclerosis. The most frequent sites are the tibia and proximal femur.[13] Although MRI is not routinely indicated for simple cases of NOF, T1-weighted MRI shows low signal intensity within the lesion compared with the skeletal muscle. T2-weighted signal intensity is variable. The lesion usually enhances avidly (Fig. 7-10).

Fibrous Bone Dysplasia

FBD is a common developmental anomaly in which the bone is centrally replaced by fibrous tissue.[14] Local bending or pathological fractures may occur. Radiologically the appearance is typically of a widened medullary cavity, bony expansion and a ground-glass appearance (Fig. 7-11). A rare condition, McCune–Albright syndrome, consists of unilateral polyostotic FBD associated with precocious puberty. The most frequent locations for FBD are the ribs, proximal femur, skull, scapula and pelvis.

Osteofibrous Bone Dysplasia

This occurs in the shaft of long tubular bones, classically the tibia. It is a cortically based multicystic lesion surrounded by sclerosis with intact cortex and no periosteal reaction (Fig. 7-12). It may be multifocal. Moth-eaten margins and complete involvement of

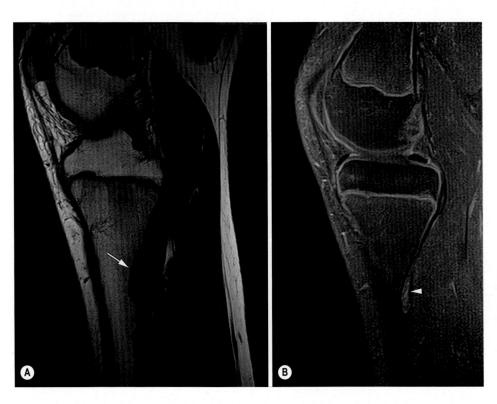

FIGURE 7-10 ■ **Non-ossifying fibroma: MRI.** Sagittal pre- (A) and (B) post-gadolinium T1-weighted MRI with fat saturation, depicting a well-defined cortical lesion with a sclerotic low signal rim (arrow) (A). The lesion avidly enhances following contrast administration (arrowhead) (B).

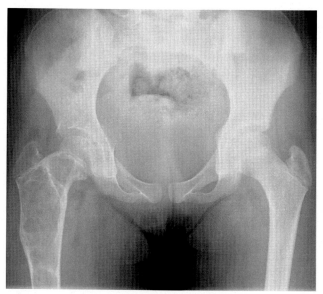

FIGURE 7-11 ■ **Fibrous dysplasia.** AP pelvic radiograph showing an expansile lytic lesion of the right proximal femur, extending to the growth plate. The internal aspect of the lesion demonstrates ground-glass appearance.

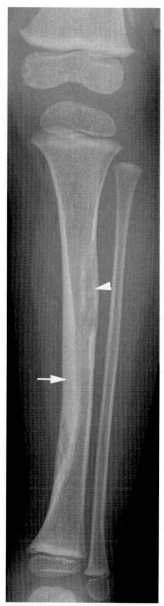

FIGURE 7-12 ■ **Osteofibrous dysplasia.** Frontal left tibial radiograph showing multifocal cortically based lesions with both sclerosis (arrow) and lucency (arrowhead). There is no periosteal reaction or cortical destruction.

the medullary cavity suggest adamantinoma rather than OFD.[15]

Cartilage-Forming Tumours

- Chondroma (enchondroma)
- Osteochondroma
- Chondroblastoma.

Osteochondroma (Exostosis)

Osteochondromas are developmental anomalies resulting from physeal cartilage displaced to the metaphyseal region, the knee being the most common site.[16] Osteochondromas are covered by a cartilaginous cap from which growth occurs. Osteochondromas may be pedunculated (Fig. 7-13) or sessile (Fig. 7-14), solitary or multiple, as seen in the autosomal dominant condition multiple hereditary exostoses (MHE). Local pressure effects on adjacent structures, deformity and shortening may result, particularly in MHE.

Plain radiography is usually diagnostic. On MRI T2-weighted sequences the hyaline cartilage appears hyperintense with a good visualisation of its structural layers. MRI demonstrates the thickness of the cartilaginous cap of the tumour. In children and adolescents, the cap may be as thick as 3 cm. Growth may continue until skeletal maturity. Growth after maturity suggests malignant degeneration, which occurs in 1% of solitary exostoses and between 3 and 5% in MHE. Persistent pain is also a worrying feature, which should prompt investigation to exclude malignant degeneration.

Chondroblastoma

This is a rare benign cartilaginous tumour found in the epiphysis or epiphyseal equivalents. It is a monostotic lesion with chondroid matrix, calcification, a sclerotic rim and commonly a periosteal reaction. Aggressive features may rarely be seen. The most common sites are the femur (proximal > distal) and proximal tibia.

The radiographic appearance is that of a well-defined radiolucent lesion. Calcified matrix may be more apparent on CT. MRI shows low (reflecting haemosiderin) to intermediate heterogeneous signal on T2 with a lobulated pattern. Bone marrow oedema may be present and ABC components may be seen.

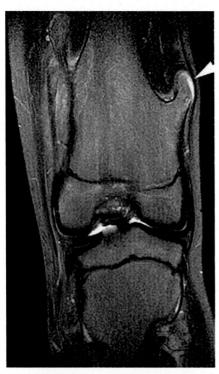

FIGURE 7-13 ■ **Pedunculated osteochondroma.** Coronal proton density MRI depicting two pedunculated osteochondromas. Note the bony medullary continuity. A thin cartilage cap is shown (arrowhead).

Vascular and Other Connective Tissue Tumours

- Bone haemangioma
- Bone lymphangioma
- Massive osteolysis (Gorham's disease)
- Myofibromatosis
- Lipoma of bone.

Myofibromatosis

Myofibromatosis presents most often in infancy, but can occur even in adults. The solitary or multiple lesions involve skin, subcutaneous tissues, muscles, bones and viscera (particularly lung, heart, gastrointestinal tract and dura). The skeletal lesions appear lytic and sharply defined, sparing the periphyseal area. Sclerotic margins appear later.[17]

Gorham's Disease

A rare disorder of unknown aetiology, typically arising in childhood, Gorham's disease presents as osteolysis, which may be dramatic ('vanishing bone disease') (Fig. 7-15). Pathologically characterised by lymphovascular proliferation, both bone and multisystem involvement can be seen.[18] The most commonly afflicted sites are the

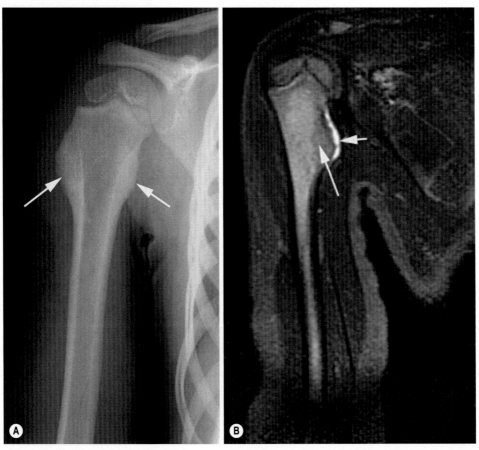

FIGURE 7-14 ■ **Sessile osteochondroma.** AP right humeral radiograph (A) and coronal STIR MRI (B) depicting sessile osteochondromas (arrows). Note the thin cartilage cap (short arrow, B).

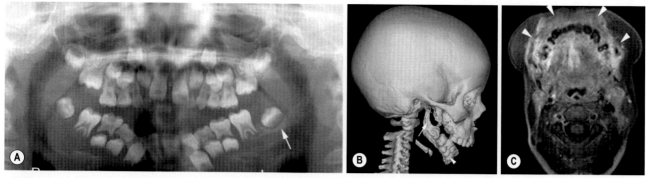

FIGURE 7-15 ■ **Gorham's disease.** Orthopantomogram (A) showing almost complete absence of the mandible, with a small remnant demonstrated (arrow). 3D surface-shaded display CT of the face (B) depicting the mandibular remnant (arrow) and 'floating teeth' (arrowhead). Post-gadolinium T1-weighted fat-saturated MRI (C) demonstrating enhancing lymphovascular soft tissue replacing the mandible.

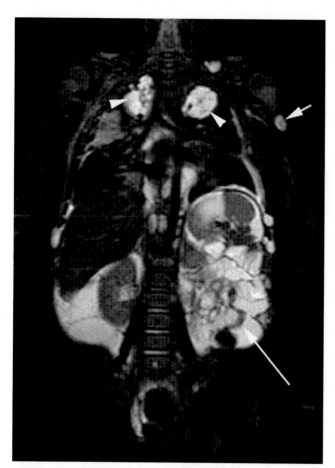

FIGURE 7-16 ■ **Multisystem lymphangiomatosis.** Coronal STIR MRI demonstrating abdominal (long arrow), left humeral (short arrow) and thoracic (arrowheads) lymphangiomatosis.

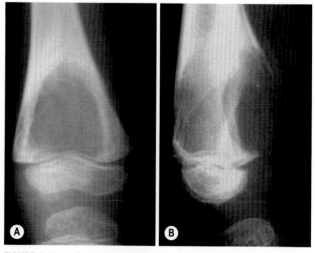

FIGURE 7-17 ■ **Chondromyxoid fibroma of the distal femoral metaphysis.** (A, B) Large osteolytic defect bulging outward.

Locally Aggressive Tumours

- Desmoplastic bone fibroma
- Chondromyxoid fibroma
- Haemangiopericytoma
- Osteoclastoma (giant cell tumour).

Chondromyxoid Fibroma

This is a rare bone tumour that accounts for only 0.5% of all bone tumours. It is mainly seen in the second decade of life, but cases have been described in the first decade. Typically, chondromyxoid fibromas are located in the metaphyseal region of the long tubular bones, near the growth plate, and can cross into the epiphysis. The lesion is well circumscribed, with an eccentric osteolytic lobulated aspect that bulges outward, thinning the cortex (Fig. 7-17). It is usually benign in character but may cause local invasion with a high recurrence rate if incompletely removed.

shoulder, face, spine and pelvis. There is no standard therapy, with interferon alpha being used successfully in some cases. Bone involvement may also be observed with diffuse multisystem lymphatic malformations (Fig. 7-16).

Tumour-Like Lesions

- Simple juvenile bone cyst
- Aneurysmal bone cyst (ABC)
- Fibrous cortical defect: see fibrous tissue tumours
- Fibrous bone dysplasia (Jaffe–Lichtenstein) (FBD)
- Osteofibrous bone dysplasia (Kempson, Campanacci) (OBD)
- Eosinophilic granuloma (Langerhans cell histiocytosis).

Simple Bone Cyst (Synonyms: Juvenile, Solitary or Unicameral Bone Cyst)

SBC is a benign lesion that develops in the centre of the metaphysis, usually of the proximal femur or humerus adjacent to the epiphyseal plate (Fig. 7-18). Most patients present with a pathological fracture, but SBC may be an incidental finding. There is cortical thinning with mild expansion. With maturity, the cyst migrates down the shaft of the bone. Following fracture, fluid–fluid levels and solid areas may be seen.

Aneurysmal Bone Cyst

This is a cystic expansile lesion, often containing haemorrhage, which occurs in the vertebral appendages, the flat bones, and most frequently in the metaphysis of the long bones in the femur, tibia and humerus (Fig. 7-19). The lesion develops eccentrically without crossing the growth plate. The lesion is frequently multilocular and may cause subtle cortical thinning. Within the vertebral column, a destructive expansile lesion is seen in the appendages and may encroach into the spinal canal. ABC can be primary or secondary to other bone tumours in up to 30% of cases. Telangiectatic OS is a mimic of ABC.

Full evaluation of ABCs requires cross-sectional imaging and biopsy. MRI demonstrates the architecture and fluid–fluid levels within the lesion, which may be haemorrhagic (Fig. 7-20). In selected cases percutaneous sclerotherapy under fluoroscopic guidance has been used with successful clinical results.[19]

Langerhans Cell Histiocytosis (LCH)

LCH is uncommon, accounting for less than 1% of bone biopsy specimens. This disorder, involving proliferation of Langerhans cell histiocytes and their precursors, may be either localised, involving one or a few bony sites (70%), or multifocal, affecting bone and extraskeletal sites. Solitary lesions (eosinophilic granuloma) frequently involve flat bones (skull, mandible, ribs and pelvis being most common) and typically appear as a geographic lytic lesion, with a variable degree of surrounding sclerosis, depending on the degree of healing (Fig. 7-21). Vertebra plana, classically, is seen within the spine; however, LCH may have variable appearances and is a great mimic of other lesions.[20]

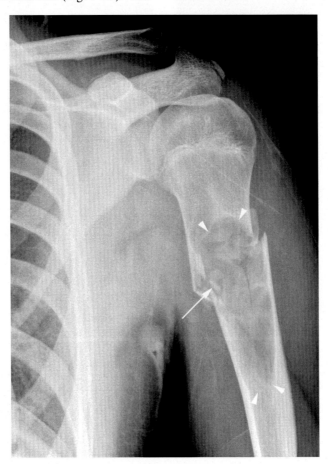

FIGURE 7-18 ■ **Simple bone cyst.** AP left humerus demonstrating a well-defined osteolytic lesion within the diaphysis (arrowheads), with a pathological fracture and internal fragments (arrow).

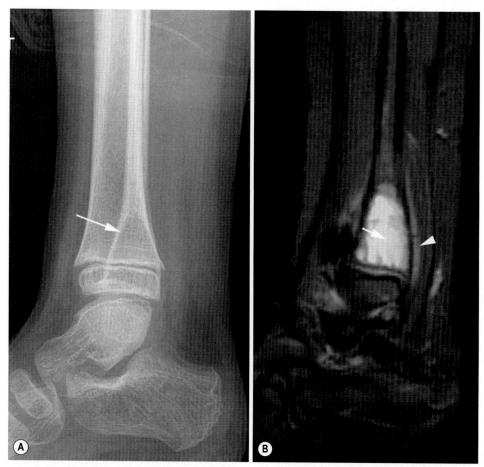

FIGURE 7-19 ■ **Aneurysmal bone cyst.** Lateral radiograph of the ankle (A) showing an expansile lytic lesion of the fibula (arrow). Sagittal STIR MRI (B) demonstrates multiple fluid–fluid levels (short arrow), with some adjacent soft-tissue oedema (arrowhead), which can be seen in association with an ABC.

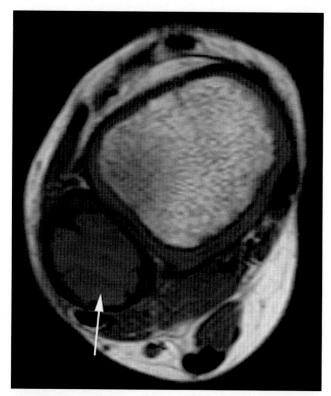

FIGURE 7-20 ■ **Axial T1-weighted MRI demonstrating the haemorrhagic nature of the fluid–fluid levels, with subtle T1 shortening observed (arrow).**

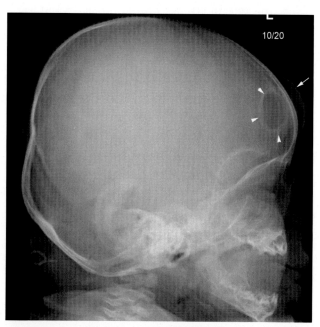

FIGURE 7-21 ■ **Langerhans cell histiocytosis.** Lateral skull radiograph showing a well-defined lytic frontal bone lesion with sclerotic margins (arrowheads) and an associated soft-tissue mass (short arrow).

NEUROBLASTOMA

Neuroblastomas (NBs)—with the less common, but more differentiated and mature ganglioneuroblastoma and ganglioneuroma (GN)—are neoplasms arising from the primordial neural crest cells. Neuroblastic tumours represent the most common extracranial solid neoplasms occurring in children, with median age at diagnosis of 2 years, and 90% of cases occurring under the age of 5 years. Overall, NBs account for 8–10% of all childhood cancers. NBs are also seen in newborns and may be detected in the fetus by antenatal imaging, most often associated with favourable prognostic features.[21] Common sites for primary NB are the adrenal glands (48%), extra-adrenal retroperitoneum (25%), chest (16%), neck (3%) and pelvis (3%). About 50% of patients have metastatic disease at diagnosis.

The signs and symptoms of NB reflect the tumour site and extent of disease. The tumours may manifest as an incidental mass, or may cause abdominal pain. Because metastases are frequently present (skeleton, bone marrow, lymph nodes, liver and, rarely, lung and brain), the clinical symptoms are often due to metastatic disease. Children may have bone and joint pain, proptosis from orbital metastases, anaemia, weight loss and fever. Horner's syndrome may be the presenting feature of cervical or thoracic NB involving the stellate ganglion. Children may also present with the effects of production of hormones such as catecholamines (hypertension) and VIP (intractable watery diarrhoea). Another paraneoplastic syndrome associated with NB is myoclonic encephalopathy of infancy (MEI). The precise pathogenesis of MEI is unknown.

NBs in infants younger than 1 year of age are often associated with extensive hepatic metastases. Hepatomegaly may be massive despite a small, sometimes not evident, primary lesion. These infants usually have bone marrow lesions and palpable subcutaneous nodules. In infants, this type of NB has a better prognosis and has a tendency to spontaneous regression, although the very young patients are at high risk because of severe respiratory complications, occurring as a result of massive hepatomegaly.

Extradural extension (dumb-bell syndrome) with possible compression of the spinal cord is relatively common with thoracic NB, but rare in abdominal tumours.

Approximately 90% of patients with NB have elevated levels of catecholamines (vanillylmandelic acid, homovanillic acid, noradrenaline, dopamine) in the urine. However, no more than 60% of newborns with NB have elevated levels of urinary catecholamines.[21] The combination of a positive bone marrow aspirate and an increase of urinary catecholamine metabolites are sufficient to confirm the diagnosis.

NB shows a broad spectrum of clinical behaviour, as in some cases it may spontaneously regress or mature, whereas in other cases it may progress despite intensive multimodality treatment. Its outcome appears to correlate with a series of well-known clinical, histological and biological features, which can be used for risk group stratification and treatment assignment, according to current treatment protocols.

GN often occurs in the posterior mediastinum and, unlike NB, does not contain neuroblastic cells. In comparison with NB, GN occurs in older patients, as the median age at diagnosis is approximately 7 years. GN often manifests as an asymptomatic mass discovered on a routine radiographic study, such as a chest radiograph. The imaging features of GN are similar to those of ganglioneuroblastoma (GNB) and NB; hence, they most often cannot be discriminated with imaging in isolation.

IMAGING

The initial diagnosis of an abdominal NB is made most frequently by ultrasound or by chest-X-ray in the case of a thoracic mass. The evaluation of the primary tumour includes CT or MRI, whereas [123]metaiodobenzylguanidine (^{123}I-mIBG) scintigraphy and ^{99m}Tc-MDP bone scintigraphy are required for the detection of metastases.

Radiographs

Radiographs may show a calcified mass in the thorax and/or in the abdomen. Erosion of vertebral pedicles may suggest an intraspinal extension. Radiographs of the long bones with metastases may be normal or may show ill-defined areas of bone destruction. A solitary lesion may appear as a lytic, moth-eaten or a permeative destructive area, interspersed with sclerotic trabeculae. New periosteal bone formation, often parallel to the shaft, may be present. The radiographic features indicate malignant growth but are not specific. The most common skeletal sites are the skull and metaphyses of long bones (humerus and femur).

Ultrasound

Ultrasound, performed to confirm the presence of an abdominal mass, often suggests the diagnosis of NB. Typical features are a retroperitoneal location, varying echogenicity with hyperechoic foci representing calcification, and usually rich vascularisation on colour Doppler. The retroperitoneal location of the mass can be confirmed by demonstration of anterior displacement of the aorta and inferior vena cava (Fig. 7-22). Hypoechoic areas secondary to haemorrhage and necrosis are frequent. Completely cystic NB has been described, especially in newborns.

Computed Tomography and Magnetic Resonance Imaging

CT of the chest, abdomen and pelvis requires a bolus intravenous administration of contrast medium. Examinations of the chest should extend from the lung apices to the lower edge of the liver during relatively early contrast enhancement; the abdominal study should cover the

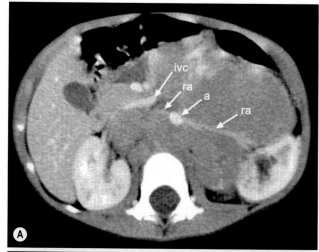

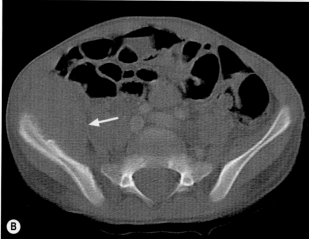

FIGURE 7-22 ■ Abdominal neuroblastoma. Contrast-enhanced CT. (A) A prevertebral tumour extends across the midline in the retroperitoneum, displaces and encases the aorta (a) anteriorly and encases the renal arteries (ra). The inferior vena cava (ivc), partially encased, is displaced anterolaterally and compressed by the tumour and nodes. The mass extends to the renal hila. (B) Infiltrative lesion to the right iliac bone with a large soft-tissue component (arrow) that projects inward as a space-occupying mass.

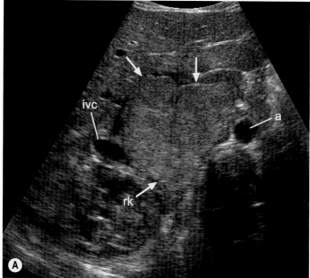

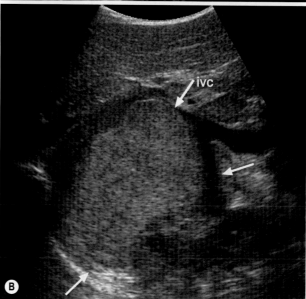

FIGURE 7-23 ■ Abdominal neuroblastoma. (A) Transverse ultrasound through the right abdomen shows a solid paraspinal mass (arrows) anterior to the right kidney (rk). The aorta (a) and inferior vena cava (ivc) are displaced by the mass. (B) Longitudinal image through the right flank shows the mass (arrows) and the stretched inferior vena cava (ivc).

liver in the portal phase and extend down to the pubic symphysis. Multiple pre- and post-contrast phases usually do not add useful information for diagnosis and staging and thus should be avoided.[22] On CT, NB appears as a large and heterogeneous mass; calcifications are detected in up to 85% of cases. Low-attenuation areas represent regions of necrosis or haemorrhage. NB usually shows mild heterogeneous enhancement, reflecting areas of vascularity alternating with areas of necrosis, haemorrhage and cystic change.

Using MRI the patient must be imaged in at least two planes by T1-weighted spin-echo (SE) and fat-saturated T2-weighted fast SE sequences, and with transverse T1-weighted gradient-echo angiographic sequences. The T1-weighted SE sequence must be repeated with fat suppression after intravenous injection of gadolinium. On MRI, NB has prolonged T1 and T2 signal. High

signal intensity on T1-weighted images represents haemorrhage. After administration of gadolinium the tumour enhancement is usually heterogeneous. MRI may also show bone marrow involvement with areas of abnormal signal intensity (low on T1- and high on T2-weighted images).

As separation of the primary tumour from adjacent enlarged lymph nodes is usually not possible, measurement must include the entire mass. The tumour may invade the spinal canal, kidney, or liver. Although intraspinal extension may be suspected at CT, it cannot be thoroughly evaluated: MRI should be performed on any paraspinal mass suspected of extending into the extradural space (Fig. 7-23).

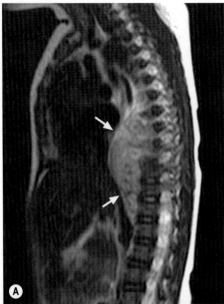

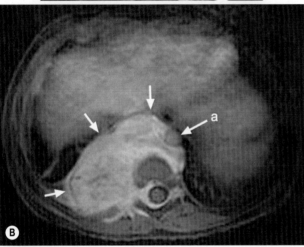

FIGURE 7-24 ■ (A) Sagittal T1-weighted images with Gd-DOTA enhancement. (B) Axial T2-weighted image. Large posterior mediastinal mass (arrows) with anterior and lateral displacement of the aorta (a), which is encased. There is massive tumour extension into the canal through the right neural foramina to displace the spinal cord to the left. Extension into the right paraspinal soft tissues is evident.

Hepatic metastases and renal atrophy (due to ischaemia secondary to encasement or compression of the renal vessels) may be seen. Indeed, NB often has an invasive pattern of growth encasing the vessels (Fig. 7-24). Therefore, with imaging it is crucial to define the extent of the tumour and its relationships to adjacent vessels, according to standardised criteria (see the section below on 'NB Staging') in order to define feasibility of a complete resection.

CT or MRI may allow the evaluation of skull and iliac bone metastases. Usually, skull metastases are located in the spheno-orbital region. They appear as an infiltrating mass causing permeative bone destruction and spiculated bony changes, which may extend into the soft tissue of the scalp or push through the inner table of the skull.

Radionuclide Radiology

[123]I-mIBG scintigraphy has a pivotal role in the diagnosis of NB: i.e. characterisation of the mass, localisation of the primary tumour in patients with MEI and evaluation of metastatic disease and in follow-up; i.e. new areas of uptake generally indicate new active disease. mIBG is a guanethidine derivative and an analogue of noradrenaline, which is specifically taken up and stored in those tumours derived from the cells of the sympathetic nervous system. In children such uptake is usually specific for NB (both primary tumour and metastases). Unfortunately, about 20% of primary lesions do not take up mIBG, and in other rare cases the uptake may stop despite the presence of persistent demonstrable disease. Furthermore, mIBG cannot differentiate bone marrow uptake from cortical bone uptake.[23] Therefore, ^{99m}Tc-MDP bone scintigraphy should be performed in all patients, as two-thirds of patients have metastatic bone disease at diagnosis.

NBs which cannot be resected at diagnosis, because of their size and/or infiltration into adjacent structures, require chemotherapy. With chemotherapy, a NB mass tends to regress in size, but the regression is frequently incomplete, leaving a small, often calcified residual mass. Determining whether this residual mass is just fibrosis or a viable tumour usually requires ^{123}I-mIBG scintigraphy.

Emerging Imaging Techniques

Recently, fluorodeoxyglucose(^{18}F) positron emission tomography (FDG-PET) coupled with computed tomography (^{18}F-FDG PET/CT) has gained a major role in the treatment of adult cancer, whereas the reported experience with childhood tumours is still limited. Preliminary reports suggest that ^{18}F-FDG-PET/CT may be useful in evaluating neuroblastoma (Fig. 7-25), contributing to disease management and even providing opportunity for modification and minimisation of treatment effect (such as in radiation treatment planning) when utilised at diagnosis for disease staging, during therapy to assess response and during follow-up after completion of therapy.[24] However, ^{18}F-FDG-PET/CT is an imaging technique carrying a high radiation exposure, which causes concern in children because of their sensitivity to ionising radiation, and especially in children with cancer, as repeated studies with ionising radiation are expected during the course of the disease.

Whole-body MRI (WBMRI) is an emerging imaging technique with great potential in paediatric oncology. Usually, T1-weighetd and short T1 inversion recovery (STIR) sequences in coronal and sagittal planes are used to image the whole body. Experience with WBMRI in NB is still limited, although preliminary studies show that WBMRI may play a role as a result of the excellent sensitivity in detecting both local disease and metastases, with no radiation burden (Fig. 7-26). However, low specificity is the main downside of WBMRI. Further studies are required to confirm the potential of WBMRI in children with NB.[25]

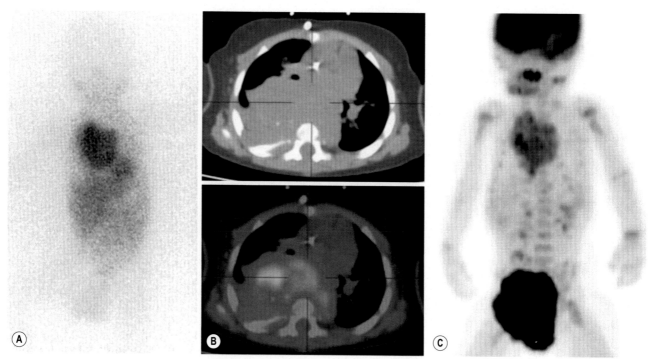

FIGURE 7-25 ■ **Infant with thoracic neuroblastoma.** ^{123}I-mIBG scintigraphy (A) shows avid uptake in the mediastinum and right hemithorax. There is no uptake within the bones. ^{18}F-FDG-PET (B) shows a similar pattern of uptake in the mediastinum and right hemithorax. Bone/bone marrow uptake is weak and diffuse, not specific for disease infiltration. (C) CT and ^{18}F-FDG-PET/CT. CT (upper image) shows a large mass in the posterior mediastinum with calcific spots, crossing the midline and spreading into the right hemithorax. ^{18}F-FDG-PET/CT (lower image) shows avid uptake in the mass. (Images courtesy of Arnoldo Piccardo, MD, Service of Nuclear Medicine, Galliera Hospital, Genoa, Italy.)

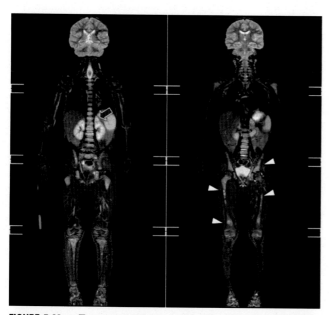

FIGURE 7-26 ■ **Two-year-old boy with left adrenal neuroblastoma.** Whole-body MRI. STIR images. Left image shows an enlarged left adrenal gland (arrow). Right image shows metastatic infiltration in both femora and left iliac bone (arrowheads).

NB STAGING

Disease staging at diagnosis relies on diagnostic imaging, which is of paramount importance for prognosis, risk group stratification and treatment, being the most statistically significant prognostic factor. Until very recently, the only staging system for NB was the International Neuroblastoma Staging System (INSS) (Table 7-2).[26] This staging system is largely based on the extent of surgical excision of the NB mass and lymph node sampling at surgery. However, some issues are evident with INSS. For example, with INSS the same tumour can be either stage 1 or 3, depending on the extent of surgical excision. Lymph node sampling is subject to the diligence of the individual surgeon. Infants with localised disease, who are just observed because tumour regression is anticipated, cannot be properly staged.[27] These difficulties can make direct comparison of clinical trials based on INSS very difficult.

Furthermore, this staging system does not address the issue of a safe and complete excision of the mass, leaving this decision to the personal evaluation of the individual surgeon. The increased awareness of this issue led the International Society of Paediatric Oncology Europe Neuroblastoma Group (SIOPEN) to classify locoregional tumors as resectable or unresectable on the basis of the presence, or absence of a series of 'image-defined risk factors' (IDRFs) detected with diagnostic imaging. This led to the new International

TABLE 7-2   **International Neuroblastoma Staging System**[26]

Stage	
1	Localised tumour confined to the area of origin; complete gross resection with or without microscopic residual disease; identifiable ipsilateral and contralateral lymph nodes negative macroscopically
2A	Localised tumour with incomplete gross excision; identifiable ipsilateral and contralateral lymph nodes negative microscopically
2B	Unilateral tumour with complete or incomplete gross resection with positive ipsilateral regional lymph nodes; contralateral lymph nodes negative microscopically
3	Tumour infiltrating across the midline with or without regional lymph node involvement; unilateral tumour with contralateral regional lymph node involvement; midline tumour with bilateral lymph node involvement
4	Dissemination of tumour to bone, bone marrow, liver, distant lymph nodes or other organs
4s	Limited to infants < 1 year of age. Localised primary tumour as defined for stage 1 or 2A or 2B with dissemination limited to liver, skin and/or bone marrow

TABLE 7-3   **International Neuroblastoma Risk Group Staging System**

Stage	
L1	Localised tumour not involving vital structures as defined by the list of image-defined risk factors and confined to one body compartment
L2	Locoregional tumour with presence of one or more image-defined risk factors
M	Distant metastatic disease (except stage MS)
MS	Metastatic disease in children younger than 18 months with metastases confined to skin, liver and/or bone marrow

Adapted from Monclair et al.[27]

Neuroblastoma Risk Group Staging System (INRGSS) (Table 7-3),[27] which now add to INSS. IDRFs and can be defined as features detected on imaging that make safe and complete tumour excision impracticable at the time of diagnosis, thus suggesting a need for preoperative chemotherapy. In INRGSS, staging of local disease—at variance with INSS—is based on imaging, as stage assignment is determined by IDRFs absence (stage L1) or presence (stage L2).[27]

A detailed description of INRGSS and IDRFs is beyond the scope of this chapter, and can be found in two recent articles by Cohn et al[28] and Monclair et al.[27] In this chapter our description will be limited to the basic principles and guidelines.

CT and/or MRI are the best-suited imaging modalities to assess the presence of IDRFs. The primary tumour should be measured with three-dimensional orthogonal measurements and the presence or absence of each individual IDRF should be systematically verified according

to tumour site. Measurement of the tumour volume is crucial for prognosis and follow-up. By definition, if the mass crosses the contralateral aspect of the vertebral body, it has crossed the midline: this determination is important for INSS staging, but not for INRGSS.

The majority of IDRFs pertain to abdominal NBs, due to their usual close relationship with major abdominal vessels. Therefore, aorta, celiac axis, mesenteric arteries, renal pedicles, inferior vena cava, iliac vessels and portal vein should be accurately assessed. Specific terms should be used to describe the relationship observed between the mass and adjacent vital structures, i.e. structures that cannot be sacrificed without impairment of normal function.[22]

- *Separation*: the interposition of a layer between the tumour and any neighbouring structure.
- *Contact*: no visible layer is present between the tumour and the adjacent structure, without obvious invasion. Contact is not an IDRF, with the exception of renal vessels as their dissection from a mass is very risky and may lead to nephrectomy or renal infarction.
- *Encasement*: a neighbouring structure is surrounded by the mass, an IDRF. With reference to a vessel, more than 50% of its circumference should be in contact with the mass.
- *Compression*: a tumour is in contact with the airway and reduces its short axis, thus representing an IDRF.
- *Infiltration*: a structure other than vessel shows ill-defined margins with the tumour, and it is an IDRF.

IDRFs are specific according to tumour site. NB arising from the paraspinal sympathetic chains in the mediastinum and abdomen may extend into the foraminal spaces, causing intraspinal involvement (the so-called 'dumb-bell' tumors) with possible cord compression. On imaging, finding invasion of more than one-third of the spinal canal diameter or loss of leptomeningeal fluid spaces is considered an IDRF. These imaging features, however, are better assessed with MRI. Intraspinal tumour extension below L2 causes radicular involvement and it does not represent a contraindication for excision of the extraspinal tumour component.[22]

A mediastinal tumour involving the costovertebral junction between T9 and T12 may cause spinal cord ischaemia during surgical excision of the mass, because of injury to the Adamkiewicz artery, which originates between T9 and T12. This should be considered an IDRF, although abundant collateral vessels are usually present due to the usual slow growth of NB located at this site. Therefore, angiography is not mandatory, although this issue is still controversial.

DIFFERENTIAL DIAGNOSIS

The differential diagnosis encompasses all paediatric abdominal masses, particularly Wilms' tumour (see Chapter 4) and neonatal adrenal haemorrhage. Concerning Wilms' tumour (WT), the mean age at onset is 3 years (for NB it is younger than 2 years). WT tends to displace the vessels, whilst NB surrounds vessels; WT may invade the renal vein and inferior vena cava and arises from the kidney with the typical 'claw sign', whereas NB classically displaces the kidney without distorting the renal collecting system. Calcifications are uncommon in NBs. In WT, lung metastases are present in 20% of cases, whereas they are very uncommon in NBs.

The diagnosis of neonatal adrenal haemorrhage is usually made by ultrasound, which identifies the mass and shows in sequential examinations, progressive decrease in size and cystic evolution. Colour Doppler is useful for showing absence of vascularisation. MRI may show the classic signal intensity pattern of ageing blood products, but diagnostic difficulties can occur because of bleeds of different ages. Other paediatric adrenal tumours, such as phaeochromocytoma and adrenal carcinoma, are much less common.

In the neck, firm/hard masses can be cysts, ectopic thymus, abscesses, inflammatory or neoplastic adenopathies, benign and malignant tumours or parotid and thyroid lesions. The most common cancers are lymphomas, thyroid cancers, rhabdomyosarcomas and NBs. In the mediastinum, NB is located in the posterior mediastinum. Other abnormalities encountered are neurofibroma, neurenteric cyst, meningocele and paraspinal inflammation due to vertebral osteomyelitis.

REFERENCES

1. Federman N, Bernthal N, Eilber FC, Tap WD. The multidisciplinary management of osteosarcoma. Curr Treat Options Oncol 2009;10(1–2):82–93.
2. Wootton-Gorges SL. MR imaging of primary bone tumors and tumor-like conditions in children. Magn Reson Imaging Clin N Am 2009;17(3):469–87.
3. Arora RS, Alston RD, Eden TO, et al. The contrasting age-incidence patterns of bone tumours in teenagers and young adults: implications for aetiology. Int J Cancer 2011;131(7):1678–85.
4. Dyke JP, Panicek DM, Healey JH, et al. Osteogenic and Ewing sarcomas: estimation of necrotic fraction during induction chemotherapy with dynamic contrast-enhanced MR imaging. Radiology 2003;228(1):271–8.
5. Franzius C, Sciuk J, Brinkschmidt C, et al. Evaluation of chemotherapy response in primary bone tumors with F-18 FDG positron emission tomography compared with histologically assessed tumor necrosis. Clin Nucl Med 2000;25(11):874–81.
6. Hayashida Y, Yakushiji T, Awai K, et al. Monitoring therapeutic responses of primary bone tumors by diffusion-weighted image: Initial results. Eur Radiol 2006;16(12):2637–43.
7. Franzius C, Sciuk J, Daldrup-Link HE, et al. FDG-PET for detection of osseous metastases from malignant primary bone tumours: comparison with bone scintigraphy. Eur J Nucl Med 2000;27(9):1305–11.
8. Gitelis S, Schajowicz F. Osteoid osteoma and osteoblastoma. Orthop Clin North Am 1989;20:313–25.
9. White LM, Kandel R. Osteoid-producing tumors of bone. Semin Musculoskelet Radiol 2000;4(1):25–43.
10. Delbeke D, Habibian MR. Noninflammatory entities and the differential diagnosis of positive three phase bone scintigraphy. Clin Nucl Med 1988;13:844–51.
11. Rosenthal D, Callstrom MR. Critical review and state of the art in interventional oncology: benign and metastatic disease involving bone. Radiology 2012;262(3):765–80.
12. Lucas DR, Unni KK, McLeod RA, et al. Osteoblastoma: clinico-pathologic study of 306 cases. Human Pathol 1994;25:117–34.
13. Smith SE, Kransdorf MJ. Primary musculoskeletal tumors of fibrous origin. Semin Musculoskelet Radiol 2000;4(1):73–88.
14. Mirra JM, Gold RH. Fibrous dysplasia. In: Mirra JM, Piero P, Gold RH, editors. Bone Tumors. Philadelphia: Lea & Febiger; 1989. pp. 191–226.
15. Khanna M, Delaney D, Tirabosco R, Saifuddin A. Osteofibrous dysplasia, osteofibrous dysplasia-like adamantinoma and adamantinoma: correlation of radiological imaging features with surgical histology and assessment of the use of radiology in contributing to needle biopsy diagnosis. Skeletal Radiol 2008;37(12):1077–84.
16. D'Ambrosia R, Ferguson AB. The formation of osteochondroma by epiphyseal cartilage transplantation. Clin Orthop 1968;61:103–15.
17. Eich GF, Hoeffel JC, Tschappeler H, et al. Fibrous tumours in children: imaging features of a heterogeneous group of disorders. Pediatr Radiol 1998;28:500–9.
18. Venkatramani R, Ma NS, Pitukcheewanont P, et al. Gorham's disease and diffuse lymphangiomatosis in children and adolescents. Pediatr Blood Cancer 2011;56(4):667–70.
19. Dubois J, Chigot V, Grimard G, et al. Sclerotherapy in aneurysmal bone cysts in children: review of 17 cases. Pediatr Radiol 2003;33:365–72.
20. Kransdorf MJ, Smith SE. Lesions of unknown histogenesis: Langerhans cell histiocytosis and Ewing sarcoma. Semin Musculoskelet Radiol 2000;4(1):113–25.
21. Granata C, Fagnani AM, Gambini C, et al. Features and outcome of neuroblastoma detected before birth. J Pediatr Surg 2000;35:88–91.
22. Brisse HJ, McCarville MB, Granata C, et al. Guidelines for imaging and staging of neuroblastic tumors: consensus report from the International Neuroblastoma Risk Group Project. Radiology 2011;261:243–57.
23. Matthay KK, Skulkin B, Ladenstein R, et al. Criteria for evaluation of disease extent by (123)I-metaiodobenzylguanidine scans in neuroblastoma: a report for the International Neuroblastoma Risk Group (INRG) Task Force. Br J Cancer 2010;102:1319–26.
24. Kaste SC. PET-CT in children: where is it appropriate? Pediatr Radiol 2011;41(Suppl. 2):509–13.
25. Goo HW. Whole-body MRI of neuroblastoma. Eur J Radiol 2010;75:306–14.
26. Brodeur GM, Pritchard J, Berthold F, et al. Revisions of the international criteria for neuroblastoma diagnosis, staging and response to treatment. J Clin Oncol 1993;11:1466–77.
27. Monclair T, Brodeur GM, Ambros PF, et al. The International Neuroblastoma Risk Group (INRG) staging system: an INRG Task Force report. J Clin Oncol 2009;27:298–303.
28. Cohn SL, Pearson ADJ, London WB, et al. The International Neuroblastoma Risk Group (INRG) classification system: an INRG Task Force report. J Clin Oncol 2009;27:289–97.

CHAPTER 8

PAEDIATRIC NEURORADIOLOGY

Maria I. Argyropoulou • Andrea Rossi • Roxana S. Gunny • W.K. 'Kling' Chong

NORMAL BRAIN MATURATION

Brain maturation is assessed by observing tissue characteristics related to myelination, as well as variations in morphology. Most of the changes associated with myelination occur in the first 2 years of life and gyral and sulcal development mainly occurs in utero or in the premature brain, while other morphological changes are observable later in life.

Normal Myelination

Myelination is the process by which brain oligodendrocytes produce layers of myelin that wrap around the neuronal axons and act as a layer of insulation for the transmission of electric action potentials down the neuronal axon. Axonal transmission is facilitated at the junctions between these myelin sheaths or nodes of Ranvier by a process known as saltatory conduction. The extent of myelination of the infant brain can be assessed by magnetic resonance imaging (MRI) according to specific milestones which are analogous to the normal milestones of clinical development. During earliest brain development none of the brain is myelinated. By term, key structures such as the ventrolateral thalami, dorsolateral putamina, posterior limb of the internal capsule, inferior colliculi, medial longitudinal fasciculus and dorsal brainstem nuclei are already myelinated. As the brain matures, there is progressive T_1 and T_2 shortening of the white matter due to an increase in the lipid content and reduced water content of developing myelin and packing of myelinated white matter tracts.[1] This follows a centrifugal posterior-to-anterior and caudal-to-cranial pattern and is virtually complete by the age of 2 years (Fig. 8-1). Advanced MRI techniques show progressive reduction in free water diffusion, increased fractional anisotropy (assessed by diffusion tensor imaging) and increased magnetisation transfer.[2-4] Brain myelination is detected in grey matter earlier on T_2-weighted fast spin-echo (FSE) and in the white matter tracts earlier on T_1-weighted spin-echo (SE) or inversion recovery (STIR) sequences. Most myelination occurs post-term in the first 8 months of life, although the final parts of this process may extend into adulthood. The brain should appear virtually fully myelinated on T_2-weighted sequences by 2 years, with almost an adult appearance on T_1-weighted sequences by 10 months (Fig. 8-2).

The newborn has limited motor function but a well-developed sensory system. Thus the myelination pattern seen at birth at full term is primarily in the sensory tracts. During the first 6 months of life the process of myelination is easiest to follow on T_1-weighted images, where the myelinated areas appear bright. T_2-weighted images are less sensitive and it takes much more myelin to produce a hypointense signal within the white matter. During this period T_2-weighted images show only subtle myelination.

At full term, T_1-weighted images should show high signal in the dorsal medulla and brainstem, the cerebellar peduncles, a small part of the cerebral peduncles, about a third of the posterior limb of the internal capsule, the central corona radiata, and the deep white matter in the region of the pre- and post-central gyrus.[5] Progression of myelination is seen in the optic radiations during the first

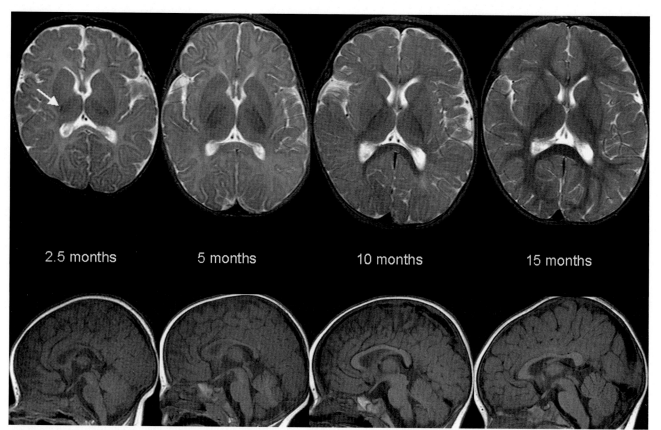

FIGURE 8-1 ■ **Normal brain development with age seen on T₂- (top row) and T₁-weighted (bottom row) MRI.** On T₂-weighted images myelination at term and at 2.5 months is seen centrally as signal hypointensity within the posterior limbs of the internal capsules. This progresses from posterior to anterior with age, as does myelination of the corpus callosum. Myelination also progresses centrally to peripherally. The sagittal T₁-weighted image shows progressive bulking up of the corpus callosum. By 6 months the corpus callosum should reach approximately its normal childhood size. The splenium is slightly enlarged with respect to the genu.

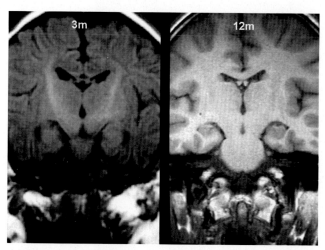

FIGURE 8-2 ■ **Normal brain myelination at 3 and 12 months.** On T₁-weighted MRI at term, T₁ shortening is seen within the posterior limb of the internal capsule. This progresses posteriorly to anteriorly and centrally to peripherally until by 12 months the brain appears fully myelinated.

months of life. The internal capsule will demonstrate T₁ shortening within the anterior limb by 3 months, while on T₂-weighted images the hypointensity due to myelin is not seen until about 8 months of age. The splenium of the corpus callosum on T₂-weighted images becomes hypointense at 3 months of age. The hypointense signal extends anteriorly along the body and genu, and the complete corpus callosum is myelinated at 6 months.[6]

After 6 months the signal pattern on T₁-weighted images becomes less precise, and after 10 months the brain is fully myelinated by T₁ criteria. T₂-weighted images are then used to assess the myelination from 6 months to 24 months of age, when the signal pattern generally is fully mature and has a completely adult pattern, though the milestones of myelination are much more imprecise than during the first 6 months of life.

On T₂-weighted images the first signs of mature subcortical white matter are found around the calcarine fissure at 4 months and in the pre- and post-central gyri at 8 months. By 10 months the occipital subcortical white matter appears isointense with the overlying grey matter and finally shows mature hypointense signal around 1 year of age. This process proceeds anteriorly and by 18 months has finally reached the most frontal parts and the frontal poles of the temporal lobes.

Regions of persistent hyperintensity on T₂-weighted sequences known as the 'terminal myelination zones'[7] may be seen within the peritrigonal areas well into adulthood. They can be distinguished from white matter disease by the presence of a rim of normal myelinated brain between these areas and the ventricular margin, and no evidence of white matter volume loss such as ventricular enlargement or irregularity of the ventricular margins. Other areas may also persist as regions of signal hyperintensity beyond 2 years, e.g. in the frontotemporal subcortical white matter and peritrigonal white matter, and should not be mistaken for disease (Fig. 8-3).

Normal Gyral Development

Gyration is the process by which the individual gyri and sulci of the cerebral hemispheres form (Fig. 8-4).

The MRI appearances lag behind the extent of gyral formation seen at the same age at post-mortem. The surface of the cerebral hemispheres is initially smooth, with the interhemispheric fissure and Sylvian fissures having already formed by 16 weeks' gestation. Other primary sulci, such as the callosal sulcus and parieto-occipital fissure, are recognisable at 22 weeks' gestation, followed by the cingular and calcarine sulci. The central sulcus is seen in most infants by 27 weeks. Gyration then continues into the post-term period in a standardised and

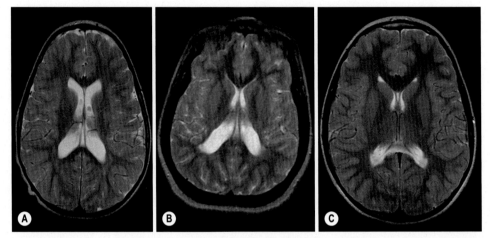

FIGURE 8-3 ■ **Normal terminal myelination zones compared to pathological states.** (A) T$_2$-weighted MRI shows signal hyperintensity adjacent to the trigones of the lateral ventricles but with a rim of darker signal between this and the ventricular margins. This is the normal appearance of the terminal myelination zones. (B) Periventricular signal hyperintensity extending down to the ventricular margin. The ventricles are dilated posteriorly and there is irregular scalloping of the ventricular margins in keeping with white matter volume loss. These are the typical features of periventricular leukomalacia due to hypoxic ischaemia. (C) Peritrigonal and splenial signal abnormality. The ventricles are not dilated. This is the typical pattern of adrenoleukodystrophy.

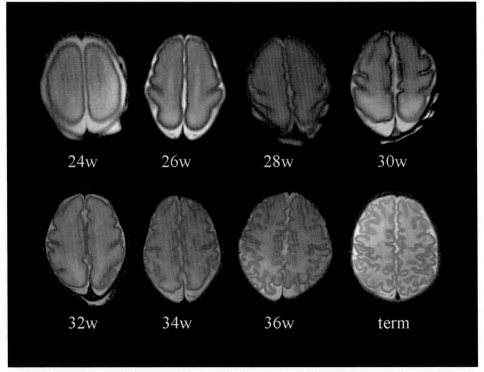

FIGURE 8-4 ■ **Normal gyral development in the fetal period seen from 24 weeks' gestational age until term on MRI.** Further sulcal development and cortical folding occurs to reach the adult gyral pattern by term. Postnatally, the sulci continue to deepen. Images are a combination of in utero fetal MRI and postnatal MRI. (Acknowledgements: Dr Cornelia Hagmann and University College Hospital, London.)

consistent sequence, beginning with the sensorimotor regions and visual pathways, areas that are also myelinating at the same time. The slowest regions of gyration are also those with the slowest myelination, such as the frontal and temporal poles. By term the gyral pattern is nearly the same as the appearance in adults, with further deepening of the sulci occurring post-term. The Sylvian fissures are also wider and vertically oriented and these continue to mature post-term.[8,9]

Other Postnatal Maturational Changes

Development of the corpus callosum begins with the posterior genu, body and splenium, and then the anterior genu and rostrum. All these components are present by 20 weeks' gestation; however, it continues to grow in length and thickness through the rest of the fetal period and post-term. The adult appearance with full thickness of the corpus callosum is achieved by 8–10 months of age, and bulking up of the splenium as the visual pathways mature occurs by 4–6 months.[10]

In the adult there are several regions where there is relative T_2 hypointensity, considered to be due to the normal deposition of iron; these are the basal ganglia, particularly the globus pallidus, substantia nigra, and red nucleus. In the infant the basal ganglia begin to appear relatively T_2 hypointense to cortex by about 6 months of age due to myelination, but the putamen and globus pallidus are isointense to each other and the internal capsule. They then become relatively bright with respect to white matter as this begins to myelinate. By 9 or 10 years there is a second stage of T_2 shortening in the globus pallidus, substantia nigra and red nucleus, which reduces further during the second decade.[11] The dentate nuclei show similar though less marked changes by about age 15 years. This phase is due to iron deposition, which continues throughout adult life.

In normal infants up to the age of 2 months the anterior pituitary gland has a convex upper border and is of relatively high T_1-weighted signal.[12] From 2 months the pituitary gland has a flat surface and is isointense with grey matter. It slowly grows during childhood and ranges from 2 to 6 mm in vertical diameter until puberty, when it enlarges again.

BRAIN MALFORMATIONS AND DEVELOPMENTAL ABNORMALITIES

Posterior Fossa Abnormalites

Cerebellar Hypoplasia

The cerebellum may be small due to lack of formation or due to cerebellar atrophy. Cerebellar hypoplasia may be due to an acquired brain injury, such as infection (especially congenital cytomegalovirus (CMV)), infarction or preterm ischaemic insult, toxins or a paraneoplastic condition, or the hypoplasia may be due to a genetic, neurometabolic or neurodegenerative condition, or a malformation. In many children (up to 50% in our series), despite extensive testing the cause remains unknown. It

has been suggested that the timing of onset is the key feature which determines whether the cerebellum is involved in isolation or whether the pons is also involved. This imaging finding may indicate an earlier disease onset with early neuronal injury to the cerebellum causing pontine hypoplasia by affecting the development of synaptic connections from the hypoplastic cerebellum or supratentorial white matter.

The inherited neurometabolic or neurodegenerative conditions causing cerebellar hypoplasia comprise an extremely wide range of aetiologies. Most are autosomal recessive, but autososomal dominant (often seen in adults), X-linked or maternally inherited forms are recognised. Clinically the child may present with progressive or intermittent hypotonia or ataxia, although there is often no clear correlation between the severity of the imaging findings and the clinical presentation. Among common causes are Friedreich's ataxia, oculomotor apraxia types 1 and 2, ataxia telangiectasia, infantile onset spinocerebellar ataxia, congenital disorders of gylycosylation and infantile neuroaxonal dystrophy (Fig. 8-5). The imaging findings in this large group of conditions are abnormal but are non-specific and include: symmetrical atrophy of the cerebellar folia with widened cerebellar fissures; progressive cerebellar atrophy on sequential images; and variable cerebellar signal changes (less common). The vermis is more frequently affected but the atrophy may be diffuse and bilateral. In most cases there are no additional imaging changes pointing to a specific imaging diagnosis. However, unilateral cerebellar atrophy is more likely to be due to an acquired insult, including

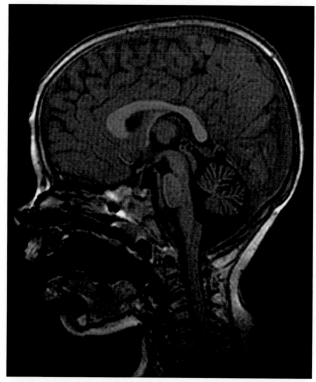

FIGURE 8-5 ■ Child with infantile neuroaxonal dystrophy. The cerebellar folia are underformed and the fissures are widened. The brainstem is also small.

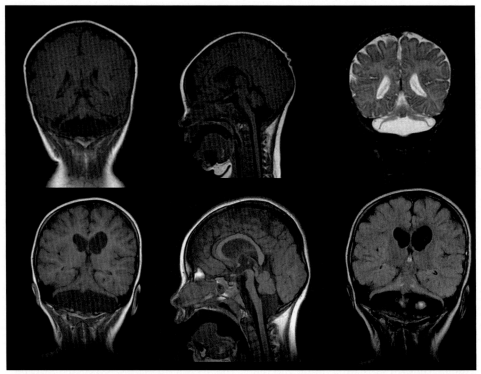

FIGURE 8-6 ■ (Top row) MRI brain images (coronal, sagittal T1W and coronal T2) at 3 months of age. (Bottow row) MRI brain images at age 4 in a child with pontocerebellar hypoplasia and confirmed TSEN54 mutation. The pons is small and there is a 'dragonfly' cerebellum with cerebellar hemisphere hypoplasia and relative sparing of the vermis. There are bilateral cerebellar hemisphere cysts.

in utero infection, stroke or germinal matrix haemorrhage. Many cases of genetic degenerative cerebellar hypoplasia are not associated with significant brainstem hypoplasia. Cerebellar white matter changes are seen in infantile Refsum's disease, adrenomyeloneuropathy and cerebrotendinosis xanthomatosis. Cerebellar grey matter signal abnormality is uncommon but may suggest diagnoses such as infantile neuroaxonal dystrophy, late infantile neuronal ceroid lipofuscinosis, mitochondrial disorders or Marinesco Sjögren's syndrome.

There is also a specific group of conditions in which the pons is more severely affected along with the cerebellum. These are known as the pontocerebellar hypoplasias (PCH) and there are six types (PCH1–6). Some are associated with a typical clinical phenotype, and others with both a classical clinical and imaging phenotype. PCH1 is associated with muscle hypotonia, joint contractures, microcephaly and breathing difficulties from birth with loss of spinal cord motor neurons. Most affected children do not survive infancy. In children with PCH2 there is lack of voluntary movements, dysphagia and absent speech as well as clonus, muscle spasms and classically dystonia, though some children may present purely with spasticity. PCH4 has a similar phenotype but is more severe. PCH3 is associated with optic atrophy. PCH6 is characterised by hypotonia, poor feeding in infancy, progressive developmental delay and seizures; typically a rapidly progressive neonatal or early infancy epileptic encephalopathy with intractabale seizures is seen.

The pontocerebellar hypoplasias may be associated with mutations in specific genes related to neuronal

development and survival. Some cases of PCH1 have a specific genetic mutation, VRK1. PCH2 is associated with three related genetic mutations: TSEN54 (the commonest), TSEN2 and TSEN34. PCH4 is also associated with TSEN54 mutation. RARS2 may be seen in PCH6, while specific genetic mutations for PCH3 and PCH5 are not yet known.

All have varying degrees of pontocerebellar hypoplasia on brain MRI. A 'dragonfly' appearances of the cerebellum is recognised typically in PCH2 commonly with TSEN54 mutations; there is marked cerebellar hemisphere atrophy with relative vermian sparing. Cerebral hemisphere cortical atrophy and cerebellar hemisphere cysts may also be seen (Fig. 8-6). In other mutations or unknown genetic mutations a more non-specific 'butterfly' appearance may be seen when there is equal involvement of the cerebellar hemispheres and vermis. Another group of conditions which can present with both cerebellar and pontine hypoplasia are the congenital disorders of glycosylation type IA.

The cerebellum may also be involved in acute presentations of neurometabolic disease or with supratentorial abnormalities and will be discussed in the context of neurometabolic disease later in the chapter.

Dandy–Walker Malformation and Its Variants

This describes a spectrum of cystic posterior fossa malformations ranging from the complete Dandy–Walker malformation to a persistent Blake's pouch and mega

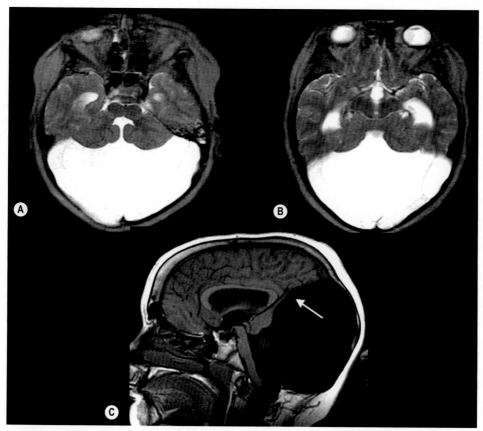

FIGURE 8-7 ■ **Dandy–Walker malformation.** (A, B) The fourth ventricle opens into a large posterior fossa cyst. There is associated hydrocephalus. (C) The cerebellum is hypoplastic and a thin rim of cerebellar tissue is seen forming the wall of the posterior fossa cyst (arrow). The vein of Galen, straight sinus and venous confluence are elevated above the level of the lambdoid suture.

cisterna magna, all of which have in common a focal extra-axial cerebrospinal fluid (CSF) collection continuous with the fourth ventricle, and variable cerebellar hypoplasia.[13] The classical Dandy–Walker malformation is the most severe posterior fossa malformation in this spectrum. It is characterised by cystic dilatation of the fourth ventricle, an enlarged posterior fossa, often with elevation of the venous confluence of the torcula above the lambdoid suture, which may be seen on plain radiography, computed tomography (CT) and MRI, and elevation of the tentorium. There is aplasia or hypoplasia of the cerebellar vermis, with vermian rotation (Fig. 8-7).[14] The Dandy–Walker malformation is associated with hydrocephalus and other midline anomalies, and can be an indicator for underlying clinical syndromes and chromosomal abnormalities. Children with any of these developmental anomalies may present as incidental findings or with developmental delay, seizures and hydrocephalus.

At the mildest end of the spectrum, the mega cisterna magna is seen as an incidental finding of no clinical significance and consists of an infracerebellar CSF collection (or normal cisternal space), with a normal cerebellum and fourth ventricle. The presence of crossing vessels and falx cerebelli favours the mega cisterna magna over a posterior fossa arachnoid cyst. Unlike the mega cisterna magna, posterior fossa arachnoid cysts are not in

continuity with the fourth ventricle. They may be associated with mass effect on the adjacent cerebellum and enlargement of the posterior fossa. Mainly these are clinically incidental findings but, like suprasellar arachnoid cysts, may occasionally increase in size in the neonatal period or infancy and cause obstructive hydrocephalus requiring surgical intervention. Arachnoid cysts do not communicate with the fourth ventricle.

Joubert's Syndrome and Related Disorders (JSRD)

These are a group of recessive congenital ataxia disorders in which typically there is neonatal hypotonia, tachypnoea, abnormal eye movements and mental retardation[15] associated with a particular pattern of cerebellar dysgenesis with a molar tooth-type malformation and vermis hypoplasia. The typical imaging findings may be seen in children without the full triad of clinical features. Cilia are found as projections from the neuron and ependyma; to date three known causative genes have been identified in primary ciliary protein genes and JSRD is, therefore, considered to be a cilopathy. Several syndromes with additional features such as renal cysts, ocular abnormalities, liver fibrosis, hypothalamic hamartoma and polymicrogyria have been classified with this anomaly, so that detection of the typical midbrain changes should prompt additional investigation for these. The cardinal feature of the Joubert malformation is the presence of a 'molar tooth' sign which is created by a combination of midbrain hypoplasia with an abnormally deep interpeduncular fossa and a failure of the superior cerebellar peduncles to decussate across the midline (Fig. 8-8). On axial imaging the fourth ventricle is abnormally shaped with a 'batwing appearance', there is cerebellar hypoplasia and there is a midline vermian cleft and dysplastic small vermis. The midbrain is small.[16]

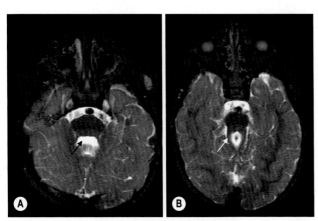

FIGURE 8-8 ■ **Child with Joubert's syndrome.** (A) Typical batwing appearance to the fourth ventricle (arrow) and (B) prominent superior cerebellar peduncles with failure of the normal midline decussation (arrow). This gives the typical 'molar tooth' appearance. The midbrain is hypoplastic in this condition.

Other Posterior Fossa Malformations or Developmental Disorders

Rhombencephalosynapsis. Rhombencephalosynapsis is a very rare cerebellar malformation in which the cerebellar hemispheres, deep cerebellar nuclei and superior cerebellar peduncles are fused across the midline and there is hypoplasia or aplasia of the vermis (Fig. 8-9).[17] It may be associated with hydrocephalus typically due to aqueduct stenosis, as well as fusion of midbrain colliculi and other midline supratentorial anomalies such as absence of the septum pellucidum, and corpus callosum.

Pontine Tegmental Cap Dysplasia. The diagnosis of pontine tegmental cap dysplasia is made on the basis of characteristic imaging findings in children presenting with multiple cranial neuropathies and evidence of cerebellar dysfunction. There is a characteristic 'cap' or projection on the dorsal surface of the pons which projects into the fourth ventricle. This is continuous with the middle cerebellar peduncles and diffusion tensor imaging studies suggest this is caused by failure of decussation and abnormal axonal pathways at this level. There is also a 'molar tooth' appearances of the superior cerebellar peduncles which fail to decussate. The cerebellar vermis and hemispheres are all small as well as the pons distal to the dorsal pontine 'cap'. The vestibulocochear nerves are absent, there is a cochlea dysplasia and there is a duplicated internal auditory canal for the facial nerve (Fig. 8-10).

Lhermitte-Duclos or Dysplastic Cerebellar Gangliocytoma. Lhermitte-Duclos or dysplastic cerebellar

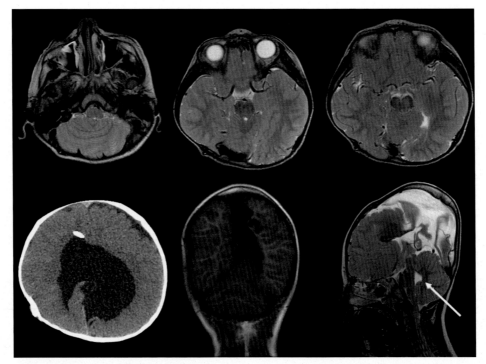

FIGURE 8-9 ■ **Child with rhombencephalosynapsis, absent septum pellucidum, initial hydrocephalus and porencephalic cyst.** Note the complete fusion across the midline of the cerebellum which herniates cranially thorough the tentorial hiatus, absent vermis and resulting abnormal configuration of the fastigial point (arrow).

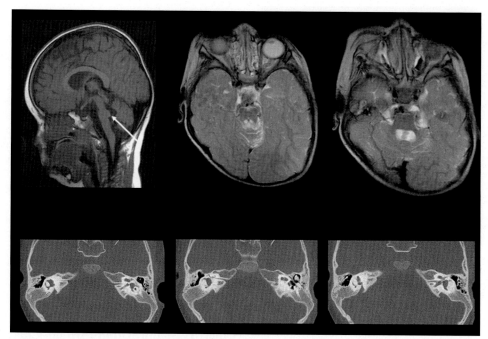

FIGURE 8-10 ■ MRI brain images in this 3-year-old with congenital sensorineural deafness as well as congenital paresis of IV, V and VII, hypotonia, vertical pendular nystagmus and developmental delay show flattened ventral pons, pontine 'cap' projecting into the fourth ventricle (arrow), very thin middle cerebellar peduncles in keeping with pontine tegmental cap dysplasia. CT petrous bones show widened bilateral vestibular aqueducts and dysplasia, small IAM on the right, which is the bony canal for the right facial nerve and on the left two bony canals instead of a single normal-sized IAM, with absence of the VIII nerves.

gangliocytoma is a developmental lesion with a distinctive radiological appearance in which there is enlargement of the cerebellar cortex, usually affecting one hemisphere. On MRI there is a non-enhancing mass with diffusely enlarged cerebellar folia.[18] Pial enhancement may be demonstrated.

There are many other forms of non-specific cerebellar dysgenesis for which as yet there are no universally accepted classification systems.

The Chiari malformations are discussed separately as they represent separate entities.

Chiari II Malformation

This is a true hindbrain malformation which is clinically, radiologically and embryologically distinct from the Chiari I malformation described below. The Chiari II malformation is aetiologically and epidemiologically intimately related to the myelomeningocele with an association that is close to 100%. It is therefore part of a spectrum of consequences of open spinal dysraphism or other failures of closure of the neural tube during fetal development. The clinical presentation is usually at birth or by earlier in utero detection of a lumbosacral meningocele. This entity is discussed in more detail in the 'Disorders of Dorsal Induction' section.

Chiari I Malformation

This may be considered a form of hindbrain deformation rather than a true malformation and is characterised by cerebellar tonsillar descent through a normal-sized foramen magnum. It may be an acquired condition and

has occasionally been observed either to improve or worsen over time without intervention. Clinical symptoms are more likely when there is greater than 5 mm descent below the foramen magnum, and therefore descent below this level is considered to be clinically significant. However, neuroimaging does not reliably predict those who are symptomatic. Children between 5 and 15 years have greater tonsillar descent up to 6 mm as a normal finding compared to children under 5 years or adults. There may be an associated syringomyelia. Symptoms including cough-induced headache, lower cranial nerve palsies and disassociated peripheral anaesthesia have been described.

Supratentorial Abnormalities

The earliest malformations to appear relate to the formation of the neural tube, and are described as abnormalities of dorsal induction or cranial dysraphism (occurring at 3–4 weeks' gestation). Anencephaly, cephaloceles and Chiari II (Arnold–Chiari) malformation are generally considered to be consequences of abnormalities of dorsal induction. The events which follow the formation of the neural tube are known as ventral induction, when the two separate cerebral hemispheres are formed (5–8 weeks). The holoprosencephalies are all abnormalities of ventral induction. The structures in the posterior fossa are also formed during this period. Neurons form and proliferate in the subependymal layer of the lateral ventricles known as the germinal matrix and subventricular zone from around 7 weeks' gestation. The neurons subsequently migrate peripherally along radially oriented microglia to form the layers of the cerebral

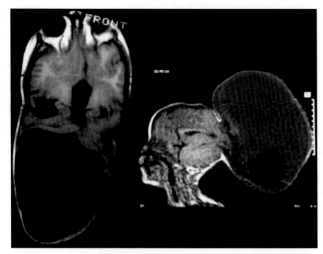

FIGURE 8-11 ■ **Parieto-occipital cephalocele with herniation of the brain and meninges through a calvarial defect.** Most of the herniated component is in the form of a cerebrospinal fluid-containing meningocele.

cortex from 2 to 5 months' gestation, the deeper layers forming first.

Disorders of Dorsal Induction

Anencephaly. Anencephaly is the most common cerebral malformation in the fetus and is incompatible with life. Most anencephalics are stillborn, but a few survive for a few days.

Cephalocele. A cephalocele is an extracranial protrusion of intracranial structures through a congenital defect of the skull and dura mater (Fig. 8-11). Some authors consider this to be a failure of neurulation or ventral induction (or primary neural tube closure) while others consider this as a post-neurulation event in which brain tissue herniates through a mesenchymal defect in the future dura and cranium.

The cephalocele may be clinically palpable. Unlike myelomeningoceles in the spine, there is usually no skin defect. When the cephalocele contains only leptomeninges and CSF it is a meningocele, and when it also contains neural tissue, typically abnormal and non-functioning with areas of necrosis, calcification and cerebral malformation, it is an encephalocele. The herniation may also include part of the ventricle when it is known as an encephalocystocele. These congenital cephaloceles mainly occur in the midline and at predictable and consistent points, assumed to be multiple closure points of the neural tube to produce frontonasal, parietal, occipital or cervico-occipital cephaloceles. As expected, the bigger the extent of herniating brain, the more microcephalic the affected child is and the more cognitive impairment is present. Occipital cephaloceles are often syndromic.

Cephaloceles are named by the bones which border the bone defect. In nasofrontal cephaloceles the bone defect lies between the frontal and the nasal bones at the level of the 'fonticulus frontalis', a small developmental communication that usually regresses during the fetal period. These lesions can be midline or just off the midline and can be associated with other midline defects such as callosal agenesis and callosal lipomas. If the communicating channel persists, there may be a cephalocele. If the more proximal part eventually obliterates, there may be a dermoid or ectopic brain tissue along the residual track but without intracranial communication. Frontoethmoidal ('sincipital'), nasoethmoidal, naso-orbital, transethmoidal, sphenoethmoidal and sphenonasopharyngeal cephaloceles are also seen, although they are less common.

The primary role of imaging is to establish the presence of neural tissue, other intracranial malformations and hydrocephalus as well as the bone defect. This requires a combination of MRI and CT. Small meningoceles that do not have an intracranial connection may not require surgery, since their size may decrease with time, producing the appearance of an 'atretic meningocele'. As well as the detection of persistent intracranial connection, the detection and localisation of vascular structures is important before any neurosurgical intervention.

Chiari II Malformation (Arnold–Chiari). This is discussed here as a congenital malformation of the hindbrain that is almost always associated with a neural tube defect, usually a lumbosacral myelomeningocele (open neural tube defect). Affected children may have hydrocephalus at birth (25%) but if not most (80%) will develop hydrocephalus following closure and repair of the lumbar myelomeningocele after birth. Other symptoms of complications of the malformation include upper airway problems, such as apnoea and stridor, and feeding problems, such as dysphagia due to brainstem compression or underdevelopment and which occur in about a third of patients. Patients can be developmentally normal or may have delay or seizures. Urinary retention may occur as well as congenital hip dislocations and feet deformities.

The Chiari II malformation is characterised by a small posterior fossa and downward displacement of the cerebellum, pons, medulla oblongata and cervical cord through an enlarged foramen magnum. Associated features include medullary kinking, an inferiorly displaced, elongated and slit-like fourth ventricle, beaking of the tectum of the midbrain, flattening of the ventral pons and low attachment of the tentorium.[19,20] The tentorial incisura is enlarged and the cerebellum herniates superiorly into the supratentorial space. The falx is partially absent or fenestrated, resulting in interdigitation of gyri across the midline, and the massa intermedia of the thalami is enlarged. The foramen magnum is enlarged and 'shield-shaped' (Fig. 8-12).

Other malformations that may be associated with the Chiari II malformation but are less consistent include a lacunar skull dysraphism (luckenschadel), disorders of neuronal migration, malformation of the corpus callosum, dorsal midline cyst and absence of the septum pellucidum.

The diagnosis can be readily made with CT by identifying the wide tentorial incisura, typical configuration of the wide foramen magnum and the small fourth ventricle and posterior fossa. Interdigitation of the cerebral hemispheres may be also identified. MRI is the

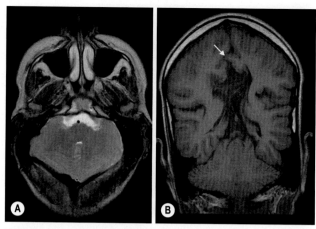

FIGURE 8-12 ■ Chiari II malformation. (A) The posterior fossa is enlarged and 'shield-shaped'. The fourth ventricle is small and slit-like. (B) The cerebellum towers superiorly through the tentorium and there is interdigitation of a cerebral gyrus through the fenestrated falx (arrow).

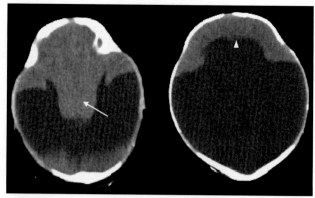

FIGURE 8-14 ■ CT brain of this infant shows that the cerebral hemispheres have failed to form and there is no interhemispheric fissure or corpus callosum. Instead there is a thin pancake of cerebral tissue crossing the midline anteriorly (arrowhead) and a single holoventricle continuous with a large dorsal cyst. The midbrain and deep grey structures are fused into a single indiscriminate mass (arrow).

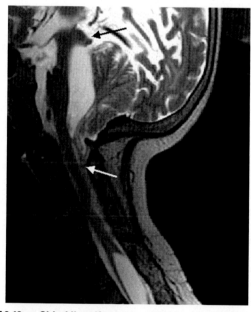

FIGURE 8-13 ■ Chiari II malformation. The fourth ventricle, which should normally be small and slit-like in this condition, is enlarged, indicating hydrocephalus. There is cascading tonsillar tissue herniating through the foramen magnum (white arrow). Beaking of the tectal plate is also seen (black arrow), as well as a cervical spinal cord syringomyelic cavity.

best investigation to show complications, which include hydrocephalus, an isolated fourth ventricle, hydrosyringomyelia and compression of the craniocervical junction. The fourth ventricle in Chiari II malformation should be slit-like: a normal or enlarged ventricle suggests hydrocephalus or that the ventricle may be isolated (Fig. 8-13). A spinal cord syrinx may be present.

The term 'Chiari III' malformation has been used by some authors to describe the association of the brain anomalies commonly seen in Chiari II malformation (inferior cerebellar, medulla and spinal cord displacement, medullary kinking and tectal beaking, etc.) plus an

occipital or cervical encephalocele with occipital bone defect.

Disorders of Ventral Induction

Holoprosencephaly. Holoprosencephaly is a relatively common structural abnormality of the human forebrain, occurring in up to 1 in 10,000 live and stillbirths. It results from a disturbance in the usual signalling pathways required for separation of the embryonic prosencephalon into two separate cerebral hemispheres. Holoprosencephaly is found in association with chromosomal abnormalities, and various teratogenic factors including maternal diabetes. At least 13 different holoprosencephaly loci on chromosomal regions, nine of which are on known holoprosencephaly genes such as sonic hedgehog, ZIC2 and TGIF are recognised. The primary pathway involved in midline developmental anomalies is the sonic hedgehog pathway. This malformation is seen in trisomy 13, 18 and in triploidy. Other abnormalities of midline development are frequently also found.

Classification of holoprosencephaly is based on the degree of separation of the cerebral hemispheres and it appears this is a continuous spectrum of failure of separation. The most severe form is alobar holoprosencephaly in which there is complete or nearly complete failure of separation of the cerebral hemispheres. Many infants are either stillborn or do not survive until term, while infants who do survive are very abnormal with abnormal reflexes, tone and seizures in the neonatal period as well as severe midline facial deformities. The facial deformities can include cyclops or a single eye on a stalk, midline clefts and hypotelorism. Only a minority of patients survive beyond the first year. The medial and ventral parts of the brain have not formed in these patients and the septum pellucidum is absent. On imaging there is a crescent-shaped holoventricle continuous with a large dorsal cyst and the cerebrum consists of a pancake-like mass of tissue with no interhemispheric fissure, corpus callosum or falx cerebri (Fig. 8-14). The hypothalamic and basal ganglia

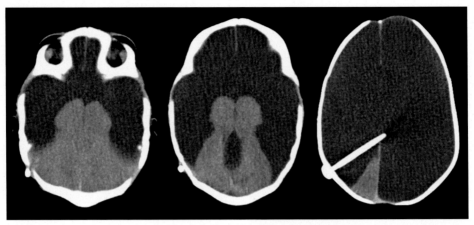

FIGURE 8-15 ■ Child with hydranencephaly in which the cerebral hemispheres are absent with the exception of some of the parieto-occipital lobes, and preservation of the thalami and posterior fossa structures.

are fused. There is no normal circle of Willis and the arterial supply comes directly from the internal carotid and basilar arteries without normal anterior, middle and posterior cerebral arteries. Despite the underlying micro-cephaly, hydrocephalus often develops and CSF diversion with a shunt may be required as a palliative procedure to help manage head size for nursing. Holoprosencephaly should be distinguished from gross hydrocephalus in which there is a very thin, barely visible cerebral cortical mantle and from hydranencephaly caused by a global early in utero insult (thought to be ischaemic) in which much of the cerebral hemisphere parenchyma is destroyed, leaving a fluid-filled cavity but with relative preservation of mesial temporal occipital lobes, deep grey matter and brainstem (Fig. 8-15). Semilobar holoprosen-cephaly is less severe; although posteriorly the interhemi-spheric fissure is partially formed, anteriorly the hemispheres fail to separate. As the brain is less dysmor-phic, the midline facial abnormalities are also mild or absent. These children present later with developmental delay or concerns over reduced or increasing head size due to hydrocephalus. The frontal lobes are fused, but the thalami are partially separated. There is still a single ventricle instead of the two lateral ventricles seen nor-mally but the failure of separation of the hypothalami, thalami and basal ganglia is less severe compared to the alobar form and there may be an indication of a third ventricle. The posterior corpus callosum is partially formed. The temporal horns are rudimentary and the hippocampi are underdeveloped.

Lobar holoprosencephaly is associated with mild (or absent) facial malformations and intellectual abilities that range from mild impairment to normal. They may have endocrine disturbance of the hypothalamic–pituitary axis. The brain is generally of normal volume and shows almost complete separation into two hemispheres, though in the depth of the frontal lobes there is continuous cer-ebral cortex between the two lobes.

Finally there is the interhemispheric variant of holo-prosencephaly, also known as syntelencephaly, which has a mild clinical presentation with mild learning and visual impairments. In this condition the interhemispheric fissure is formed anteriorly at the level of the anteroir frontal lobes, and posteriorly at the level of the occipital lobes but in the middle the posterior frontal and parietal lobes are fused and there is no interhemispheric fissure, falx and corpus callosum (Fig. 8-16). This results in an unusual callosal malformation in which the genu and splenium are present but the body is absent

Malformations of Commissural and Related Structures

Agenesis of the Septum Pellucidum. Absence of the septum pellucidum is not a severe malformation, but should be recognised as an indicator of other cerebral malformations. Associated malformations include septo-optic dysplasia, agenesis of the corpus callosum, holo-prosencephaly, Chiari II malformation, schizencephaly and other migration disorders. Septo-optic dysplasia or de Morsier's syndrome describes the triad of hypopitui-tarism, hypoplasia of the optic nerves and absence of the septum pellucidum (Fig. 8-17). Less than 1% are associ-ated with mutations in the HESX1 gene. However, the the clinical manifestations are quite variable. Neuroimag-ing may show absence of the septum pellucidum with a typical box-like configuration of the frontal horns, small optic nerves and chiasm, small anterior pituitary gland and ectopic 'bright spot' of the posterior pituitary gland on T1W imaging. Isolated absence of the septum pel-lucidum may also occur and it is important to look for other associated brain anomalies such as callosal agenesis, holoprosencephaly, cobblestone cortical malformations and bilateral polymicrogyria. The septum pellucidum may also be absent as an acquired lesion in the context of hydrocephalus.

Commissural Agenesis or Dysgenesis. The major interhemispheric commissural connections are the corpus callosum and anterior and hippocampal commissures. The corpus callosum consists of the rostrum, genu, body and splenium with the isthmus defining a normal point of narrowing between the body and the splenium of the corpus callosum. The corpus callosum may be partially

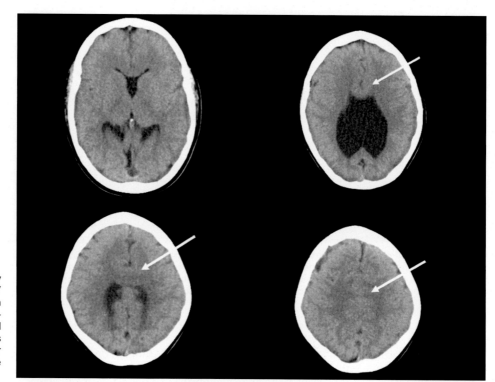

FIGURE 8-16 ■ Syntelencephaly or 'middle interhemispheric' variant of holoprosencephaly in which the anterior interhemispheric fissure is present and frontal lobes and occipital lobes are separate, but the posterior frontal and parietal lobes have failed to separate (arrows).

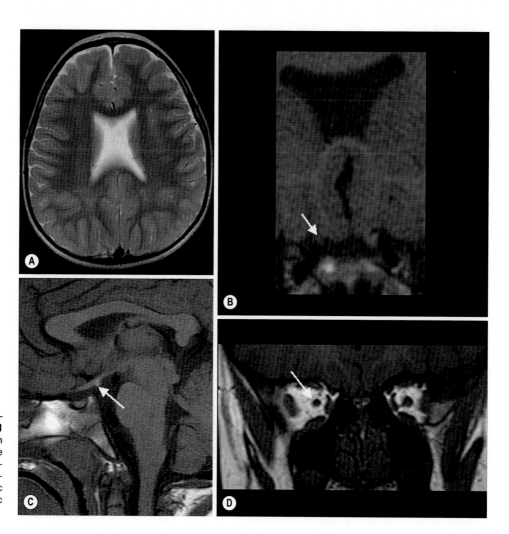

FIGURE 8-17 ■ **Septo-optic dysplasia in a child with HESX1 gene mutation.** (A) The septum pellucidum is absent and the frontal horns have a typical box-like configuration. (B) The posterior pituitary gland is ectopic (arrow). (C, D) The right optic nerve is small (arrows).

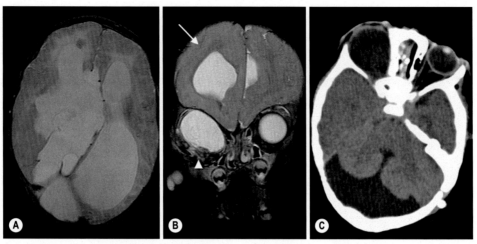

FIGURE 8-18 ■ **Child with skin lesions and right orbital cyst in oculocerebrocutaneous syndrome.** (A) There is callosal agenesis with dorsal interhemispheric cysts. (B) The right cerebral hemisphere is dysplastic with thickening of the cortex and an indistinct grey–white matter junction (arrow). There is a cyst expanding the orbit with a small calcified globe seen inferiorly (arrowhead). (C) An associated Dandy–Walker posterior fossa malformation is also present.

formed (dysgenesis) or completely absent (agenesis). The anterior part (posterior genu and anterior body) is formed before the posterior part (posterior body and splenium). Hence a small or absent genu or body, with an intact splenium and rostrum, is more likely to suggest secondary destruction rather than abnormal development. The structure develops between about 7 and 20 weeks' gestation, which parallels the development of the rest of the cerebrum and the cerebellum; abnormalities of the corpus callosum are therefore commonly associated with other congenital malformations of the brain, such as Chiari II malformation, Dandy–Walker malformation, lipoma, abnormalities of neuronal migration and organisation, dysraphic anomalies, encephaloceles, septo-optic dysplasia, ocular anomalies and other midline facial anomalies.[21]

There are many well-defined syndromes in which callosal abnormalities feature, including Aicardi's syndrome which is X-linked dominant occurring in females and characterised by seizures, intellectual impairment, chorioretinal lacunae seen at fundoscopy examination and brain malformations such as polymicrogyria, ectopic grey matter and cortical dysplasias. Callosal agenesis is a feature of oculocerebrocutaneous syndrome or Delleman's syndrome (Fig. 8-18), Alport's syndrome, orofacial-digital syndrome and many other syndromes. Dysgenesis of the corpus callosum is also frequently seen in fetal alcohol syndrome.

Agenesis of the Corpus Callosum. On axial imaging the lateral ventricles have a parallel orientation and a typical posterior dilatation known as colpocephaly. The third ventricle extends more superiorly than normal within the interhemispheric fissure between the bodies of the lateral ventricles and the normal convergence of the bodies of the ventricles towards the midline is absent. On sagittal imaging, partial or complete absence of the corpus callosum must be distinguished from a generally

thinned one (which is more likely to be an acquired abnormality). In callosal agenesis the vertically oriented sulci extend right down to the ventricle without formation of the cingulate gyri which normally run parallel to the corpus callosum and there is no horizontally running cingulate sulcus. On coronal imaging the corpus callosum is absent in the midline, the third ventricle is high-riding and there is a characteristic indentation on the medial aspect of the lateral ventricles caused by the bundles of Probst, which are the white matter tracts that are no longer able to cross the midline in the corpus callosum (Fig. 8-19). Presence of one midline anomaly, such as callosal agenesis, should prompt the reporting radiologist to look carefully for other midline anomalies that are frequently associated, such as midline lipomas and cephaloceles.

Agenesis of the Corpus Callosum with Interhemispheric Cyst. In some cases the interhemispheric cyst frequently seen with this malformation originates from the herniated third ventricle and is in continuity with it and the rest of the ventricular system, while in others continuity between the cyst and the third ventricle is lost. In both cases progressive increase in head circumference with hydrocephalus may occur in the neonate and infant, requiring shunting/drainage.

Malformations of Cortical Development— Histogenesis, Neuronal Migration and Cortical Organisation

Abnormalities of the cerebral cortex are a common finding in children with developmental delay and children with partial epilepsy. After neurulation, the process by which the neural tube is formed, has occurred, an important stage in the development of the brain is the formation of the cortex. The cortex is formed from neuroblasts that are generated in the germinal matrix,

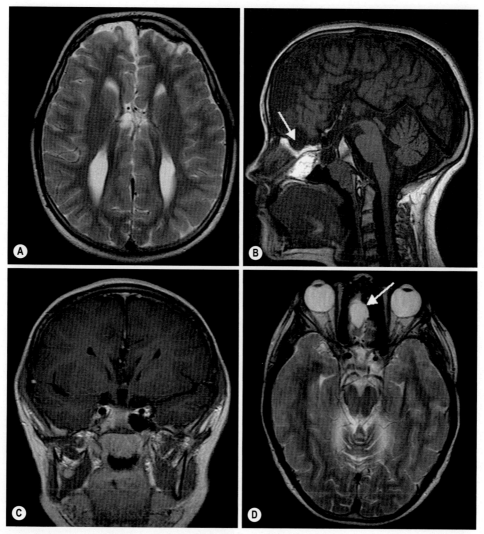

FIGURE 8-19 ■ **Callosal agenesis.** (A) Axial T$_2$-weighted MRI shows separated ventricles with parallel orientation. The superior part of the third ventricle is just seen. (B) Sagittal T$_1$-weighted MRI through the midline confirms callosal agenesis. There is no cingulate sulcus and the vertically oriented cerebral sulci extend right down to the third ventricle. This finding is associated with other midline anomalies such as a frontoethmoidal cephalocele (arrow), seen also on the axial T$_2$-weighted MRI (arrow, C). (D) The optic chiasm is absent.

located at the ependymal border of the ventricular wall. There is a migration of excitatory glutaminergic neurons by radial migration from the ventricular zone at the ependymal surface. These neuroblasts migrate to the surface of the brain along radially oriented glia, passing neurons previously laid down to form the layers of cortex. Thus the six layers of the cortex are formed, with the youngest neurons on the surface and the oldest ones adjacent to the subcortical white matter. The migration of the neuroblasts starts at about week 7 of gestation, is most intense during weeks 15–17 and is largely complete by weeks 23–24. In parallel with this, another process of tangential migration occurs involving inhibitory GABA-ergic interneurons which migrate from the ganglionic eminences. There organise in a precise manner with the radially migrating neurons described earlier.

Malformations of cortical development result from disorders of cell proliferation (or histogenesis), cell migration or cell organisation. Based on this neuroembryology, it is convenient to attempt to classify malformations of cortical development broadly according to these embryological principles.[22] For the purposes of this chapter, these malformations will be described by radiological pattern, starting with disorders of neuronal organisation, then migration, then histogenesis.

Polymicrogyria

This is considered to be a disorder of neuronal organisation, occurring after neuronal migration. The extent of polymicrogyric cortex may vary from small, isolated, unilateral areas to larger areas of bilateral disease (Fig. 8-20). The key pathological feature to identify on imaging is an

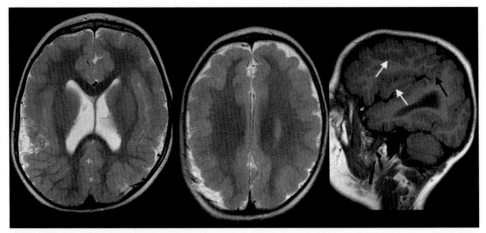

FIGURE 8-20 ■ **Extensive bilateral cerebral hemisphere polymicrogyria.** Virtually no normal cortex is seen. At first glance the cortex appears thickened, but closer inspection reveals an overconvoluted gyral pattern and a 'lumpy bumpy' grey–white matter interface (including regions marked by white arrows). The Sylvian fissure is abnormally oriented with a parietal cleft that extends posteriorly (black arrow).

overconvoluted and fused cortex of normal thickness. The appearances on imaging may vary from apparently broad, thickened gyri mimicking pachygyria (particularly when examined with relatively thick imaging slices), to clearly overconvoluted multiple gyri with irregular outer and inner cortical surfaces.

The identification of polymicrogyria assists with genetic counselling. There are recessive and dominant forms that are often bilateral and symmetrical, as well as disease believed to be acquired from intrauterine infection such as CMV infection or an underlying neurometabolic disorder, which may often be asymmetrical in distribution. There may be associated dystrophic calcification in these lesions, which typically may only be visible on CT.

Schizencephaly

Schizencephaly is a defect that involves the complete cerebral mantle and connects the calvarium and the outer surface of the brain with the lateral ventricles. The defect is a cleft lined by grey matter and leptomeninges, which differentiates it from a transmantle infarction in which the defect is lined by white matter. The schizencephaly may have an 'open lip' with a wide open defect (Fig. 8-21), or a 'closed lip' when the cleft is closed but lined with grey matter entirely into the ventricle. The convolutional pattern of the cortex adjacent to the clefts is abnormal and consists of polymicrogyria.

The clinical features are variable, depending on the size and location of the lesion. Severe seizures are quite common, as is spasticity. Children with bilateral clefts have severe mental and psychomotor developmental delay. Wide clefts usually correlate with moderate-to-severe developmental delay, while children with narrow or closed-lipped lesions may only have hemiplegia and/or seizures. The location of the lesion is typically central, involving the pre- and post-central gyri. However, the clefts may also be found in parasagittal, frontal or occipital sites when the clinical manifestations are often mild.

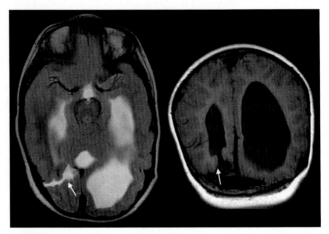

FIGURE 8-21 ■ Schizencephaly with a grey matter-lined cleft (arrows) extending from the leptomeningeal surface through the brain parenchyma to the ventricular margin.

In most cases the diagnosis can be made with CT, but this may not detect all cases of closed lip schizencephaly, which are best detected using coronal T_1-weighted MRI, preferably a three-dimensional (3D) volume acquisition. MRI also shows the abnormal appearance of the cortical mantle along the cleft and the cortex appearing thicker than normal owing to the presence of polymicrogyria. The contralateral hemisphere may also have developmental abnormalities, such as polymicrogyria and subependymal heterotopia. CT may show subependymal or parenchymal calcification in many cases, which suggests that one cause of schizencephaly may be intrauterine infection such as CMV infection.

Lissencephaly–Agyria–Pachygyria

The lissencephaly–agyria–pachygyria group includes the severest forms of abnormal neuronal migration. Lissencephaly literally means 'smooth brain'. The classical or

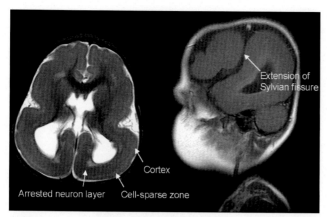

FIGURE 8-22 ■ **Classical with lissencephaly.** This child was 'floppy' at birth and then had developmental delay, seizures and strabismus. MRI shows a smooth gyral pattern which is slightly more developed frontally in keeping with classical lissencephaly (*LIS1* mutation). The cerebral cortex is generally thin and there is a band of arrested neurons deep to the 'cell-sparse zone'. The Sylvian fissures are vertically oriented and extend into a vertical cleft.

type 1 Lissencephaly will be discussed first. The cortex is thickened and the brain has very few or no gyri, opercularisation (development of the Sylvian fissures) is abnormal, and the Sylvian fissures are shallow and wide. Other associated features are agenesis or hypoplasia of the corpus callosum or septum pellucidum. Agyria refers to the total or almost total absence of a convolutional pattern, i.e. there are no gyri or sulci, and is synonymous with 'complete lissencephaly'. In pachygyria, the gyri are relatively few and are unusually broad and flat. The entire brain is not affected and therefore it is sometimes referred to as 'incomplete lissencephaly'. Macroscopically and on standard thick-slice MRI, the thickened cortex of pachygyria may be difficult to differentiate from the overconvoluted, fused and normal-thickness cortex of polymicrogyria, but the latter may be distinguished more easily on higher-resolution imaging, e.g. with volumetric T_1-weighted imaging (e.g. MPRAGE, SPGR, FLASH).

In complete lissencephaly the brain surface is smooth and the Sylvian fissures are wide and vertically orientated. The posterior fossa structures are typically spared and appear normal. The cortex has a thin outer layer, an underlying 'cell-sparse zone' and a thicker broad band of grey matter, the 'arrested neurons' that have failed to migrate to the cortex, deep to it (Fig. 8-22). The gyral pattern of the brain resembles the appearance of the 23- to 24-week normal fetal brain. The implication of this is that lissencephaly is unlikely to be reliably diagnosed on early fetal MRI (before 24 weeks), though there may be clues to the diagnosis before this, such as the immature appearance of the Sylvian fissures, cell-sparse zone and the broad band of arrested neurons.

With incomplete lissencephaly there is an antero-posterior gradation of disease severity. In the *LIS1* mutation (chromosome 17) the frontotemporal gyri are more developed than the parieto-occipital gyri and in the X-linked form (*DCX* a.k.a. *XLIS* mutation) the posterior gyri are more developed. Subcortical band heterotopia is

a feature of these mutations and is therefore discussed here. On imaging, band heterotopia appears as a homogeneous band of grey matter between the lateral ventricle and the cerebral cortex, separated from both by a layer of white matter. The overlying cortex is usually of normal thickness but has shallow sulci. *DCX* mutations result in subcortical band heterotopia or 'double cortex' that is predominantly seen in girls (> 90%), as boys with these mutations usually develop lissencephaly. Impairment to neuronal migration is more severe anteriorly, so the band heterotopia is typically seen symmetrically in the frontal regions. Although the imaging appearances may be severe, the degree of developmental delay may be quite variable. Some children may even be normal except for a relatively mild seizure disorder.

Variants of classical lissencephaly are now increasingly recognised. They account for a minority of cases and may demonstrate additional findings on imaging. These include X-linked lissencephaly with abnormal genitalia (XLAG) demonstrating agenesis of the corpus callosum and associated with *ARX* mutations, lissencephaly with cerebellar hypoplasia (LCH) associated with *RELN* or *VLDLR* mutations and tubulin mutations such as *TUBA1A* which result in a per-Sylvian pachygyria, absent anterior limbs or the internal capsules and dysplastic basal ganglia (Fig. 8-23).

Type 2 or Cobblestone lissencephaly is distinct from the above, the result of overmigration of neurons and is characterised by thick meninges adherent to the smooth cortical surface. There is disordered lamination of the cortex on histological examination. Extensive subcortical heterotopia are a feature and delay in myelination is frequently present. The posterior fossa structures are usually abnormal with the appearance of dysplasia with microcysts of the cerebellar hemispheres, a flattened shape of the pons in the AP dimension with a midline cleft or with a Z-shaped brainstem in the sagittal plane. The congenital muscular dystrophies (CMDs) are a heterogeneous group characterised clinically by hypotonia at birth, muscle weakness and joint contractures, developmental delay and seizures. The cobblestone lissencephaly in these cases may range from the severe clinical phenotype of the Walker–Warburg syndrome with coexistent ocular abnormalities to the milder phenotype of Fukuyama CMD with relatively normal eyes. In parallel with these clinical phenotypes, several genes have been identified with these clinical syndromes, including *POMT1, POMT2, FKRP, POMGnT1* and *LARGE*.

Grey Matter Heterotopia

Grey matter heterotopia refers to the occurrence of grey matter in an abnormal position anywhere from the subependymal layer to the cortical surface, but the term is usually reserved for ectopic neurons in locations other than the cortex. Its most common clinical presentation is as a seizure disorder. However, small isolated areas of heterotopia may be seen occasionally as incidental findings in normal patients.

Heterotopia can be subependymal, focal subcortical or band formed, or parallel to the ventricular wall (double cortex). They are isointense with cortical grey matter on

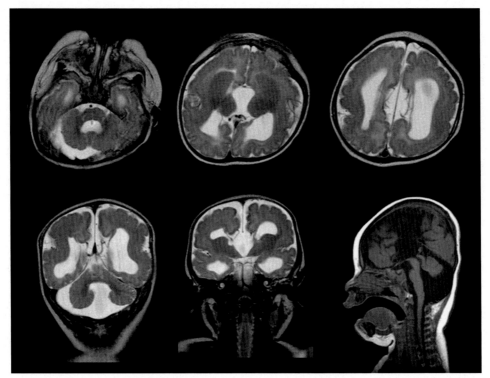

FIGURE 8-23 ■ MRI brain of a child with confirmed *TUBA1A* mutation shows frontal and peri-Sylvian pachygyria with more normal gyral differentiation anteriorly and posteriorly, absent corpus callosum, cerebellar vermian hypoplasia and rotation, small pons and absent anterior limb of internal capsule.

all imaging sequences and do not enhance after the intravenous infusion of paramagnetic contrast agents. Subcortical band heterotopia has already been discussed with classical lissencephaly.

Subependymal heterotopia are smooth and ovoid, with their long axis typically parallel to the ventricular wall, quite different from subependymal hamartomas in tuberous sclerosis which are irregular and have their long axis perpendicular to the ventricular wall (Fig. 8-24). In contrast, hamartomas seen in tuberous sclerosis are more heterogeneous depending on the presence of calcification, gliosis, etc., and do not have signal characteristics of grey matter. They may also enhance after the intravenous infusion of a paramagnetic contrast agent.

Focal subcortical heterotopia produces variable motor and intellectual impairment, depending on the size and location of the lesions. The overlying cortex is thin with shallow sulci. The foci may be isolated or may coexist with other malformations such as schizencephaly, microcephaly, polymicrogyria, dysgenesis of the corpus callosum, or absence of the septum pellucidum.

Hemimegalencephaly

This is a structural malformation due to defective neuronal proliferation, migration and organisation, leading to hamartomatous overgrowth of all or part of one hemisphere. It may occur in isolation or in association with syndromes such as Proteus, epidermal naevus and Klippel–Trénaunay–Weber syndromes, neurofibromatosis type 1

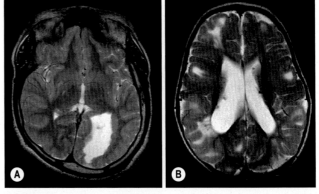

FIGURE 8-24 ■ **Subependymal grey matter heterotopia (A) and subependymal hamartomas of tuberous sclerosis (B).** (A) Multiple subependymal continuous 'nodules' running along the ventricular margin with signal intensity isointense to grey matter. (B) Scattered nodules which project into the ventricles and with variable signal intensity. Some are markedly hypointense in keeping with calcification. Note also the multiple regions of cortical and subcortical white matter abnormality with slight mass effect in keeping with cortical tubers.

(NF1) and tuberous sclerosis. The affected hemisphere contains regions of pachygyria, polymicrogyria, heterotopia, as well as dysmyelination and gliosis. Usually (but not always) the hemisphere is enlarged, there is diffuse cortical thickening, white matter signal abnormality and there may be calcification. The ipsilateral lateral ventricle is enlarged and there is a very characteristic configuration of the

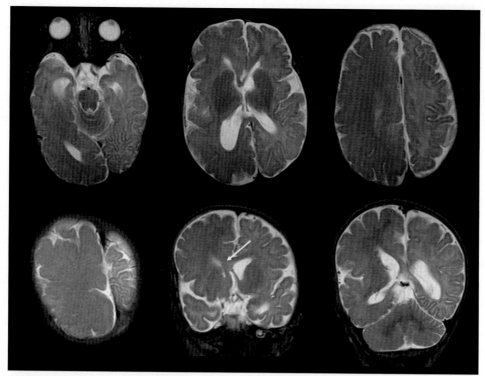

FIGURE 8-25 ■ **Enlargement of the right cerebral hemisphere in keeping with hemimegalencephaly.** There is thickening of the cortex with broad, thickened gyri, underdeveloped sulci and extensive white matter signal abnormality. Note the straightening of the right frontal horn and thickening of the genu of the corpus callosum and right anterior fornix (arrow).

frontal horn which is straight and pointed (Fig. 8-25) and associated thickening of the septum pellucidum. Occasionally this may be the only imaging clue to an underlying malformation.

Focal Cortical Dysplasia (FCD)

These are localised regions of malformed cerebral cortex and are frequently associated with epilepsy in children and adults. They are the commonest lesion found in paediatric epilepsy surgical series and were first described by Taylor et al. in 1971. This term is now used for a wide spectrum of lesions including cortical dyslamination, cytoarchitectural lesions and underlying abnormalities of white matter. Classification may be imaging-based[22] or pathologically based and the challenge remains to identify discriminating imaging features to differentiate the different histopathological subtypes of FCD. A recent classification produced by the ILAE describes FCD I (a–c), II (a, b), both isolated, and III (associated with a principal lesion such as hippocampal sclerosis, glioneuronal tumour, vascular malformation or adjacent to an early acquired insult).[23] Overall they can be located in any part of the cortex, have variable size and location and can affect more than one lobe. If seizures become resistant to medical treatment, patients with these lesions may be considered for epilepsy surgery and lesion resection. Neuroimaging is a crucial part of the clinical assessment of these children in order to identify and localise lesions which may be resectable.

FCD type IIB is a particular subtype of FCD that is characterised by the presence of balloon cells. On imaging there are features which are commonly seen with these lesions: subcortical white matter signal abnormality, blurring of the grey-white matter junction, well-defined margins, single lobe involvement, abnormal gyration/sulcation, 'transmantle sign', in decreasing order of frequency (Fig. 8-26). The key point about these lesions is that they may be a group associated with a better seizure-free outcome as they are often small, well-defined and more frequently completely resectable than other FCDS.

Imaging is ideally performed in the epilepsy surgical centre and focuses on multiplanar, multisequence imaging, including thin-section volumetric T_1- and T_2- weighted imaging. Some centres obtain surface views of the cortex to detect abnormal gyral patterning, though this can often be seen without using this technique. There is a correlation between abnormal venous drainage and dysplastic cortex, so it can be useful to look for large cortical vessels on MRI in the search for the abnormal area of cortex. The lesion may sometimes be calcified and this may be detected more easily on CT. The detection of FCDs depends largely on the conspicuity of the lesion and relative differences in signal intensity between the FCD and adjacent brain. FCDs may appear different or may be easier to detect at different ages—for example, it can be easier to detect the lesion by the presence of signal change suggesting accelerated myelination in the unmyelinated brain (so the lesion will appear dark on T_2, bright

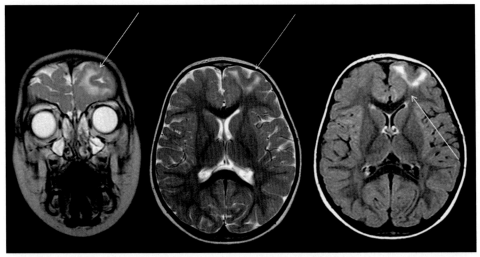

FIGURE 8-26 ■ **Child with focal epilepsy and type 2B focal cortical dysplasia.** There is abnormal gyral patterning, apparent cortical thickening and abnormal subcortical signal change extending towards the lateral ventricle ('transmantle' sign—arrow).

on T_1 images compared to the adjacent white matter). Sometimes the lesion may be very difficult to see on later imaging acquired when the brain is completely myelinated as the signal contrast between the lesion and the adjacent brain tissue is much less, giving rise to the so-called 'disappearing' lesion. Therefore when reviewing the imaging as part of the epilepsy surgery assessment, it is important to review all imaging acquired at different ages and to have a low threshold for repeating the imaging, using different sequences and tissue contrasts, optimising sedation/anaesthesia and considering higher field strength imaging.

NEUROCUTANEOUS SYNDROMES

The neurocutaneous syndromes or phakomatoses are congenital malformations affecting particularly structures of ectodermal origin, i.e. the nervous system, skin and eye. The most frequently seen are NF1, tuberous sclerosis, neurofibromatosis type 2 (NF2), von Hippel–Lindau disease and Sturge–Weber syndrome.[24,25]

Neurofibromatosis Type 1

The most common neurocutaneous syndrome is NF1, with an incidence of 1 in 3000–4000 births. As well as being one of the most common inherited central nervous system (CNS) disorders, it is the most common autosomal dominant condition, due to a mutation on chromosome 17 which encodes for the tumour suppressor gene product neurofibromin, and the most common inherited tumour syndrome. Half of children affected have new mutations. The diagnosis is made on the basis of at least two major criteria (Table 8-1).[26] Minor criteria are supportive of the diagnosis.

CNS tumours in NF1 include visual pathway gliomas, plexiform neurofibromas and cranial and peripheral nerve gliomas. These may be diagnosed radiologically

TABLE 8-1	Diagnostic Criteria for Neurofibromatosis Type 1	
Major Criteria		**Minor Criteria**
Café-au-lait spots		Small stature
Freckling in the inguinal or axillary areas		Macrocephaly
		Scoliosis*
One plexiform neurofibroma or two neurofibromas of any type*		Pectus excavatus*
Visual pathway glioma*		'Hamartomatous lesions' of NF1*
Two or more Lisch nodules of iris		Neuropsychological abnormalities
Distinctive osseous lesion, e.g. sphenoid dysplasia or thinning of cortex*		
First-degree relative with neurofibromatosis type 1 (NF1)		

*Radiologically detectable features.

without recourse to biopsy and the diagnostic criteria allow the diagnosis of NF1 to be made purely on neuroimaging or as an adjunct to clinical findings. Visual/optic pathway gliomas (OPGs) are usually WHO Grade I pilocytic astrocytomas and are the most common brain abnormality in NF1, occurring in up to 15% of patients. Most of these are diagnosed in childhood but only half are symptomatic. OPGs in NF1 are more likely to affect the optic nerves rather than the chiasm and post-chiasmatic pathways, as opposed to non-NF1 OPGs, and are also associated with a better prognosis. Once the tumour involves the chiasm and hypothalamus there is a risk of precocious puberty and a greater risk of visual deterioration.[27] They have a wide spectrum of biological behaviours, ranging from static or minimal growth in most to rapidly increasing size in a minority.

Fusiform expansion of the optic nerve and widening of the optic foramen may be detected on CT, along with the very characteristic sphenoid wing dysplasia and plexiform neurofibroma which are frequently associated. Although CT can detect the intraorbital involvement of OPG, this involves irradiating the eye and is less sensitive than MRI for delineating tumour within the chiasm and intracranial extension. Other orbital features seen in NF1 include dilatation of the optic nerve sheaths due to dural ectasia and intraorbital extension of plexiform neurofibroma. Variable extension into the chiasm, the lateral geniculate bodies or optic radiations is best detected on MRI. A suggested NF1 imaging protocol includes orbital MRI with axial and coronal dual-echo STIR, coronal and T_1-weighted pre- and fat-saturation post-gadolinium images, all with a slice thickness of 3 mm or less. Images obtained with a fat-saturation pulse allow elimination of chemical shift artefact at the interface of the optic nerve sheath complex and intraorbital fat, making assessment easier, and contrast medium improves visualisation of the normal intraorbital optic nerves.

The whole of the optic nerve may be expanded or there may be subarachnoid extension of tumour around a normal-sized nerve. Tumour infiltration within the nerve is detected as expansion of the nerve within the optic nerve sheath, often but not always with enhancement following a paramagnetic contrast agent, whereas if the tumour is predominantly subarachnoid, a rim of tumour around a minimally enhancing nerve is sometimes detected. It is important to identify the expanded nerve within the optic nerve sheath in order to distinguish it from NF1-associated dural ectasia in which the optic nerve sheath is expanded by CSF rather than tumour. Generally these optic pathway tumours are kept under observation unless symptomatic or progressive ($\leq$ 5%). Spontaneous involution of tumour is also well recognised.

There is an increased risk of other CNS tumours in NF1 with OPG. These are usually WHO Grade I pilocytic astrocyomas occurring in 1–3% of patients, particularly within the cerebellum and brainstem, although other low-grade and higher-grade tumours also occur. In the brainstem they are usually less aggressive than non-NF1 brainstem astrocytomas and are more likely to be seen in the medulla and midbrain (e.g. tectal plate gliomas) than the pons. A tectal plate tumour may cause aqueduct stenosis and hence hydrocephalus. These brainstem NF1 tumours are often biologically benign and may regress spontaneously, and therefore clinical management is generally not aggressive unless clinical/radiological tumour progression is seen.

Another characteristic lesion of NF1 is the so-called 'hamartomatous' changes of NF1, also known as 'unidentified bright objects (UBOs)', 'neurofibromatosis bright objects (NBOs)' or areas of myelin vacuolation. These are seen in 60–80% of NF1 cases, depending on the age at which the child is imaged, and in 95% of children with NF1 and OPG, and may have an impact on cognitive function.[28] They are few in number before the age of 4 years, increase in number and volume between 4 and 10 years and then decrease in the second decade, being rare over the age of 20. Therefore, they are rarely seen in the adult NF1 population. Multiple hyperintense lesions are seen on T2W images. They have normal signal on T_1-weighted images, apart from lesions in the basal ganglia which are often slightly hyperintense on T1W images. They have minimal mass effect and no contrast enhancement and occur in typical sites such as the pons, cerebellar white matter, internal capsules, basal ganglia, thalami and hippocampi (Fig. 8-27). Their lack of growth, eventual regression and lack of contrast enhancement distinguish them from gliomas. Astrocytomas, however, may develop in the areas involved by UBOs and radiologically it can be difficult to distinguish them without serial imaging. Enhancement and increasing mass effect are suspicious for tumour development, in which case the involved areas should be kept under regular imaging review. Other non-CNS neoplasia recognised in NF1 include phaeochromocytoma, carcinoid, rhabdomyosarcoma and childhood chronic myeloid leukaemia.

Plexiform neurofibromas are one of the main diagnostic criteria of NF1. These are multinodular lesions formed when tumour involves either multiple trunks or

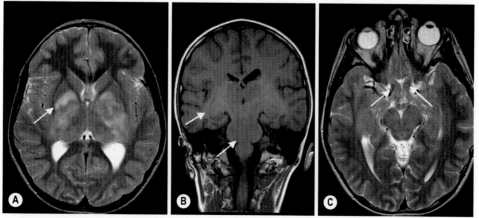

FIGURE 8-27 ■ **Child with neurofibromatosis type 1 (NF1).** (A, B) There are very characteristic lesions within the lentiform nuclei, brainstem and midbrain, the so-called 'hamartomatous' lesions or 'unidentified bright objects' of NF1 (arrows). They are hyperintense on T_2-weighted imaging, with minimal mass effect. Basal ganglia lesions may demonstrate some T_1 shortening, as in this case, or are hypointense on T_1-weighted imaging. (C) There are also bilateral optic nerve gliomas extending into the optic chiasm (arrows).

multiple fascicles of a large nerve. A typical location is the orbit where the tumour grows along the ophthalmic division of the trigeminal nerve in association with sphenoid wing dysplasia. They are hypodense on CT and generally do not enhance with contrast agents. On MRI they have a more heterogeneous appearance, of low signal intensity on T_1 images and hyperintensity on T_2 images, with variable contrast enhancement, although at least part of the tumour normally enhances. Extension occurs along the nerve pathways into the pterygomaxillary fissure, orbital apex/superior orbital fissure and cavernous sinus (Fig. 8-28). Other characteristic sites include the lumbosacral and brachial plexi. There is a malignant potential with transformation to fibrosarcoma quoted at between 2 and 12%, though probably within the lower range. Neurofibromas are more homogeneous and well-defined lesions which cause diffuse expansion of nerves. It may be possible to distinguish plexiform from other types of neurofibroma radiologically, as the former are more diffuse lesions. Neurofibromas appear on MRI as nodules seen along the spinal nerves of the cauda equina and, as they enlarge, they extend out through the neural exit foramina, enlarging them. They may have a central region of hypointensity on T_2 images, producing

a target appearance. NF1 is associated with some characteristic bone dysplasias, including lambdoid sutural dysplasia, thinning of long bone cortices and kyphoscoliosis with a high thoracic acute curve. One of the most common is sphenoid wing dysplasia marked by a bone defect which allows herniation of the temporal lobe through the orbit. On plain radiography this produces the 'empty' or 'bare' orbit (Fig. 8-28A). Clinically there may be pulsatile exophthalmos due to transmission of CSF pulsations. The globe may also be affected with proptosis or enlargement.

As well as kyphoscoliosis due to a primary skeletal dysostosis, there may be dural ectasia with vertebral scalloping and lateral meningoceles containing CSF. Scoliosis may be seen in association with an intrinsic spinal cord tumour or peripheral nerve neurofibroma.

Tuberous Sclerosis

Tuberous sclerosis (TS) is a multisystem genetic neurocutaneous syndrome characterised by hamartomas, cortical tubers and benign neoplastic lesions (giant cell astrocytomas), with an incidence of around 1 in 5800 live births. The most frequently affected organs are the skin,

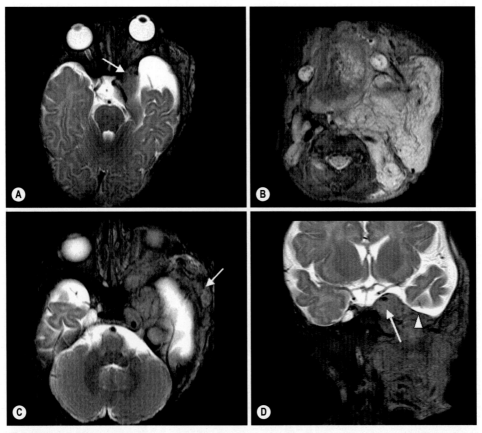

FIGURE 8-28 ■ **Infant with neurofibromatosis type 1.** The diagnosis was made from these images. (A) There is sphenoid wing dysplasia causing expansion of the middle cranial fossa (arrow) and absence of the lateral orbital wall, which causes the 'bare orbit' sign (arrow) on AP plain radiographs. (B) There is an associated extensive plexiform neurofibroma involving the deep and superficial fascial spaces of the neck, tongue and orbit. (C, D) This is almost indistinguishable on imaging from multiple cranial nerve fibromas involving the left cavernous sinus (arrows) and middle cranial fossa. Note the neurofibroma has extended through the foramen ovale and is elevating the dura, seen as a black line (arrowhead).

brain, retina, lungs, heart, skeleton and kidneys, but the few manifestations that are associated with the reduced life expectancy seen in this condition are, in order of highest to lowest frequency, neurological disease (seizures and subependymal giant cell tumour), renal disease (angiomyolipoma and renal cell carcinoma), pulmonary disease (lymphangioleiomyomatosis and bronchopneumonia) and cardiovascular disease (rhabdomyosarcoma and aneurysm). TS is autosomal dominant with a high level of penetrance and variable phenotypic expression; 60–70% of cases are sporadic and two gene mutations have been identified, TSC1 and TSC2, encoding protein products with a tumour suppressor function.

The classical clinical presentation of TS is the triad of intellectual impairment, epilepsy and adenoma sebaceum, but there is a wide phenotypic range. There are a large number of diagnostic primary, secondary and tertiary criteria for TS, some of which are radiological and which categorise TS as 'definite', 'probable' or 'possible'. Radiological primary criteria are the presence of calcified subependymal nodules, while non-calcified subependymal nodules and tubers, cardiac rhabdomyoma and renal angiomyolipoma are secondary criteria.[29,30] In 80% of patients with TS, infantile spasms or myoclonic seizures are the presenting symptom. Conversely, 10% of children with infantile spasms will have evidence of TS, so structural MR neuroimaging is indicated in these children.

Ocular manifestations of TS include retinal hamartomas seen near the optic disc in 15% and are often bilateral and multiple. On CT they appear as nodular masses originating from the retina and when calcified may be difficult to distinguish from retinoblastomas unless there are also calcified subependymal nodules. Subretinal effusions may also be detected. Micro-ophthalmia and leukocoria are other features.

The intracranial manifestations include subependymal hamartomas or nodules (SENs), subependymal giant cell astrocytomas (GCAs), radially oriented linear bands and cortical tubers (Fig. 8-29). SENs are the most common lesion and are seen in 88–95% of individuals with TS. They may be calcified, which is a useful diagnostic feature on CT or T_2^* MRI; calcification increases with age and

is rarely detected under the age of 1 year.[30] Histologically, they are indistinguishable from GCAs. The latter are determined by location in the caudothalamic groove adjacent to the foramen of Monro, progressive growth on serial imaging and the presence of hydrocephalus. Contrast enhancement may be seen in both SENs and GCAs. The lack of myelination in infants helps to identify white matter anomalies, which become less visible as myelination progresses.[31] SENs and linear parenchymal tuberous sclerosis lesions in infants under 3 months old are hyperintense on T_1-weighted images and hypointense on T_2-weighted images as opposed to the reverse pattern of signal intensity in older children and adults.

Sturge–Weber Syndrome

Sturge–Weber syndrome is a congenital syndrome characterised by a port-wine naevus on the face and ipsilateral leptomeningeal angiomas with a primarily parieto-occipital distribution.[32] Bilateral involvement may occasionally occur. The clinical manifestations include the onset of focal seizures, appearing during the first year of life, and developmental delay with progressive hemiparesis, hemianopsia and intellectual impairment. The seizures progressively become refractory to medication.

The leptomeningeal angiomas cause abnormal venous drainage with chronic ischaemia, leading ultimately to cortical atrophy and calcification, the latter feature being usually very prominent. By 2 years of age, skull radiographs may reveal 'tramline calcifications' within the cortices.

In early imaging the brain may look normal on CT as well as on MRI even with intravenous contrast enhancement as the pial angioma may not be conspicuous until after 2 years of life. The involved hemisphere progressively becomes atrophied and the pial angioma is seen as diffuse pial enhancement of variable thickness (Fig. 8-30).[33] The ipsilateral white matter appears hypointense on T_1-weighted images and hyperintense on T_2-weighted images. Other findings include enlargement of the ipsilateral choroid plexus and dilatation of transparenchymal veins that communicate between the superficial and deep cerebral venous systems. In 'burnt out' cases the pial angioma may no longer be detected after contrast enhancement, leaving only a chronically shrunken and calcified hemisphere.

Neurofibromatosis Type 2

This is located to an abnormality on chromosome 22 and occurs in 1 in 50,000 live births. Nearly all have bilateral vestibular schwannomas, other tumours such as meningiomas and other cranial and peripheral nerve schwannomas and ependymomas, including spinal tumours (Fig. 8-31). While in adults hearing loss is a common presentation, seizures and facial nerve palsy are more common in children.

Other Neurocutaneous Syndromes

These include hypomelanosis of Ito in which hypomelanotic skin lesions are associated with polymicrogyria,

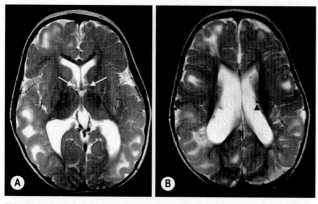

FIGURE 8-29 ■ **Intracranial manifestations of tuberous sclerosis.** (A) Multiple tubers involving the cortex and subcortical white matter. Bilateral lesions are seen at the foramina of Monro, in keeping with giant cell astrocytomas (arrows). (B) Subependymal nodules project into the ventricles, some of which are markedly hypointense, in keeping with calcification (arrowhead).

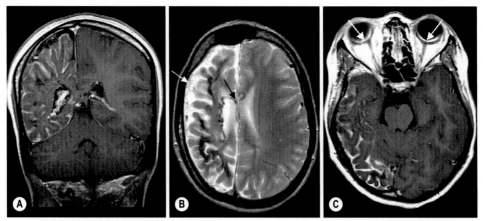

FIGURE 8-30 ■ **Sturge–Weber syndrome.** (A) Coronal T₁ post-contrast image shows an enhancing pial angioma overlying the right cerebral hemisphere which is atrophic. The right choroid plexus is enlarged. Foci of signal hypointensity within the gyri and adjacent white matter are due to calcification. (B) Axial T₂-weighted image shows in addition prominent superficial cortical veins and ependymal veins (arrows). (C) Axial post-contrast T₁-weighted image shows bilateral choroidal angiomas (arrows) in addition to the pial angioma.

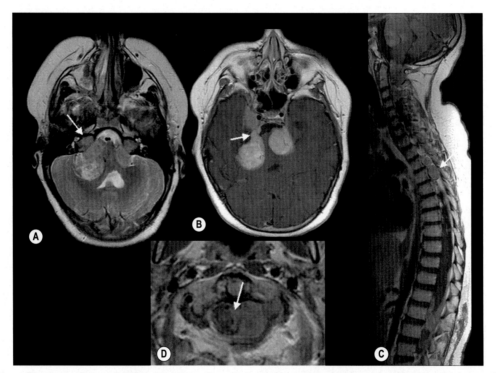

FIGURE 8-31 ■ **Neurofibromatosis type 2 (NF2).** (A) Bilateral cerebellopontine angle masses extending into the internal auditory meati and causing expansion (arrow) in a child with NF2 and bilateral acoustic neuromas. (B) Trigeminal schwannomas extending into the cavernous sinus on the right. The arrow indicates the cisternal segment of the right trigeminal nerve. (C) Sagittal T₁-weighted images show expansion of the neural exit foramina by enhancing nerve or nerve sheath tumours (arrow). (D) Axial image shows a mainly dural mass extending out through the neural foramen with a small intradural component (arrow).

heterotopias and callosal dysgenesis, basal cell naevus syndrome and PHACES (posterior fossa malformations, facial haemangiomas, arterial anomalies, cardiac and eye anomalies and sternal cleft) syndromes. Neurocutaneous melanosis is a rare syndrome in which giant congenital melanocytic naevi on the skin are associated with intracranial melanosis (Fig. 8-32). Neuroimaging detects the clusters of melanocytes by the melanin that they are associated with, therefore appearing as regions of T₁ shortening on MRI in characteristic locations: the anterior and mesial temporal lobe, cerebellum and pons. CT may detect areas of increased density but these are much more difficult to appreciate. Diffuse melanosis with intracranial and intraspinal leptomeningeal spread may occur and therefore hydrocephalus. Degeneration into malignant melanoma is rare.

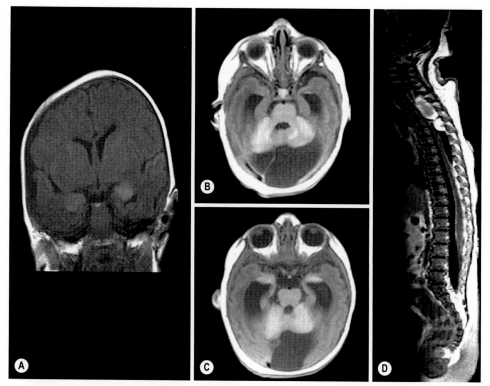

FIGURE 8-32 ■ **Child with giant pigmented naevus and neurocutaneous melanosis.** (A) Initial coronal T₁-weighted MRI shows the typical regions of T₁ shortening within the amygdalae of the mesial temporal lobes. (B, C) Axial T₁-weighted MRI obtained 2 years later shows hydrocephalus in addition to the regions of melanin deposition within the mesial temporal lobes and cerebellum. These do not show any enhancement. There is a posterior fossa arachnoid cyst, a described association. (D) Within the spine there is diffuse pial enhancement over the spinal cord in addition to focal haemorrhagic and partly enhancing extramedullary lesions, indicating malignant melanoma, which was subsequently confirmed histologically.

SPINAL MALFORMATIONS

Normal Development

The spinal cord forms during three embryological stages known as gastrulation (at 2–3 weeks of gestation), primary neurulation (3–4 weeks) and secondary neurulation (5–6 weeks). During gastrulation the embryonic bilaminar disc consisting of epiblast and hypoblast is converted to a trilaminar disc by migration of cells from the epiblast through Hensen's node, a focal region of thickening occurring at the cranial end of the midline 'primitive streak' of the disc. This results in the midline notochord and a layer that will form the future mesoderm. During primary neurulation the notochord induces the overlying ectoderm to become neurectoderm and form the neural plate. Subsequent folding and bending occurs until the margins unite to form the neural tube. The cranial end closes at day 25, while the caudal end closes a couple of days later. Finally the caudal cell mass arises from the primitive streak and undergoes retrogressive differentiation with cavitation. This is the origin of the foetal neural tissue and vertebrae distal to S2, and will become the conus medullaris. A focal expansion of the fetal canal known as the terminal ventricle occurs as a result of incomplete retrogressive differentiation. This may be seen as a normal asymptomatic finding in young children and may persist in a small minority into adulthood. It is seen on all post-mortem studies but is bigger in those

detectable on MRI. Spinal dysraphisms can result from abnormalities occurring during any of these periods.[34–36]

Definitions

Spinal dysraphisms may be open, in which case nervous tissue is exposed, or closed, in which case the defect is covered by skin, although a cutaneous lesion such as a dimple, sinus, hairy naevus or haemangioma may be seen as a marker of an underlying defect in 50% of these cases.[35,36] Spina bifida refers to the failure of fusion of the posterior spinal bony elements. The neural placode is a flat segment of un-neurulated nervous tissue that may be seen at the end of the spinal cord or at an intermediate position along its course.

The normal level of the spinal cord termination has a normal or Gaussian distribution. It is a popular misconception that the spinal cord lies lower in the neonate and continues to rise as the vertebral column grows during childhood. In fact most authors agree that it has already reached its adult position by term, and in 98% lies above L2/3, the majority lying between T11/12 and L1/2.[37,38] The spinal cord termination should be considered unequivocally abnormal if seen at or below L3. Tethered cord syndrome is a clinical diagnosis of progressive neurological deterioration (usually leg weakness, deformities such as scoliosis or foot abnormalities, loss of bladder and bowel function), presumed to be due to traction damage on the tethered cord. Although there may be some suggestive features such as a low positioned conus and associated spinal cord syrinx, this is not a diagnosis made radiologically; and the position of the conus or neural placode following successful surgical 'untethering' typically remains unchanged.

Open Spinal Dysraphism

Most open spinal dysraphisms (OSDs) are myelomeningoceles and these are virtually always associated with Chiari II malformation The neural placode protrudes beyond the level of the skin and there is an expanded CSF-containing sac lined by meninges.[35,36] A small proportion of OSDs are myeloceles where the placode is flush with the surface and there is no meningocele component. Both disorders result from defective closure of the primary neural tube and persistence of un-neurulated nervous tissue in the form of the neural placode, usually at the lumbosacral level at the spinal cord termination. Nerve roots arising from the everted ventral surface of the placode cross the widely dilated subarachnoid spaces of the meningocele to enter the neural exit foraminae. The posterior elements of the vertebral column and any other mesenchymal derivatives, such as the paravertebral muscles, remain everted. Hemimyelomeningoceles and hemimyeloceles may occur with diastematomyelia (split cord syndrome) and may be associated with an asymmetric skin abnormality and clinical presentation. These can be hypothesised to occur as the result of an embryological failure of primary neurulation of one hemicord in addition to a gastrulation abnormality.

Myelomeningoceles are operated on soon after birth; if untreated, the exposed neural tissue is prone to ulceration and infection. In some centres, in utero repair has been correlated with subsequent failure to develop the typical hindbrain malformation of Chiari II, although other abnormalities such as the enlarged massa intermedia and falx fenestration persist. The advocates of this technique suggest that hydrocephalus and the need for surgical drainage may also be delayed and even reduced in these children Hydrocephalus usually develops 2–3 days post-neonatal repair of the myelomeningocele but may occur preoperatively. Other causes of postoperative deterioration include re-tethering of the spinal cord and the development of a syrinx, which may, later, be associated with scoliosis.[39] The Chiari II malformation is described in more detail with brain malformations in the 'Disorders of Dorsal Induction' section.

Closed Spinal Dysraphism

Closed spinal dysraphisms (CSDs) are often associated with midline cutaneous stigmata or a mass.[40,41] This may be a subcutaneous lipomatous mass overlying the spinal defect, as in lipomyeloceles and lipomyelomeningoceles. In these conditions there is an intraspinal lipoma. In a lipomyelocele the junction between the placode and the lipoma lies within the spinal canal (Fig. 8-33), while in lipomyelomeningoceles it lies outside. Typically the placode is rotated to one side while the lipoma rotates on the other. McClone's hypothesis is that during primary neurulation there is premature disjunction of the cutaneous ectoderm from the adjacent neuroectoderm, allowing mesenchymal elements to come into contact with the open neural tube and then differentiate into fat. These lipomas may be dorsal, with a normal conus below, or transitional where the lipoma extends caudally along the conus. In both these situations the lipoma–placode junction is dorsal, well-defined and complete removal of the lipoma at surgery is feasible. A third form exists, known

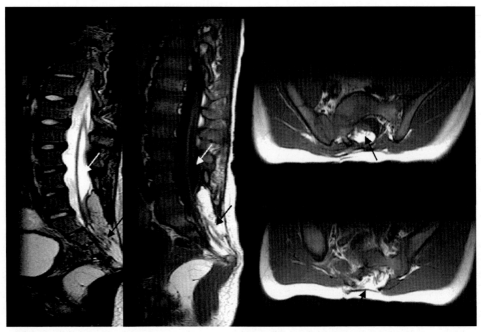

FIGURE 8-33 ■ **Closed spinal dysraphism.** The spinal cord is too low and the neural placode terminates at the lumbosacral junction in a lipomyelocele (black arrows). There is an associated spinal cord syringomyelic cavity (white arrows). The posterior elements are deficient and everted.

as 'chaotic' where the lipoma extends ventrally around the neural placode and the lipoma is much more difficult to resect.[42] These are less common conditions but are more commonly seen with sacral agenesis. It is harder to explain these by the premature disjunction theory, given the ventral fat, and it may be that these are disorders of caudal cell mass development. The terminal lipoma and filum terminale lipoma are also considered to arise from a disturbance of caudal regression. Other examples of these are described in a separate section below.

A posterior meningocele consists of herniation of a CSF sac lined by dura and arachnoid through a posterior spinal defect, resulting in a clinically apparent mass covered by skin. These are mainly lumbosacral but may be seen at any level. Anterior meningoceles are typically presacral, are seen with caudal agenesis and are present in older children and adults with low back pain and bladder/bowel disturbance. The terminal myelocystocele is a rare condition associated with syndromes such as VACTERL in which the central canal is dilated by a hydromyelic cavity that herniates into a posterior meningocele through the posterior spinal bony defect. Sometimes it can be difficult to see the communication with the central canal of the spinal cord which is the key finding of the terminal cystocele cavity. The cystocele cavity is seen at the most caudal aspect of the spinal canal, with a myelomeningocele seen ventrally and posteriorly around the neural placode, giving rise on MRI to two fluid-filled sacs (Fig. 8-34).

CSDs without a mass include simple intramedullary and intradural lipomas. These typically occur along the posterior midline in a subpial juxtamedullary location at the cervicothoracic level. Embryologically they are also the result of premature disjunction and the lipoma fills in the gap between the unopposed folds of the neural placode. On MRI they have the signal characteristics of fat, including signal suppression on STIR sequences.

Fatty change within the filum terminale is detected on MRI, and may be more easily seen on axial T_1-weighted sequences extending caudally from the conus. This is estimated to occur in 1.5–5% of the normal adult population and may be considered a normal variant in the absence of the clinical tethered cord syndrome. The 'tight' filum terminale, also due to abnormal retrogressive differentiation, is a short, thick filum greater than 2 mm in diameter associated with clinical tethering and a low-lying spinal cord.

Dorsal Dermal Sinus

A dermal sinus is an epithelial-lined opening on the skin with variable fistulous extension to the dural surface, typically seen in the lumbosacral region and often associated with cutaneous stigmata, such as hairy naevus and capillary haemangioma.[40,41] Embryologically it arises from a failure of disjunction of neuroectoderm from cutaneous ectoderm. Dermal openings seen at the sacrococcygeal level are directed inferiorly below the thecal sac and are known as sacrococcygeal pits. They do not require further imaging unless there are neurological features to suggest additional spinal dysraphism, as there should be no risk of CNS infection in the absence of a

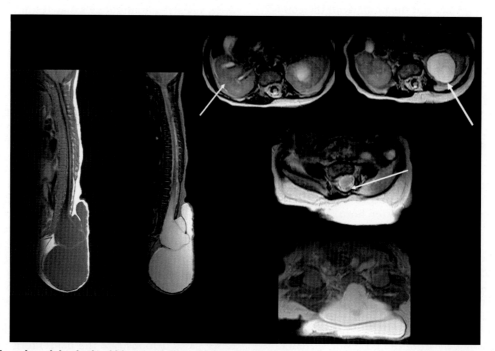

FIGURE 8-34 ■ **There is a right duplex kidney and dilated left pelvicalyceal system (axial top images).** The termination of the spinal cord is very low and the neural placode is seen at the sacrum. The distal bony lumbosacral spine is deficient. The placode splits in two, forming a disastemyelia (middle axial image) and two cystic structures are identified. At surgery there was an inner sac (myelomeningocele) with nerve roots seen within it and an outer sac (the cystocele cavity), into which the neural placode opened.

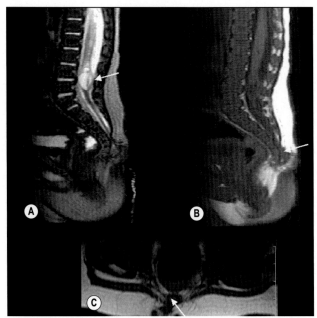

FIGURE 8-35 ■ **Dorsal dermal sinus.** (A) The termination of the spinal cord is very low and there is a syringomyelic cavity with internal septations. In addition there is a more focal cyst within the conus confirmed at surgical untethering to be a dermoid cyst (arrow). (B, C) There is an associated dermal sinus track (arrows).

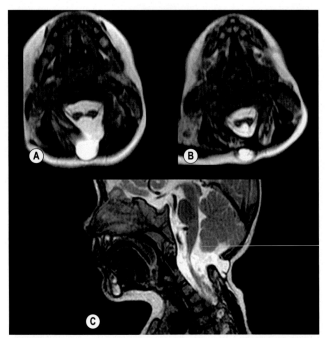

FIGURE 8-36 ■ **Cervical spinal cord diastematomyelia type II with associated craniocervical meningocele.** (A) Sagittal T₂-weighted MRI appears to show signal abnormality and thinning of the spinal cord, and is the clue to the diastematomyelia seen on the axial images. (B, C) Axial T₂-weighted MRI shows that the cord has split into two hemicords. The apparent signal abnormality is in fact normal cerebrospinal fluid interspersed between the two hemicords. These reunite inferiorly. The meningocele is seen herniating through a bony defect in the vertebral posterior elements.

connection with the thecal sac. Those seen above the natal cleft have a more cranial direction and may form a fistulous connection with the dural sac and warrant further investigation as they may need to be resected to prevent future CNS infection. Ultrasound (US) may provide useful information about the intradural extension of the dermal sinus tract and the mobility of the conus.[43] MRI is more sensitive for additional intraspinal findings such as spinal cord syrinx and intraspinal dermoid. On MRI the dermal sinus is seen as a thin linear strip of tissue hypointense to adjacent fat but MRI is not particularly reliable for determining whether there is continuity with the thecal sac and surgical exploration may be required (Fig. 8-35).

Diastematomyelia

The split notochord syndromes are disorders of notochord midline integration. In diastematomyelia the spinal cord is split in two, with each hemicord having one anterior and one posterior grey matter horn.[44,45] In type I diastematomyelia there are two complete dural sacs. There is a craniocaudal gradient of division, ranging from partial clefting cranially to two complete dural sacs separated by an osteocartilaginous spur inferiorly. There may be plain radiographic features, including scoliosis or hemivertebrae or bifid/fused vertebrae at the level of the bony spur. The bony spur in type I diastematomyelia is completely extradural, usually midline, though it may be seen coursing obliquely from the posterior vertebrae to the laminae, and may be complete or incomplete. It is seen at the caudal end of the split and the hemicords fuse tightly just below it. On MRI marrow signal may be

detected within it and this distinguishes it from a simple fibrous band. Above it the split is much longer. In rare cases, the separate dural sacs may terminate distally with different fates, one as an OSD and the other as a CSD. In diastematomyelia type II (Fig. 8-36) there is a single dural sac in which the two hemicords lie, and a fibrous septum, seen as a band of hypointensity, may be seen passing intradurally between the two hemicords. There may be no septum or there may only be partial clefting of the cord. The conus is often low and there may be a tight or fatty filum. Both forms of diastematomyelia may be associated with hydromyelia within the spinal cord.

Neurenteric Cysts

The severest and rarest form of notochordal midline integration anomaly occurs with dorsal enteric fistulas and neurenteric cysts.[46] The cysts are usually seen intradurally anterior to the spinal cord and are derived from endodermal remnants trapped between a split notochord. They have signal characteristics of CSF or of proteinaceous fluid with T shortening (Fig. 8-37). The commoner variants of these involve cysts that extend through a ventral bony defect through abnormally formed vertebral bodies, called the canal of Kovalevsky (Fig. 8-38). Rarer cases demonstrate the neurenteric cyst extending between a split cord malformation. It is possible for such a fistula to connect the dorsal skin with bowel across duplicated spinal elements.

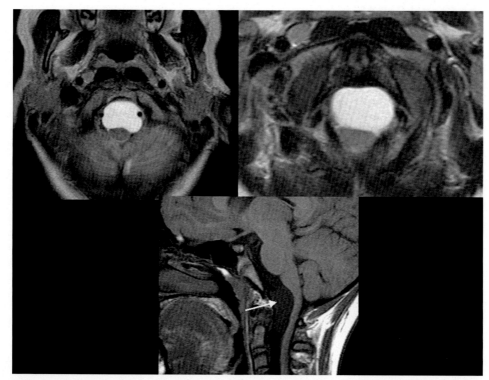

FIGURE 8-37 ■ **Neurenteric cyst ventral to the medulla and upper cervical spinal cord, displacing them posteriorly, and with the vertebral arteries displaced around it.** The cyst is hyperintense on the T_2-weighted images and there is also some mild T_1 shortening (arrow).

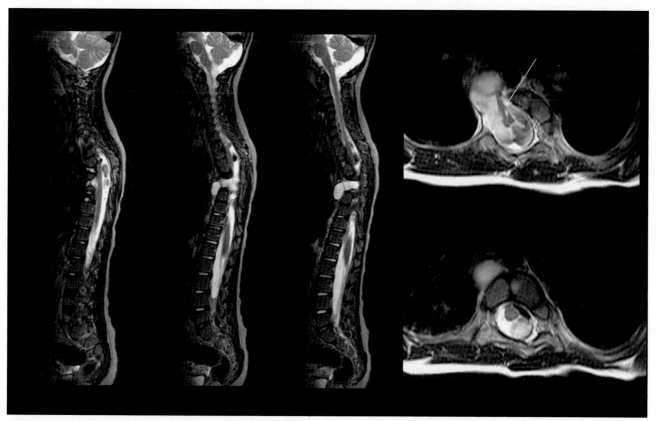

FIGURE 8-38 ■ **Sagittal and axial T2W images show ventral herniation of a sac through a thoracic bony defect (the canal of Kovalevsky) at the level of a verterbal segmentation anomaly.** The spinal cord appears stretched and a ventral component extends into the sac (arrow). There is a small syrinx cavity within it.

Disorders of the Caudal Cell Mass/ Caudal Regression Syndrome

The last group of developmental spinal abnormalities affects development of the caudal cell mass.[47] Caudal agenesis and the rarer condition of segmental spinal dysgenesis are considered to occur as a result of apoptosis of notochordal cells which have not formed in their correct craniocaudal position. In caudal agenesis there is a severe abnormality which results in absence of the vertebral column at the affected level, as well as a truncated spinal cord, imperforate anus and genital anomalies. It may be seen with OEIS (omphalocele, exstrophy, imperforate anus, spinal defects), VACTERL and the Currarino triad in which there is partial sacral agenesis (or sometimes a 'scimitar'-shaped sacrum), anorectal malformation and a presacral mass which may be a teratoma or anterior meningocele[48–50] (Fig. 8-39). In type I caudal agenesis, which affects secondary neurulation and formation of the caudal cell mass, there is a high (often at T12) abrupt spinal cord termination with a characteristic wedge-shaped configuration and variable coccygeal to lower

thoracic vertebral aplasia (Fig. 8-40). Clinically the neurological deficit due to absence of the distal spinal cord is stable. In type II caudal agenesis the true notochord is not affected and only the caudal cell mass is involved. The vertebral aplasia is less extensive, with up to S4 present as the last vertebra. It may be difficult to detect partial agenesis of the conus because it is stretched and tethered to a fatty filum terminale, lipoma, lipomyelomeningocele, or anterior sacral meningocele.

Segmental Spinal Dysgenesis

These represent a segmental abnormality affecting the spinal cord, segmental nerve roots and vertebrae, and are associated with a congenital paraparesis and lower limb deformities. A short segment of the spinal column is deficient and the spinal canal may be obliterated. On imaging there may be an acute angle kyphus, and the spine and spinal cord in the most severe cases may appear 'severed', but with functioning spinal cord neural tissue anatomically present above and below the affected segment. In less severe cases the cord is focally

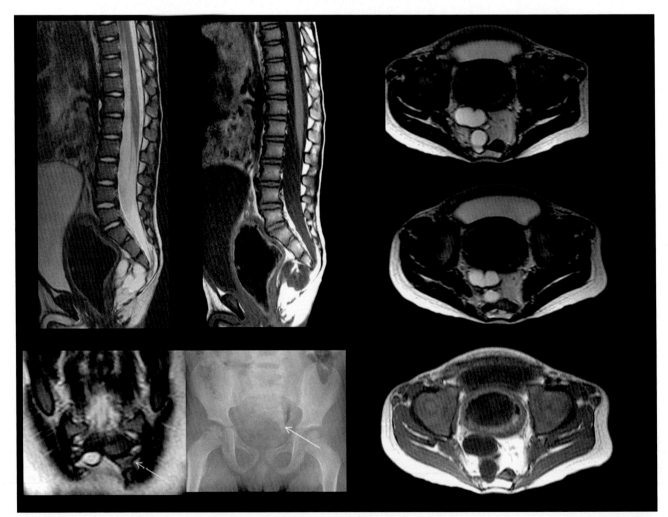

FIGURE 8-39 ■ **There is a presacral cystic lesion in continuity with the thecal sac at the level of the sacrum.** A small solid component is seen in keeping with a benign teratoma with associated meningocele. The conus is seen at the L2/3 level and the spinal cord was untethered at surgery. The left side of the sacrum has a scimitar configuration, with the meningocele seen on the right. These are the features of the Currarino triad.

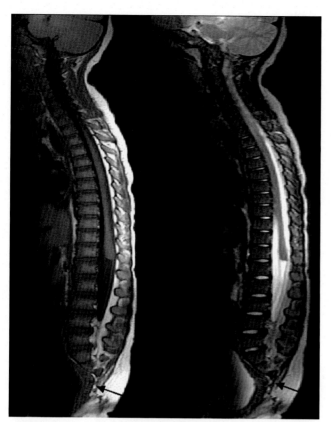

FIGURE 8-40 ■ **Caudal regression syndrome.** The spinal cord is truncated with a typical blunt edge seen at the inferior margin of T12. The thecal sac terminates at the superior margin of L4. The sacrum distal to S2 is agenetic (arrows).

hypoplastic. These anomalies may be a result of a post-neurulation insult.

INBORN METABOLIC BRAIN DISORDERS

Metabolic disorders may be inborn or acquired. Inborn errors of metabolism may result from an enzyme deficiency leading to the build-up of a directly toxic metabolite, or have an indirect toxic effect by activation or inhibition of another metabolic pathway, leading to increased levels of a different toxic metabolite.

The inborn errors of metabolism may be subdivided according to a number of different classification systems, one of which is radiological. One system classifies them by cellular organelle involvement into mitochondrial (usually meaning disorders of mitochondrial energy metabolism), lysosomal and peroxisomal disorders. Another scheme classifies them by the biochemical enzyme pathway affected, e.g. the organic acidaemias, aminoacidopathies or disorders of heavy metal metabolism. In the radiological approach, neuroimaging can be used to help classify them according to white or grey matter involvement, by anatomical distribution of disease, contrast enhancement and other radiological features, mostly by MRI characteristics. Interested readers can also

refer to Van der Knaap and Valk[51] and Patay.[52] With each of these methods, advances in molecular genetics and genetic classifications are leading to a deeper understanding of specific gene defects in the manifestation of disease.

There are some general principles that may be helpful in detecting and characterising the radiological features. The abnormalities of metabolic disease are characteristically bilateral and symmetrical. Assessment on MRI should include analysis of the selective involvement and/or sparing of deep grey, cortical grey and white matter structures. When describing white matter abnormalities it is helpful to describe them in terms of general location (lobar involvement, centripetal/centrifugal distribution and AP gradient), juxtacortical U-fibre involvement, involvement of deep white matter structures such as the internal capsule, corpus callosum and white matter tracts such as the pyramidal tracts as they descend from the motor strip (pre-central gyrus) through the posterior limbs of the internal capsules and cerebral peduncles to the decussation within the medulla and then into the spinal cord.

Assessment of the grey matter should include analysis of the cerebral and cerebellar cortex and basal ganglia and thalami for signal abnormality, swelling and volume loss. Signal changes include T_2 and T_1 prolongation, but faint T_1 shortening within the basal ganglia may be seen also when there is calcification. Other deep grey matter structures include the red nuclei, and subthalamic and dentate nuclei. Calcification is much better assessed on CT. Macrocephaly is a useful clinical pointer to diseases such as megalencephalic leukodystrophy with subcortical cysts (MLC), Canavan's and Alexander's leukoencephalopathies, glutaric aciduria type I, GM2 gangliosidosis and L-2-hydroxyglutaric aciduria.

An assessment of the degree of myelination is useful as delay or hypomyelination is frequently seen in metabolic disorders. Although often non-specific, it is a helpful clue to an underlying neurometabolic condition. Myelination requires active energy-dependent metabolism and therefore may also be seen with cardiorespiratory illness. However, hypomyelination may also be seen as a general marker of developmental delay and correlates well with clinical developmental milestones. In premature infants the appropriate MRI markers for corrected age should be assessed before deciding that myelination is immature. There are also specific inherited hypomyelination disorders that may be detected on MRI as a myelination pattern which is immature for the child's age. These include Pelizaeus–Merzbacher disease, in which T_2-weighted imaging often shows more severe hypomyelination compared to T_1-weighted imaging (Fig. 8-41).

Serial imaging should be assessed for progressive cerebral atrophy. This may involve white matter, shown as ventricular enlargement and thinning of the corpus callosum, cortical grey matter, shown as sulcal widening, or deep grey matter with atrophy of the specific basal ganglia and thalamic structures.

Pathognomonic imaging patterns are seen in X-linked adrenoleukodystrophy (ALD), Alexander's disease, glutaric aciduria type I, Canavan's disease, L-2-hydroxyglutaricaciduria, neonatal maple syrup urine disease and MLCs.

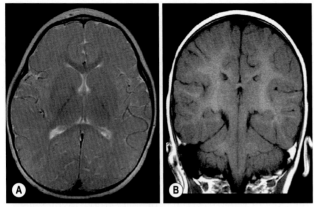

FIGURE 8-41 ■ **Pelizaeus–Merzbacher disease in a 2-year-old child with nystagmus and developmental delay.** (A) Axial T$_2$-weighted image shows dark regions of myelination in the posterior limbs of the internal capsules, splenium and genu of the corpus callosum, and within the parieto-occipital lobe white matter. The rest of the cerebral hemispheres are not myelinated (the white matter is too bright). This pattern is severely delayed and equivalent approximately to an age of 6 months. (B) Paradoxically coronal T$_1$-weighted MRI shows much more advanced myelination, which appears virtually complete, with T$_1$ shortening extending right out into the subcortical white matter.

Classic X-linked adrenoleukodystrophy is the most common leukodystrophy of children and affects 1 in 20,000 boys. It is due to a defect in a peroxisomal membrane protein leading to defective incorporation of fatty acids into myelin. Screening of family members of affected cases for the specific gene defect should be considered. Clinically, boys present between the ages of 5 and 10 years with learning difficulties, behavioural problems, deteriorating gait and impaired visuospatial perception. Adrenal insufficiency may precede the CNS presentation or may be absent. Without bone marrow transplantation (which replaces the defective gene), the disease progresses to spastic paraparesis, blindness and deafness. Lorenzo's oil may also delay disease progression. Imaging features are of low attenuation on CT and hyperintensity on T2W images in the posterior central white matter, specifically the splenium and peritrigonal white matter progressing to the corticospinal tracts and visual and auditory pathways. The regions of T$_2$ signal abnormality show increased diffusion. The leading edge of the demyelination enhances where there is active inflammation and disruption of the blood–brain barrier (Fig. 8-42). MR spectroscopy may detect early changes

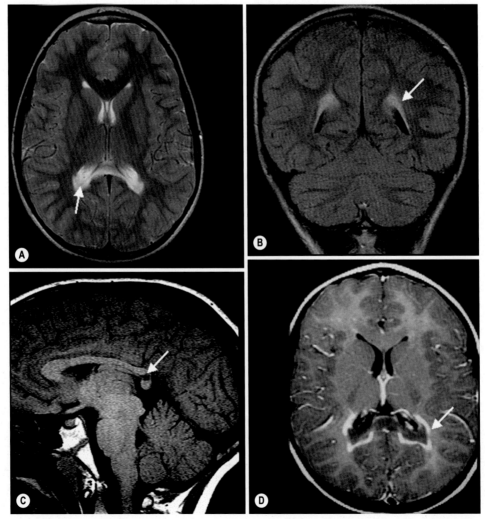

FIGURE 8-42 ■ **Adrenoleukodystrophy.** MRI of a 6-year-old boy with increasing gait disturbance and impaired vision demonstrates peritrigonal and splenial signal abnormality (increased signal on T$_2$-weighted images and low signal on T$_1$-weighted images), and (A–C, arrows) marginal enhancement at the leading edges where there is active inflammation, typical of adrenoleukodystrophy (D, arrow).

and may, in the future, guide early bone marrow transplantation before overt and irreversible changes in the white matter have occurred. Adrenomyeloneuropathy is a variation on ALD which presents in young adults or adolescents, usually boys, with progressive paraparesis and cerebellar signs. It has a less specific radiological pattern causing diffuse disease of the white matter, and it more commonly involves the cerebellum and less frequently the cerebral hemispheres.

In **Alexander's disease**, which has a neonatal, juvenile and adult form, imaging shows extensive white matter abnormality beginning in the frontal and periventricular white matter (Fig. 8-43). Large cystic cavities are seen within the frontal and temporal regions. The basal ganglia may also be involved. Contrast enhancement or garland appearance may be seen along the ventricular ependyma. Less typical forms can show symmetrical or nodular lesions in the brainstem (Fig. 8-44).

L-2-Hydroxyglutaricaciduria is a slowly progressive disorder which is usually discovered in childhood or early adulthood, although it is likely to have started earlier than this. The clinical presentation is non-specific with learning difficulties, epilepsy and pyramidal and cerebellar signs. The MRI findings show white matter involvement with peripheral involvement, particularly of the subcortical U fibres, internal, external and extreme capsules, sparing of the periventricular white matter and corpus callosum, and with a slight frontal predominance. There is macrocephaly. There is also grey matter involvement affecting the basal ganglia, especially the globus pallidi, and sparing the thalami (Fig. 8-45).

Maple syrup urine disease (MSUD) is an autosomal recessive disorder presenting in the neonate in which an enzyme deficiency leads to an accumulation of amino acids (leucine, isoleucine and valine) and their metabolites. A characteristic feature at acute presentation is marked swelling and oedema of the white matter tracts and brainstem often best appreciated in the corticospinal tracts as they course through the internal capsules (Fig. 8-46).

Megalencephaly with leukoencephalopathy and cysts (MLC) is a recently identified autosomal recessive

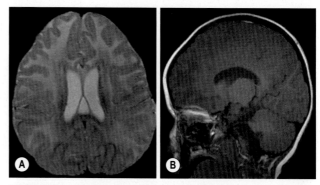

FIGURE 8-43 ■ **Child with Alexander's disease.** Head circumference charts showed the child had macrocephaly. (A) Axial T$_2$-weighted MRI shows extensive bilateral symmetrical deep and subcortical white matter signal hyperintensity with a frontal predominance and mild swelling. (B) Sagittal T$_1$-weighted MRI shows corresponding low signal in the affected areas without evidence of cavitation but in keeping with oedema.

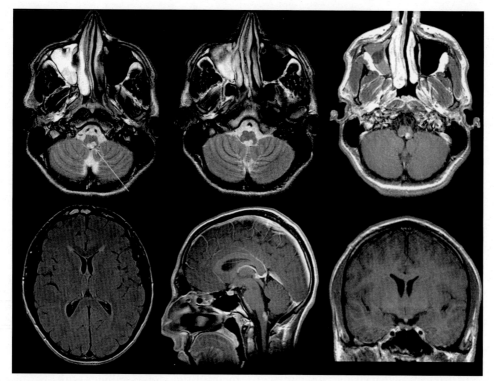

FIGURE 8-44 ■ **A 15-year-old with a 3-year history of progressively worsening nausea, vomiting and hiccups, triggered by exercise.** The MRI images show asymmetrical enhancing nodular lesions in the dorsal medulla and pituitary infundibulum. Very subtle periventricular white matter changes were seen. A de novo GFAP mutation for Alexander's disease was confirmed.

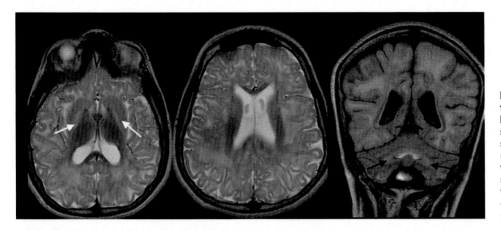

FIGURE 8-45 ■ L-2-Hydroxyglu-taricaciduria axial T₂-weighted MRI. Coronal FLAIR images show extensive white matter signal hyperintensity involving mainly deep and subcortical white matter but with relative sparing of the periventricular white matter, and bilateral palli-dal involvement. The dentate nuclei are also abnormal.

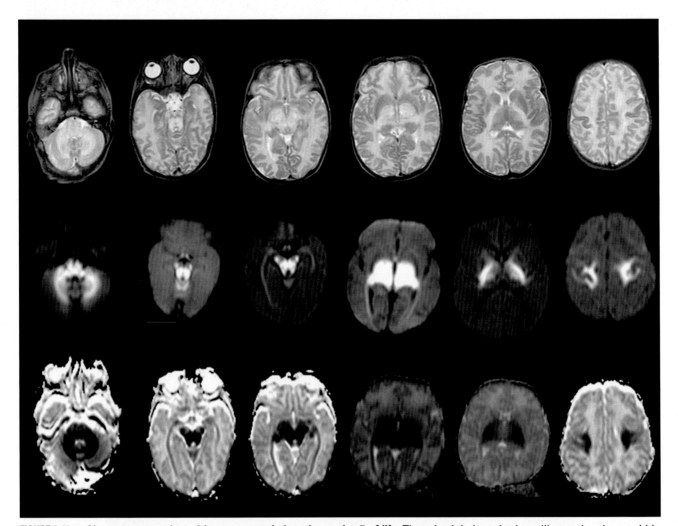

FIGURE 8-46 ■ **Neonate presenting with acute encephalopathy on day 5 of life.** There is global cerebral swelling and oedema within the white matter. There is also oedema and swelling with restricted diffusion (bright on diffusion-weighted images and dark on ADC maps) within the basal ganglia, thalami, internal capsules and perirolandic cortex/white matter along the course of the corticospinal tracts as well as the midbrain, pons and both cerebellar hemispheres.

leukodystrophy with macrocephaly. A characteristic feature is the relatively mild clinical course despite very abnormal findings of extensive signal change and rarefac-tion of white matter, particularly in the parietal and ante-rior temporal lobe regions.

Suggestive MRI patterns include methylmalonicaci-daemia in which there is bilateral symmetrical involve-ment of the globus pallidus with sparing of the thalami and the rest of the basal ganglia (Fig. 8-47). The cerebral cortex is also normal. In the acute stage there is swelling

CRANIOSYNOSTOSIS **251**

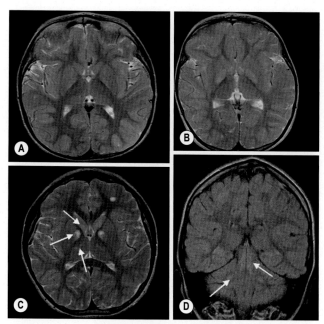

FIGURE 8-47 ■ **Examples of signal abnormality affecting both globus pallidi.** (A) Kernicterus. (B) Methylmalonicacidaemia. (C) Kearns–Sayre syndrome. This child also has hyperintense signal in both caudate nuclei and thalami, left frontal white matter and (D) dorsal midbrain and cerebellar dentate nuclei (arrows).

and oedema of these structures, while in the chronic phase there is imaging evidence of atrophy and gliosis. Bilateral pallidal involvement is also seen in other rarer inborn errors of metabolism, such as GAMT (guanidinoacetate methyltransferase deficiency), Kearns–Sayre syndrome and some acquired and toxic disorders, such as kernicterus and carbon monoxide poisoning (Fig. 8-47).

Disorders of heavy metal metabolism include Wilson's and Menkes' diseases, both disorders of copper metabolism, molybdenum cofactor deficiency and disorders of magnesium and manganese metabolism. **Wilson's disease** results from defective extracellular copper transport and leads to multiorgan copper deposition. Hyperintensities on T_2-weighted MRI are seen in the basal ganglia, midbrain and pons, thalami and claustra, and there is T_1 shortening in the basal ganglia and thalami, as in other hepatic encephalopathies. **Menkes' disease** is X-linked and affects transcellular copper metabolism at the level of the cell membrane. There is a systemic failure of copper-requiring enzymes, particularly those of the cytochrome-c oxidase system. Affected children have connective tissue defects with 'kinky hair', inguinal herniae, hyperflexible joints and bladder diverticula. In the brain there is progressive cerebral atrophy, which may allow subdural collections of CSF or subdural haematomas (and therefore this is a mimic of non-accidental head injury). The basal ganglia may also show T_1 shortening. Children develop a severe cerebral vasculopathy in which vessels are tortuous and prone to dissection.

Another cause of neonatal encephalopathy is **molybdenum cofactor deficiency** in which acutely there is global cerebral swelling and oedema with many features similar to the brain infarction seen in hypoxic-ischaemic injury, but in addition focal symmetrical, selective changes

within the globus pallidi and subthalamic nuclei (mocod paper).

Disorders of cellular organelle function include mitochondrial, lysosomal and peroxisomal disorders. Mitochondria are involved in energy metabolism; lysosomes in the degradation of macromolecules, e.g. those involved in the maintenance of cell membrane integrity such as lipids and lipoproteins; and peroxisomes have a role in both catabolic and anabolic metabolism. Mitochondrial disorders include those of mitochondrial energy metabolism affecting oxidative phosphorylation, fatty acid oxidation and ketone metabolism. Respiratory chain disorders affect the respiratory chain, an enzyme pathway mostly located on complex proteins on the inner membrane of the mitochondria. This has an integral role in oxidative phosphorylation and these disorders tend to be multisystem or organ diseases. In the brain they may result in multiple cerebral infarcts in non-vascular territories.

Leigh's disease is not one single entity and can be caused not only by respiratory chain defects but also by enzyme disorders such as those of pyruvate and tricarboxylic acid metabolism. It is characterised by a typical radiological pattern. Bilateral, typically symmetrical, signal change is seen within the brainstem, deep cerebellar grey matter, subthalamic nuclei and basal ganglia (Fig. 8-48). The midbrain changes have been described as a 'panda face' with involvement of the substantia nigra and tegmentum, and the medulla is frequently involved and may account for the apnoeic episodes often seen clinically. Cerebral grey matter infarction may also be seen. MELAS (mitochondrial encephalomyopathy with lactic acidosis and stroke-like episodes) is another mitochondrial disease, typically occurring between the ages of 4 and 15 years but which can occur at any age. Acute metabolic decompensation may be provoked by any insult which causes increased metabolic demand, e.g. febrile illness. Patients may also have a cardiomyopathy and endocrinopathies. Imaging features are those of cerebral infarcts in non-vascular territories and symmetrical basal ganglia calcification.

Lysosomal disorders include Krabbe's disease and metachromatic leukodystrophy. Imaging features which might suggest Krabbe's disease are white matter changes, more severely posteriorly and centrally; basal ganglia and thalamic involvement, specifically dark signal in the thalami on T2W images; cerebellar white matter abnormality, sparing the dentate nuclei; and involvement of the pyramidal tracts within the brainstem. Peroxisomal disorders include Zellweger's syndrome and X-linked ALD. Imaging features of Zellweger's syndrome include severely delayed myelination, periventricular germinolytic cysts, peri-Sylvian polymicrogyria and grey matter heterotopias. When this combination is seen in the clinical context of severe hypotonia with visual and hearing deficits, seizures, hepatomegaly and jaundice, the pattern may be considered pathognomonic.

CRANIOSYNOSTOSIS[53]

Craniosynostosis is a disorder of growth, one of the manifestations of which is premature closure of one or more

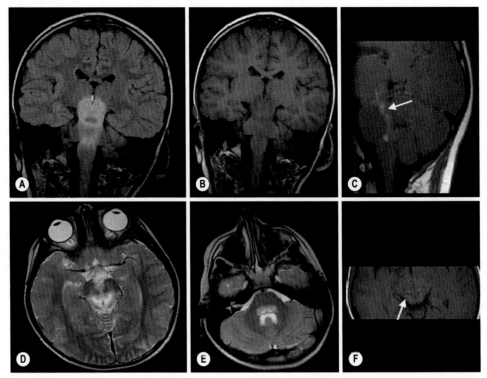

FIGURE 8-48 ■ **Leigh's disease.** There is bilateral symmetrical signal hyperintensity on the coronal FLAIR (A) and axial T_2 images (D, E) matched by hypointensity on the coronal T_1-weighted MRI (B) affecting the midbrain, pons and medulla. Symmetrical contrast enhancement (C, F) indicates breakdown of the blood–brain barrier in keeping with active disease.

calvarial or skull base sutures. The three broad categories of craniosynostosis are the simple non-syndromic type, usually involving one suture; complex syndromic forms involving many sutures; and secondary craniosynostosis due to disrupted growth caused by a wide range of insults such as drugs and metabolic bone disease or secondary to an underlying small brain, as in chronic, treated hydrocephalus or any other cause of microcephaly. The most common type of primary craniosynostosis is simple sagittal synostosis.

The diagnosis is made initially by clinical assessment of the skull shape. Imaging provides confirmatory evidence and information regarding the skull base and orbits, and is important in the assessment of intracranial complications of craniosynostosis, such as hydrocephalus and visual failure. Standard radiographs will allow assessment of the coronal, sagittal, lambdoid and metopic sutures on the AP view; lambdoid and sagittal sutures on the Towne's view; and coronal and lambdoid sutures on the lateral view in addition to assessment of the skull shape, foramen magnum and fontanelles. The affected suture may be absent, indistinct, show bridging sclerosis or a heaped-up or beaked appearance, but also may appear normal if the synostosis is fibrotic not bony. Skull growth decreases perpendicular to the suture and increases parallel to it. Therefore, greater weight is given to the skull shape than the radiological evidence of direct sutural involvement on plain film or CT. Conversely, if the sutures are not clearly visualised but the skull shape is normal, then primary craniosynostosis is unlikely.

Sagittal synostosis produces an elongated head shape called scaphocephaly (Fig. 8-49). Bicoronal synostosis

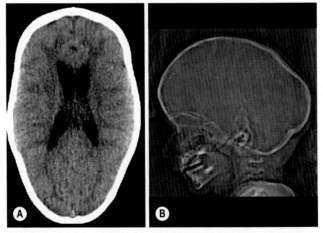

FIGURE 8-49 ■ **Sagittal synostosis.** (A) Brain CT and (B) lateral scout view showing the typical 'boat-shaped' skull or scaphocephaly of sagittal synostosis.

causes brachycephaly or foreshortening in the AP direction, which is accompanied by lateral elevation of the sphenoid wings producing the characteristic 'harlequin' deformity, upward slanting of the petrous apices and hypertelorism. Unicoronal synostosis causes anterior plagiocephaly or asymmetrical skull deformity and may be associated with compensatory growth on the unaffected side, resulting in frontoparietal bossing (Fig. 8-50). Metopic synostosis causes trigonocephaly or 'keel deformity' and an AP view may show parallel, vertically oriented medial orbital walls. True unilateral lambdoid

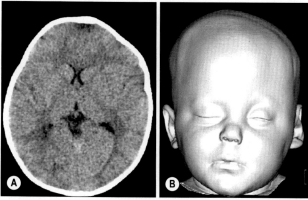

FIGURE 8-50 ■ **Unicoronal synostosis.** (A) Axial CT and (B) 3D surface-shaded reformat show the asymmetrical head shape of left frontal plagiocephaly due to unicoronal craniosynostosis, with bossing seen on the right side.

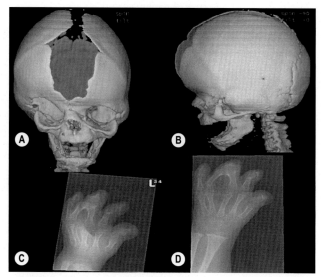

FIGURE 8-51 ■ **Apert's syndrome.** (A, B) 3D CT surface-shaded display shows the wide open defect of the sagittal suture and brachycephaly with bicoronal synostosis typical of Apert's syndrome. The coronal sutures appear fused and are ridged. (C, D) Plain radiographs of the hands show the 'mitten' hand appearance with syndactyly and shortened metacarpals.

synostosis, the rarest form of monosutural synostosis, causes posterior plagiocephaly. This should be distinguished from the much more common positional or deformational plagiocephaly in which the suture is normal, and which is seen more often since the 1992 recommendation of the American Academy of Pediatrics to place newborns supine rather than prone in their cots to reduce the incidence of sudden infant death. In this case the skull deformity is caused by the child lying on one side in preference to the other, and may also be seen in children with torticollis or developmental delay. On plain radiographs and CT the lambdoid sutures appear open. Imaging of the spine may reveal segmentation anomalies, e.g. C5 and C6 in Apert's syndrome, and atlanto-occipital assimilation and basilar invagination in Apert's and Crouzon's syndromes.

CT is more sensitive and specific than plain radiographs for detecting radiological evidence of craniosynostosis, such as sclerosis and bony bridging, and CT venography may be helpful to assess the jugular foramina, variations in venous anatomy and patency of the venous sinuses. Three-dimensional CT surface-shaded bone and soft-tissue reconstructions or maximum intensity projections (MIPs) with a low milliampere technique may also be acquired, preferably in the craniofacial unit where treatment is being considered. The sutures should be assessed on both the axial 2D CT and 3D CT as either technique may miss relevant diagnostic features. There is also increasing prenatal diagnosis of craniosynostosis, particularly the syndromic forms, by ultrasound and fetal MRI.

In Apert's syndrome there are features of brachycephaly due to bicoronal synostosis, a wide open midline calvarial defect from the root of the nose to the posterior fontanelle in what would normally be the sagittal and metopic sutures and anterior fontanelle (Fig. 8-51). The sutures never form properly and, instead, bone islands appear within the defect, eventually coalescing to bony fusion by about 36 months. There is also hypertelorism with shallow anterior cranial fossae, depressed cribriform plate, as well as maxillary hypoplasia causing midface retrusion with exorbitism. Indeed, the globe may actually

sublux onto the cheek. The hand and feet deformities distinguish this condition from most other syndromic craniosynostoses and include syndactyly, phalangeal fusion and a short radially deviated thumb producing the 'mitten' or more severe 'hoof' hand. Children with Crouzon's syndrome demonstrate a more complex syndromic synostosis involving the coronal, sagittal, metopic and squamosal sutures, with early rather than late fontanelle closure. There is no midline calvarial defect but there is maxillary hypoplasia, hypertelorism, exorbitism and dental malocclusion. The limbs are usually clinically normal.

CT will detect any underlying structural brain abnormality. Although the brain usually appears structurally normal, midline anomalies such as callosal and septum pellucidum agenesis, limbic system abnormalities in Apert's, ventriculomegaly or distortion of the posterior fossa and skull base causing Chiari I malformations (tonsillar descent) may be detected. Tonsillar herniation is more frequently seen in Crouzon's syndrome, probably because there is more frequent skull base sutural synostosis in these conditions compared to Apert's.

Predicting raised intracranial pressure is known to be difficult by imaging, and correlation with clinical assessment is extremely important. Sometimes, however, direct invasive intracranial pressure (ICP) monitoring will be required. Hydrocephalus, seen in 4–25% of craniosynostosis and more commonly in the syndromic forms, may be multifactorial; possible aetiologies include tonsillar herniation and altered craniocervical junction CSF dynamics and venous hypertension due to venous foraminal narrowing, such as the jugular foramina, which ultimately may lead to venous occlusion and the development of venous collateral pathways such as enlargement of the stylomastoid emissary veins. Hydrocephalus is the most sensitive radiological indicator (see below) but only detects 40% of these children with raised ICP.

Finally CT may also be useful to assess the airway. Midface hypoplasia, small maxilla with dental overcrowding and basilar kyphosis may contribute to nasopharyngeal obstruction. Deviation of the nasal septum and choanal atresia may also be detected.

NEONATAL NASAL OBSTRUCTION: NASAL CAVITY STENOSIS/ATRESIA

The most common cause of neonatal nasal obstruction is mucosal oedema, followed by choanal atresia, skeletal dysplasias and congenital dacrocystocele due to distal nasolacrimal duct obstruction.

Choanal Atresia and Pyriform Stenosis

Choanal atresia/stenosis, a congenital malformation of the anterior skull base characterised by failure of canalisation of the posterior choanae, is the most common form of nasal cavity stenosis. It may be bony and/or fibrous in nature, unilateral presenting in later childhood with chronic nasal discharge and bilateral presenting in newborns with respiratory distress, particularly during feeding and which is a surgical emergency. Bilateral forms are more likely to be syndromic (50%) than unilateral forms and common associations are Crouzon's, Treacher Collins, CHARGE and Pierre Robin syndromes. The CHARGE syndrome describes the association of colobomas of the eye, heart defects, atresia of the choanae, retardation of growth and development,

genitourinary anomalies and ear anomalies. The atresia is best evaluated on CT by direct axial and direct coronal imaging on a bone algorithm after administration of a nasal decongestant. The nasal cavity appears funnel shaped with a fluid level proximal to the obstruction. The posterior vomer is thickened and the nasal septum is deviated to the side of the stenosis. A bony, fibrous or membranous bridging bar across the posterior choana is seen (Fig. 8-52). There is also congenital nasal pyriform aperture stenosis in which there is focal stenosis of the nasal aperture anteriorly caused by medial displacement of the nasal process of the maxilla assessed on axial bone CT at the level of the inferior meatus, often associated with a single central maxillary incisor (Fig. 8-53).

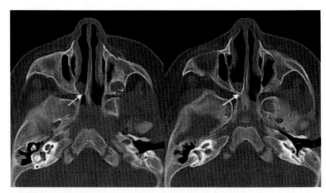

FIGURE 8-52 ■ **Choanal atresia.** Axial skull base CT in a child with chronic nasal discharge shows right-sided choanal atresia. There is bony narrowing of the funnel-shaped posterior right choana down to a bony bridging bar (arrows) and pooling of secretions proximally.

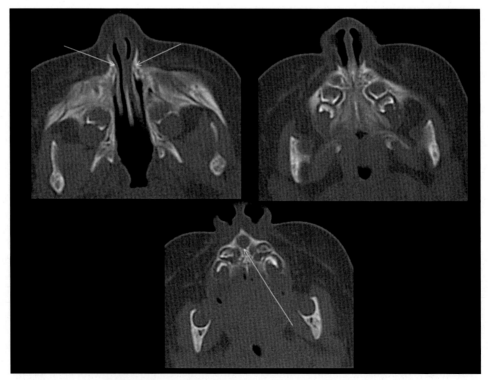

FIGURE 8-53 ■ **Pyriform stenosis and single central incisor.**

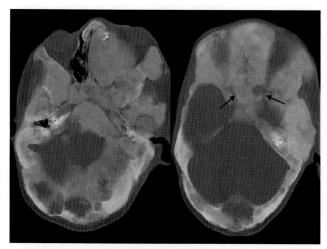

FIGURE 8-54 ■ **Polyostotic fibrous dysplasia with diffuse calvarial expansion, mixed lytic lesions and sclerosis.** The optic nerve canals are markedly narrowed (arrows).

Skeletal Dysplasias

Fibrous dysplasia is a benign congenital disorder in which bone is gradually replaced by fibrous tissue. McCune–Albright syndrome is a subtype of polyostotic fibrous dysplasia in which there is pituitary hypersecretion (hence precocious puberty but also Cushing's syndrome, etc.) and café-au-lait spots. Cherubism refers to fibrous dysplasia of the mandible and maxilla, and unlike the other forms of fibrous dysplasia is an inheritable condition. Typically the mandibular condyles are spared. The teeth may be displaced, impacted, resorbed or appear to be floating.

Clinical symptoms other than cosmetic deformity relate to the site of bony involvement; hence, cranial nerve impingement caused by narrowing of the skull base foramina, exophthalmos and optic foraminal narrowing caused by orbital involvement are all seen. On CT the typical lesion is a region of bony expansion with a 'ground-glass' appearance, but lesions may be lytic or sclerotic, or a combination of all three (Fig. 8-54).

BRAIN TUMOURS[54]

The Children's Cancer and Leukaemia Group (CCLG) Guidelines[55]

At initial presentation all paediatric brain tumours should have brain and whole-spine MRI, including contrast-enhanced images. A suggested protocol includes T_2-weighted FSE axial coronal FLAIR, T_1-weighted SE pre- and post-contrast imaging in three orthogonal planes for the brain (axial, coronal, sagittal), diffusion-weighted imaging and post-contrast imaging of the whole spine. Ideally spine imaging should be performed at the outset, but if the need for surgery is immediate, then postoperative spinal imaging (pre- and post-contrast T_1-weighted MRI to allow exclusion of T_1 shortening due to post-surgical blood products) should be performed.

The immediate postoperative MRI should be performed within 48 h (or 72 h maximum, according to the CCLG guidelines), the rationale being that post-surgical nodular enhancement which mimics tumour will not be seen before then. Post-surgical linear enhancement may be seen within this time period and, indeed, intraoperatively, and should therefore be interpreted with caution. The management strategy and frequency of subsequent surveillance imaging is determined by the tumour histology and presence of residual or recurrent tumour.[56–58] There remain regional differences in outcome in the UK, emphasising the importance of managing children with these tumours in a paediatric neuro-oncology centre with multidisciplinary support of neurosurgery, radiology and pathological condition.

Posterior Fossa Tumours

The most common intra-axial cerebellar tumours in children are medulloblastoma (generically known as infratentorial primitive neuroectodermal tumour or PNET), pilocytic astrocytoma, ependymoma and atypical teratoid/rhabdoid tumour, of which medulloblastoma and astrocytoma are the most common. Cerebellar haemangioblastoma may be seen in the context of von Hippel–Lindau disease but otherwise is an unusual tumour in the paediatric age group. Other posterior fossa tumours include brainstem gliomas and extra-axial tumours, such as dermoid and epidermoid cysts, schwannoma, neurofibroma, meningioma and skull base lesions, such as Langerhans' cell histiocytosis, Ewing's sarcoma and glomus tumours.

Clinically all of these tumours may present as a 'posterior fossa' syndrome with lethargy, headache and vomiting due to hydrocephalus and/or direct involvement of the brainstem emetic centre. Before the fontanelles have closed, infants may present with macrocephaly and sun-setting eyes. Truncal and gait ataxia is seen more often in older children and adults.

Infratentorial PNET (medulloblastomas) are highly malignant small, round cell tumours. They are slightly more common than pilocytic astrocytomas in most pathological series, are more common in boys, and account for 30–40% of posterior fossa tumours. They are also associated with some rare oncogenetic disorders such as Li–Fraumeni syndrome, Gorlin's or basal cell naevus syndrome (with falcine calcification), Turcot's and Cowden's syndromes. They are aggressive, high-grade tumours (WHO Grade IV) and tend to have a shorter onset of symptoms, typically shorter than 1 month, compared to other cerebellar tumours. The peak age of presentation is 7 years but they have a wide age range and may be seen from the neonatal period to late adulthood. There is a second peak in young adults presenting with the 'desmoplastic', less-aggressive type of medulloblastoma, which is seen more frequently in the cerebellar hemisphere than the vermis. Closely related to this is the medulloblastoma with extensive nodularity found in young children and also with a better prognosis than standard medulloblastoma (Fig. 8-55). Occasionally there may be symptoms and signs or imaging evidence of intracranial or intraspinal leptomeningeal metastatic disease at presentation, a

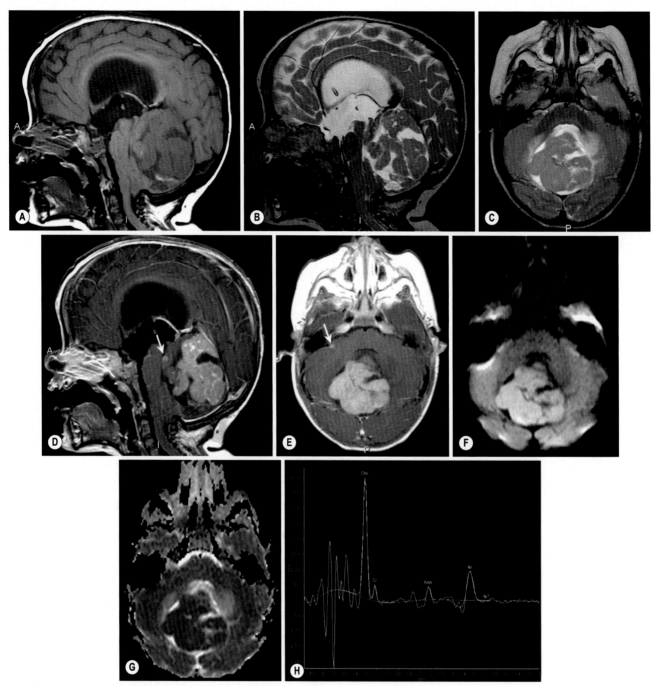

FIGURE 8-55 ■ Medulloblastoma with extensive nodularity (MB-EN). (A) Sagittal T1-weighted image and (B, C) sagittal and axial T2-weighted images show a large, cerebellar mass predominantly involving the vermis, composed of a macronodular conglomerate. There is marked supratentorial hydrocephalus. (D, E) Post contrast T1-weighted images show enhancement of the macronodules as well as secondary lesions in the cerebral acqueduct and right cerebellopontine cistern (arrows). Note the mass is superficially located in the cerebellar vermis and abuts the pial surface posteriorly, whereas the fourth ventricle is compressed. (F, G) Diffusion-weighted image and corresponding ADC map show restricted diffusion consistent with hypercellularity. (H) MR spectroscopy (PRESS, TE 144 ms) shows markedly elevated choline, reduced creatine and NAA, and an abnormal lipid peak, consistent with a high-grade lesion.

feature observed more commonly than with other posterior fossa tumours.

The typical appearance of the childhood medulloblastoma on CT is of a hyperdense midline vermian mass abutting the roof of the fourth ventricle, with perilesional oedema, variable patchy enhancement and hydrocephalus. The brainstem is usually displaced anteriorly rather than directly invaded. Cystic change, haemorrhage and calcification are frequently seen. On MRI, the mass is hypointense or isointense compared to grey matter. The CT finding of hyperdensity and MRI finding of T_2 hypointensity, supported by the presence of restricted diffusion on diffusion-weighted imaging, are the most reliable observations in prospectively differentiating

TABLE 8-2 ■ Differential Diagnosis of Posterior Fossa Tumour with CT Hyperdensity and T₂ Hypointensity

- Infratentorial PNET (medulloblastoma) or atypical teratoid/rhabdoid tumour
- Choroid plexus carcinoma
- Ewing's sarcoma
- Chondrosarcoma
- Chordoma
- Lymphoma
- Langerhans' cell histiocytosis

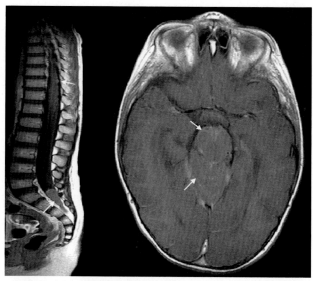

FIGURE 8-57 ■ Medulloblastoma. Same patient as described in the legend to Fig. 8-56, with posterior fossa medulloblastoma, has evidence of disseminated metastatic disease. There is nodular enhancement over the conus medullaris and a mass within the thecal sac in addition to pial enhancement over the midbrain and cerebellar folia (arrows).

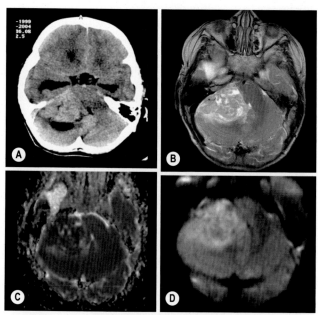

FIGURE 8-56 ■ Medulloblastoma. (A) CT and (B–D) axial T₂, ADC and diffusion MRI show a mixed solid and cystic mass within the right cerebellopontine angle encroaching on the pons and fourth ventricle and causing hydrocephalus. The solid component is hyperdense on CT, is hypointense on the T₂-weighted sequence and demonstrates restricted diffusion in keeping with a cellular tumour. Despite some less typical features, such as lateral site (more usually seen in older patients and associated with the desmoplastic variant) and cystic components, on the basis of the signal characteristics this was correctly diagnosed as a medulloblastoma.

medulloblastoma (and atypical rhabdoid tumour which on imaging appears identical to medulloblastoma) from ependymoma or other posterior fossa tumours (Fig. 8-56, Table 8-2).[59] Both the CT hyperdensity and MRI T₂ signal hypointensity reflect the increased nuclear-to-cytoplasmic ratio and densely packed cells of the tumour, and are particularly useful in differentiating medulloblastomas with 'atypical' features, such as a lateral site involving the foramen of Luschka or extrusion through the foramen of Magendie, which are more commonly seen with ependymomas. Medulloblastomas demonstrate restricted diffusion and reduced *N*-acetyl asparatate (NAA) peak with an increased choline-to-creatine ratio, and occasionally lactate and lipid peaks on MR spectroscopy.

In medulloblastoma, both intracranial and intraspinal subarachnoid dissemination should be actively looked for, and is seen in a third of cases at presentation, most often occurring as irregular, nodular leptomeningeal enhancement (Fig. 8-57). Imaging is reported as being more sensitive than CSF cytology and false positives can be avoided by preoperative imaging of the brain and spine. Occasionally, enhancement may not always be detected or may be very mild, making the detection of both disseminated disease and residual or recurrent tumour on surveillance imaging more difficult. Other features of leptomeningeal disease include sulcal and cisternal effacement and communicating hydrocephalus; thickening, nodularity and clumping of nerve roots; and pial 'drop' metastases along the surface of the spinal cord.

Standard treatment for infratentorial primitive neuro-ectodermal tumour (PNET) (medulloblastoma) is by surgical resection, with adjuvant craniospinal radiotherapy for those over 3 years of age (as the infant brain is more susceptible to radiation effects) and chemotherapy. The 5-year survival varies from 50% to 80%. Favourable prognostic factors include complete surgical resection, lack of CSF dissemination at presentation, onset in the second decade, female gender and lateral location within the cerebellar hemisphere, while poor prognostic factors include specific oncogene expression. Surveillance imaging detects recurrences earlier than clinical presentation, allows earlier therapeutic intervention and correlates with increased survival.

Atypical teratoid/rhabdoid tumours are unusual malignant tumours with a poor prognosis. For practical purposes, the imaging features are indistinguishable from medulloblastoma/PNET. They are more aggressive tumours, are often large at the time of presentation and occur in slightly younger children, typically under the age of 2 years.

The next most common cerebellar tumour in children after medulloblastoma, and accounting for 30–40%, is the cerebellar low-grade astrocytoma (CLGA), which in most cases (85%) is a pilocytic tumour (WHO Grade I) and in up to 15% is a more diffuse fibrillary type with a higher histological grade. The 5-year survival for cerebellar pilocytic astrocytoma is in excess of 95% in most reported series, including the original description by Cushing in 1931. The CLGA is a well-circumscribed, slowly growing lesion of children and young adults, though it is occasionally seen in older people. There is an association with NF1, as there is for other neuro-axis pilocytic astrocytomas. The duration of symptom onset is more insidious than that of medulloblastomas, typically being intermittent over several months.

On CT and MRI the tumour is typically a cerebellar vermian or hemispheric tumour which is cystic with an enhancing mural nodule. The solid component is hypointense to isodense on CT, hyperintense on T_2-weighted FSE and hypointense on T_1-weighted sequences reflecting the hypocellular and loosely arranged tumoural architecture.[60] The solid component is highly vascular with a deficient blood–brain barrier and therefore enhances avidly and homogeneously (Fig. 8-58).

Occasionally the pilocytic astrocytoma may present with diffuse nodular enhancement of the leptomeninges, indicating intracranial or intraspinal pial dissemination. This is typically seen with WHO Grade I tumours, does not imply a higher-grade tumour and, like the tumour primary, tends to grow slowly.

Ependymomas (WHO Grade II) account for approximately 10% of paediatric posterior fossa tumours and the posterior fossa is the most common site for ependymomas in children. Their mean age at presentation is 6.4 years, with a range of 2 months to 16 years. They are well-defined tumours which typically originate from the floor or the roof of the fourth ventricle, extend into the cerebellopontine angle and extrude through the foramina of Luschka and Magendie (Fig. 8-59). Perivascular pseudorosettes and ependymal rosettes are the cardinal histopathological features. They are more cellular than CLGAs but usually demonstrate CT and MRI features consistent with a greater water content than medulloblastomas. Therefore they are still hypodense or isodense on CT, hypointense on T_1 and isodense to hyperintense on MRI. Foci of microcystic change, haemorrhage and calcification are common features. They can also disseminate throughout the neuro-axis by leptomeningeal spread, although this is much less common than for medulloblastoma, and tends to occur later in the disease rather than at initial presentation. Incomplete resection, age under 3 years and anaplastic histopathological features correlate with a worse prognosis. The 5-year progression-free survival is 50% but worse under the age of 2 years.

Children with von Hippel–Lindau disease may occasionally present with cerebellar haemangioblastoma (WHO Grade I), which in the sporadic form is usually a tumour of adults. It consists of a rich capillary network in addition to large vacuolated stromal cells. On imaging, haemangioblastomas may mimic a CLGA with an intensely enhancing mural nodule and a cystic component. The tumour abuts the pial surface, but unlike the CLGA it may be associated with prominent vascular flow

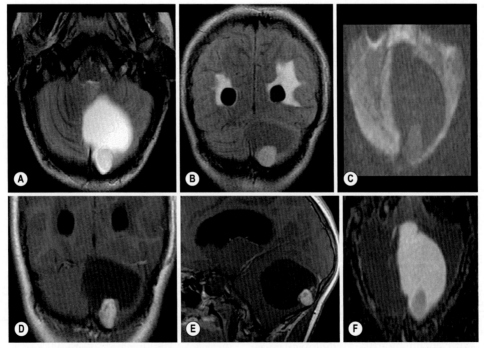

FIGURE 8-58 ■ **Cerebellar hemispheric tumour in a child with a history of ataxia, nausea and vomiting over several months.** (A, B, D, E) Axial T_2, coronal FLAIR, coronal and sagittal T_1-enhanced MRI show a left cerebellar hemispheric tumour with a large cystic component and solid homogeneously enhancing component which is bright on T_2-weighted sequences (compare with the images of posterior fossa medulloblastoma, Figs. 8-56 and 8-57). The solid component is not restricted on the diffusion-weighted image (C) and ADC map (F) compared to medulloblastoma and there is free diffusion in the cystic component.

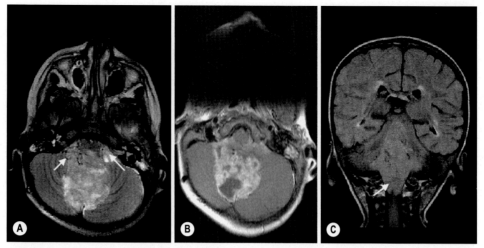

FIGURE 8-59 ■ **Ependymoma.** (A–C) Axial T₂, enhanced T₁ and coronal FLAIR images showing a solid and microcystic fourth ventricular tumour extending out through the foramina of Luschka, Magendie and the foramen magnum (arrows), the typical features of an ependymoma.

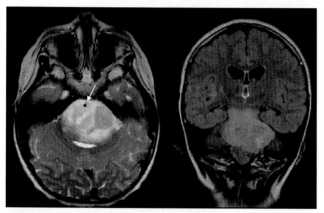

FIGURE 8-60 ■ **Diffuse brainstem astrocytoma.** Note the mass effect within the pons distorting the fourth ventricle and the encasement of the basilar artery (arrow).

voids. Haemorrhage and frank necrosis may occur but are less common.

Most brainstem tumours in children are astrocytomas. Medullary tumours may present with symptoms and signs of raised intracranial pressure and cranial nerve dysfunction. The two major groups are diffuse tumours and focally exophytic tumours.[61] Diffuse tumours extend up and down the brainstem and are seen best as ill-defined signal hyperintensity on T₂-weighted (including FLAIR) images in association with expansion of the brainstem. Their enhancement if present is usually minimal unless the tumour has been irradiated (Fig. 8-60). Focal exophytic tumours are usually dorsally exophytic, well-defined tumours, which do not extend along white matter tracts in the same ways as diffuse astrocytomas (hence their exophytic growth), but often enhance. They are usually Grade I pilocytic or Grade II astrocytomas and are associated with a better prognosis than diffuse astrocytomas, particularly focal tumours within the midbrain tectum.[62] Occasionally, however, anaplastic gangliogliomas or PNET tumours may appear like this.

TABLE 8-3	Differential of Enhancing Infundibular Lesions

- Germinoma
- Langerhans' cell histiocytosis
- Lymphocytic hypophysitis
- Granuloma (tuberculosis, sarcoid)

Suprasellar Tumours

Some knowledge of the typical clinical presentation of certain suprasellar tumours can be very helpful in differentiating them even before imaging. For example, hypopituitarism is more likely to be seen with craniopharyngioma, delayed puberty with hypothalamic astrocytoma or Langerhans' cell histiocytosis and occasionally pituitary adenoma, precocious puberty due to hypothalamic infundibular lesions, such as Langerhans' cell histiocytosis, germinoma, craniopharyngioma, hamartoma and non-neoplastic granulomatous disease, such as sarcoidosis and tuberculosis (Table 8-3). Large suprasellar mass lesions have the ability to produce hydrocephalus by obstruction at the foramen of Monro, and visual field defects by compression or involvement of the optic chiasm.

Craniopharyngioma

Although histologically benign (WHO Grade I), this tumour is associated with significant morbidity and mortality because of its site and often large size at presentation. It is the most common suprasellar tumour in children, accounting for 1–3% of intracranial tumours of all ages, but usually occurring from age 5 to 15 years. Most craniopharyngiomas have a suprasellar mass and a smaller intrasellar component. In 5% of cases it is purely intrasellar and may be difficult to distinguish from a Rathke's cleft cyst. Classically it appears as a calcified, mixed cystic and solid tumour with enhancement of the solid component and the cyst wall (Fig. 8-61). Large

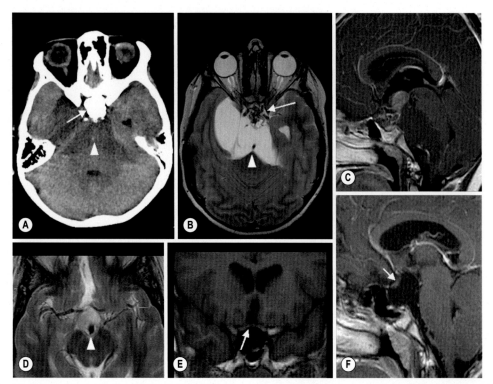

FIGURE 8-61 ■ Craniopharyngiomas in two children. (A–C) The first child has a large suprasellar, pre-pontine and middle cranial fossa tumour which is causing considerable mass effect on the brainstem and is encasing the basilar artery (arrowheads). There are solid enhancing and calcified components (arrows). The cystic components are of higher density on CT and there is T_1 shortening on MRI in keeping with proteinaceous contents. (D–F) The second child has a smaller suprasellar lesion, which is also calcified (arrowhead). The optic chiasm is clearly separate from the lesion and is draped over the top (E, F).

tumours may cause hydrocephalus and compression and distortion of the optic chiasm. The cystic components may extend behind the clivus and into any of the cranial fossae. On T_1-weighted sequences the cyst may demonstrate T_1 shortening due to proteinacaeous components, which have been described macroscopically as appearing like 'machine oil'. The cystic components are of increased signal on T_2-weighted FSE. MR spectroscopy demonstrates high lipid peaks. Surgical resection is often incomplete (in > 20%) because of the close adherence of the tumour to the optic chiasm; despite this, long-term survival is good (> 90% in children). Partial surgical resection with adjuvant radiotherapy with preservation of the hypothalamic–pituitary axis is a considered treatment strategy which aims to maximise outcome and reduce long-term endricological morbidity. This is advocated in the UK, while more aggressive surgical resection may be the strategy pursued in other centres.

Hypothalamic–Optic Pathway Glioma

Astrocytomas of the optic chiasm and hypothalamus account for 10–15% of supratentorial tumours in children. Optic chiasm tumours often extend into the hypothalamus and vice versa; hence they are discussed here together. Optic nerve tumours are usually pilocytic astrocytomas with a very indolent course, while hypothalamic/chiasmatic tumours may be of slightly higher histological grade (for example, WHO Grade II tumours) and more aggressive biological behaviour.

CT and MRI both define involvement of the optic nerves. CT can detect expansion of the optic canal. However, MRI is the best technique for delineating expansion of the chiasm and hypothalamus and involvement of the posterior visual pathways (Fig. 8-62). Tumour appears isointense to hypointense on T_1 weighted imaging and hyperintense on T_2-weighted imaging. There may be diffuse fusiform expansion of the nerve from subarachnoid dissemination of tumour around the optic nerve. Enhancement is variable. The main differential diagnosis is from craniopharyngioma, which tends to present later, is usually calcified and is adherent to the chiasm rather than arising from it and causing expansion.

Infundibular Tumours

These include germinomas and Langerhans' cell histiocytosis, both of which cause expansion and enhancement of the pituitary infundibulum (Fig. 8-63). Onset of diabetes insipidus appears to correlate with absence of high T_1 signal in the posterior pituitary gland. The hypothalamic hamartoma (by definition a hypothalamic mass rather than a tumour) presents either with precocious puberty or with gelastic seizures. These may be sessile or pedunculated and are well-defined lesions arising from the floor of the third ventricle and extending inferiorly into the suprasellar or interpeduncular cistern. They are typically isointense to grey matter on T_1- and T_2-weighted MRI and do not enhance (Fig. 8-64).

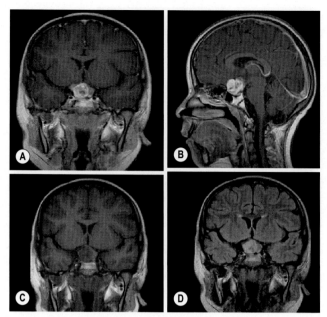

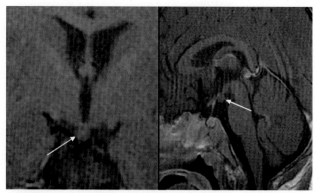

FIGURE 8-64 ■ **Hypothalamic hamartoma.** Coronal T$_1$ and sagittal T$_1$-weighted post-contrast MRI shows a non-enhancing lesion arising from the floor of the third ventricle posterior to the pituitary infundibulum and projecting inferiorly into the suprasellar cistern (arrows).

FIGURE 8-62 ■ **Hypothalamic–optic pathway glioma.** (A) Coronal T$_1$-weighted, (B) sagittal and (C) coronal enhanced T$_1$-weighted MRI and (D) coronal FLAIR show an optic chiasm glioma. The chiasm is not identified separately from the tumour.

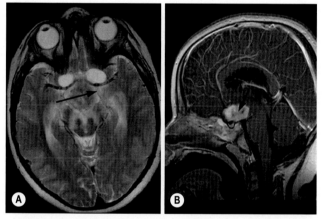

FIGURE 8-63 ■ **Langerhans' cell histiocytosis.** (A) Axial T$_2$-weighted image. (B) Sagittal T$_1$-weighted post-contrast image. Suprasellar T$_2$ hypointense and enhancing mass (arrows) with associated oedema extending superiorly along white matter tracts in a child with multisystem Langerhans' cell histiocytosis.

Pituitary Tumours

Pituitary adenomas are uncommon in children but may present in adolescents, and account for 2% of all pituitary adenomas. The most common functional tumours are prolactinomas and corticotrophin- and growth hormone-secreting tumours. A quarter of paediatric pituitary tumours are non-functioning. The imaging appearances are the same as in adults. Rathke's cleft cysts are also rare in children.

Pineal Region Tumours

The pineal region is a descriptive term and encompasses the posterior third ventricle and its contents, including the pineal gland itself, the tectal plate and aqueduct, the posterior septum pellucidum, corpus callosum and thalami, internal cerebral veins in addition to the quadrigeminal cistern containing the posterior cerebral arteries, vein of Galen and straight sinus. Lesions may arise from any of these components and therefore the differential diagnosis of a pineal region tumour is wide. The most common lesions are germ cell tumours (GCTs), followed by primary pineal gland masses. Gliomas are also relatively common lesions at this site, usually derived from adjacent brain parenchyma. Pineal region tumours can cause hydrocephalus by obstruction of the cerebral aqueduct. Direct compression or invasion of the tectal plate, specifically the colliculi, may cause failure of upward gaze and convergence (Parinaud's syndrome). They may also cause precocious puberty.

Central Nervous System Germ Cell Tumours

CNS GCTs are primarily tumours of the young, over 90% occurring in the under-20 age group and with a peak incidence from age 10 to 12 years. They are more common in Asia but in the West account for 1% of intracranial neoplasms in children. Germinoma is the most common type of CNS GCT, followed by non-secreting teratoma. Other GCTs include rarer secreting forms such as yolk sac, embryonal and choriocarcinoma, and may be of mixed cellular types, the latter associated with the worst prognosis.

Germinomas are characteristically found in the midline, in the pineal or suprasellar regions. A minority of lesions may be found in the basal ganglia, thalami, or cerebellum. Pineal and suprasellar lesions may be synchronous, and when so, are pathognomonic. Most pineal region GCTs occur in boys and suprasellar GCTs in girls. Pathologically the tumour is solid and consists of large, glycogen-rich germ line cells with variable desmoplastic stroma and lymphocytic infiltrate. Necrosis and haemorrhage are unusual, with the exception of lesions seen in the basal ganglia.

Germinomas are classified as malignant tumours but respond extremely well to radiotherapy and may melt away over just a few days of treatment. Overall they are

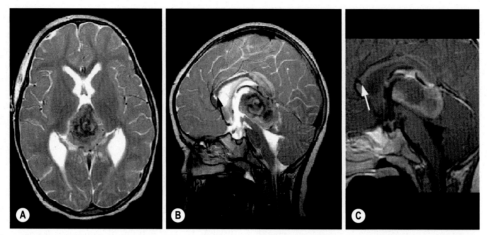

FIGURE 8-65 ■ **Pineoblastoma.** (A) Axial, (B) sagittal T$_2$-weighted fast spin-echo and (C) enhanced sagittal T$_1$-weighted MRI in a 2-year-old girl show a pineal region tumour effacing the tectal plate. The hydrocephalus is treated by a frontal extraventricular drain (track through the genu of the corpus callosum marked by the arrows). The tumour is hypointense on the T$_2$-weighted images with rings of lower signal consistent with calcification and haemorrhagic products, and peripheral rim enhancement, and was confirmed as a pineoblastoma.

more common in young adolescent males. On CT they appear as a hyperdense, solid mass within the posterior third ventricle and enhance avidly and homogeneously. They tend to engulf the pineal gland, which may be calcified. Occasionally this may be difficult to differentiate from intrinsic tumoural calcification more suggestive of a teratoma or primary pineal gland tumour, such as a pineoblastoma, although both of these lesions are typically more heterogeneous with haemorrhage and cyst formation. On MRI the cellularity of the tumour is reflected by T$_2$ hypointensity relative to grey matter. The tumour may be less homogeneous than on CT and cystic change may be detected, although enhancement remains a marked feature. Germinomas demonstrate restricted diffusion. Synchronous germinomas in typical midline sites, such as the suprasellar region, and evidence of early CSF dissemination should be actively looked for.

Benign teratomas are very heterogeneous, mixed cystic, solid and well-defined masses characterised by calcification and fat. Enhancement is not usually seen unless there are areas of malignant degeneration. Other GCTs are also heterogeneous in appearance and do not contain fat, but the individual tumour types are not distinguishable radiologically.

Primary Pineal Tumours: Pineoblastoma and Pineocytoma

Pineoblastomas are malignant (WHO Grade IV), small, round cell tumours which histologically are similar to medulloblastomas and share similar imaging characteristics in terms of hyperdensity on CT and are hypointense to isointense signal on T$_2$-weighted FSE relative to grey matter. They may contain areas of calcification and rarely haemorrhage. The solid parts of the tumour enhance intensely. They may be distinguished from Grade II pineocytomas by the age at presentation, as they occur most frequently in the first two decades of life compared to pineocytomas, which are tumours of young adults; by

their size (> 3 cm); and by their relative T$_2$-weighted hypointensity (Fig. 8-65).

Supratentorial Hemispheric Tumours

Overall, supratentorial tumours occur as frequently as posterior fossa tumours in the paediatric age group but are more common under the age of 2 and over the age of 10, while posterior fossa tumours are more common from the ages of 2 to 10. The presenting symptoms are due to a large mass-occupying lesion and include headaches and vomiting. In the under 2-year-old age group the tumour may be very large at the time of presentation; the fontanelles are open so that infants present with increasing head size as often as they do with hydrocephalus. Seizures are seen more particularly with temporal and frontal cortex lesions.

Astrocytomas

The most common paediatric cerebral hemispheric tumour is the astrocytoma, accounting for 30% of supratentorial brain tumours in children. In children under 2 years, other diagnoses should be considered; teratomas and desmoplastic infantile gangliogliomas are seen in neonates and PNET, atypical teratoid/rhabdoid tumours, and ependymomas are seen in slightly older infants. Some children who present with a longer history and refractory epilepsy may have low-grade, indolent glioneuronal tumours, including the dysembryoplastic neuroepithelial tumour.

As with cerebellar astrocytomas, hemispheric astrocytomas may be cystic with an enhancing mural nodule, entirely solid with variable enhancement or solid with a necrotic centre. On CT the solid part of the hemispheric astrocytoma is isodense or hypodense and on MRI T$_2$-weighted sequences it is hyperintense, helping to distinguish these tumours from small, round cell tumours such as supratentorial PNET. They may rarely be multicentric. The histological grade cannot be reliably determined by the radiological features. Contrast enhancement can be seen in both low- and high-grade tumours. A simple cyst with non-enhancing walls, minimal surrounding oedema and a single enhancing mural nodule is more likely to be a pilocytic astrocytoma. Lesions containing haemorrhage and associated with marked adjacent oedema are more likely to be of higher grade. Glioblastoma is seen in children and in children is associated with a better prognosis than in adults. The pleomorphic xanthoastrocytoma is an uncommon astrocytoma of children and young adults. It is usually a WHO Grade II lesion, though it may have anaplastic features. Typically it has a superficial location within the temporal lobe and consists of a cyst and enhancing mural nodule with minimal adjacent oedema. Radiologically it is often indistinguishable from ganglioglioma and some other glioneuronal tumour subtypes.

Ependymomas

Supratentorial ependymomas occur more commonly in boys, with a peak incidence between the ages of 1 and 5 years, and again are similar to the posterior fossa ependymoma. However, they are more usually extraventricular in site and therefore CSF dissemination is less common than with their posterior fossa equivalent. They are iso-dense to hyperdense, well-defined lesions on CT with variable enhancement of the solid component. Tumour heterogeneity with cystic areas and foci of calcification are common (Fig. 8-66). Haemorrhage may also be seen.

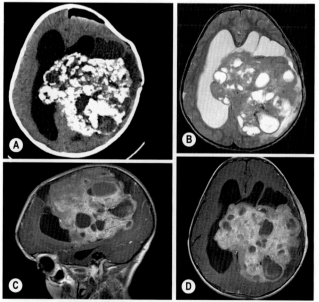

FIGURE 8-66 ■ **Supratentorial Grade II ependymoma.** The left cerebral hemisphere tumour extends across the midline into the right ventricle. (A) CT (post partial debulking) shows it is heavily calcified and (B–D) MRI (axial T_2-enhanced, sagittal T_1 and axial T_1-weighted MRI) show a mixed cystic and solid heterogeneously enhancing tumour. There is associated hydrocephalus.

Supratentorial Primitive Neuroectodermal Tumours

PNET (WHO Grade IV) is a cellular tumour of primitive cell types and may be seen in children as young as 4 weeks to 10 years, with a mean age of 5.5 years. A rare subtype that includes more neuronal cells is known as cerebral neuroblastoma. PNET is found more frequently in the posterior fossa (where it is also known as medulloblastoma) than in the supratentorial compartment. Poor prognostic factors for PNET include age under 2 years and a supratentorial location. The 5-year survival drops from 85% for tumours in the posterior fossa to 34% for supratentorial tumours. They are frequently haemorrhagic, necrotic and have foci of calcification. The solid parts of the tumour are hyperdense on CT and hypointense on T_2-weighted FSE. There is always some enhancement, although the degree is variable. Although the tumour may appear well-defined radiologically, tumour cells are likely to extend beyond the apparent margins. Widespread dissemination of tumour, both through the CSF space and to the lungs, liver and spleen, is not infrequent.

Medulloepithelioma is a rare, highly malignant tumour usually affecting children between the ages of 6 months and 5 years. Solid components are hypercellular; therefore, the density and signal characteristics may be similar to PNET. They are large at the time of presentation with extensive areas of haemorrhage and necrosis but may be distinguished from other tumours, including PNET, by their lack of contrast enhancement.

Desmoplastic Infantile Gangliomas

These typically present as a massive cyst with an enhancing cortically based mural nodule in an infant with increased head size and bulging fontanelle. Adjacent dural enhancement may also be seen. The cyst, which is hypointense on T_1, hyperintense on T_2 and may contain septations, usually does not enhance.

Choroid Plexus Tumours

These are 'cauliflower-like' tumours arising from the epithelium of the choroid plexus and are more frequently benign (papilloma) than malignant (carcinoma). Both types may disseminate within the CSF space. They are the most common brain tumour in children under 1 year and present with hydrocephalus, possibly due to CSF hypersecretion or obstructive hydrocephalus due to haemorrhage, arachnoiditis or carcinomatosis in carcinomas. For papillomas the 5-year survival approaches 100%, while for carcinomas it ranges from 25 to 40%, with a higher survival if the tumour is completely resected.

On CT they are seen as hyperdense or isodense, lobulated 'frond-like', avidly and homogeneously enhancing masses with punctate calcifications, occasionally with haemorrhage and with hydrocephalus. The typical site is the trigone of the lateral ventricle, while in older children the cerebellopontine angle or fourth ventricle

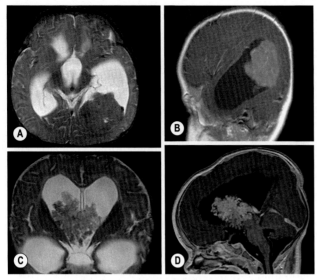

FIGURE 8-67 ■ **Choroid plexus tumours.** (A, B) Axial T₂, enhanced sagittal T₁-weighted MRI in a boy aged 6 months demonstrate a lobulated homogeneously enhancing intraventricular tumour with relative T_2 hypointensity, in keeping with a highly cellular tumour closely related to the choroid plexus. The ependyma is enhancing and the interface between tumour and adjacent brain is indistinct. Histology confirmed the tumour to be a choroid plexus carcinoma and this was subsequently embolised before surgery. There is a communicating hydrocephalus which may be due to increased cerebrospinal fluid production or to proteinaceous/haemorrhagic exudate. (C, D) A different child with choroid plexus papilloma. Choroid plexus tumours, although commonly seen within the trigone of the lateral ventricle, may arise from anywhere within the ventricular system. This child has a frondy choroid plexus papilloma arising within the third ventricle and extending superiorly through the foramina of Monro. In this case the hydrocephalus was obstructive.

may be involved (Fig. 8-67). On MRI the papillary appearance is more readily appreciated: they are more mottled and isointense or hypointense on T_1-weighted imaging with intense enhancement. Vascular flow voids, usually from choroidal arteries, are often seen in association, and arterial embolisation may be considered before surgery in an attempt to reduce the vascularity of the tumour. Haemorrhage and localised vasogenic oedema are suggestive of carcinoma with invasion but the two histological types cannot be reliably distinguished on imaging.

Other intraventricular tumours include meningiomas, which are rare in children outside NF2 and ependymomas.

Dysembryoplastic Neuroepithelial Tumours

Dysembryoplastic neuroepithelial tumour (DNT) is a WHO Grade I benign tumour which classically presents with complex partial seizures in children and young adults under the age of 20. It is a cortically based lesion which may have associated foci of cortical dysplasia.

On imaging it appears as a well-defined cortically based lesion with a characteristic 'bubbly' internal structure, minimal mass effect and no associated vasogenic oedema (Fig. 8-68). There may be some adjacent bony scalloping consistent with a long-standing lesion and a

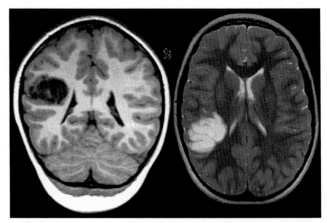

FIGURE 8-68 ■ **Dysembryoplastic neuroepithelial tumour (DNT) in a child with long-standing refractory focal epilepsy referred to the epilepsy surgical programme.** Several MRI examinations over 3 years had shown no change in the appearances of this right inferior parietal lobe lesion. The lesion is well-defined and cortically based, extends towards the ventricular margin and has the typical lobulated internal architecture of DNT.

third of lesions demonstrate calcification. On MRI they are hypointense on T_1 and have a hyperintense rim on FLAIR or proton density-weighted imaging. Most tumours do not enhance and, if present, enhancement is faint and patchy.

CEREBROVASCULAR DISEASE AND STROKE

Stroke is an important paediatric illness, with an incidence of around 2 cases per 100,000 children per annum. The aetiology of paediatric stroke is significantly different from adult stroke, as large artery atherosclerosis, cardio-embolic and small vessel disease combined account for only 10% of cases in children.[63]

There have been several misconceptions regarding stroke in children. Paediatric stroke was said to be idiopathic, associated with a good prognosis with low recurrence rates and good recovery of motor function and school performance, and was minimally investigated on the assumption that this would not affect management. Recent work has shown that there are many different aetiologies associated with stroke in children and a single episode may be multifactorial. Associated factors, some of which may be amenable to treatment, include congenital heart disease, anaemias, prothrombotic disorders such as protein C and S deficiencies, hyperhomocystinaemia, lipid abnormalities, recent infections and respiratory chain disorders (Fig. 8-69). Equally, long-term follow-up has shown a poor outcome with some degree of dependency in 60% of affected children. Although difficult to quantify due to selection bias, the risk of recurrence for ischaemic stroke ranges from 5 to 20%. Children who have a stroke at a young age have a worse physical and intellectual outcome and behavioural problems may be significant. Hence children with acute stroke should be referred to, or have their management discussed with, a paediatric neurologist, and thoroughly investigated on

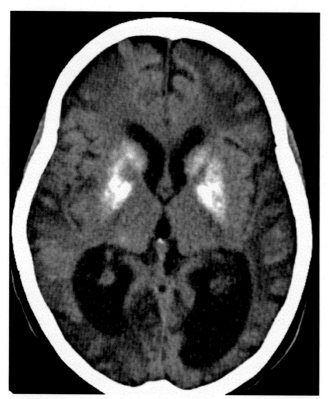

FIGURE 8-69 ■ **Strokes occurring in mitochondrial cytopathy.** Bilateral symmetrical lentiform and caudate calcification and extensive cerebral infarction crossing arterial territories in a child with a mitochondrial disorder (MELAS).

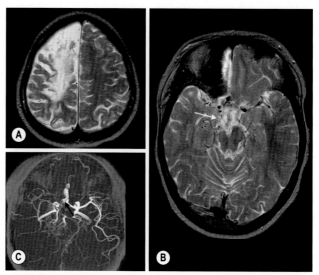

FIGURE 8-70 ■ **Sickle cell disease and moya moya syndrome.** Child with extensive frontal, deep and posterior watershed infarction (A). (B) Extensive perimesencephalic 'moya moya' collaterals (arrow) and attenuated right middle cerebral artery (MCA) flow voids. (C) Compressed maximum intensity projection image shows narrowed terminal internal carotid artery (ICA), reduced filling of right MCA, and A1 segment of the anterior cerebral artery. There is an aneurysm at the A1/anterior communicating artery (ACOM) junction (arrow).

each occasion to detect all potential risk factors. Cross-sectional brain imaging is mandatory in children presenting with clinical stroke. Brain MRI is recommended and should be performed as soon as possible after presentation. If MRI is not available within 48 h, CT is an acceptable initial alternative. Imaging should be undertaken urgently in those who have a depressed conscious level or whose clinical status is deteriorating.[64]

The purpose of neuroimaging is to confirm the diagnosis and exclude alternative treatable lesions, as well as to help understand the underlying cause, guide treatment and monitor progression of the disease. The radiological findings of brain parenchymal involvement in stroke are not significantly different from findings in adults. There is, however, some evidence that restricted diffusion may occur for a shorter time in younger children and pseudonormalisation may occur earlier than in adults. Vascular abnormalities in paediatric ischaemic stroke are common.[65] These are more frequently intracranial than extracranial, involve the anterior rather than posterior circulation and typically consist of occlusion of proximal large arteries, i.e. middle cerebral artery (MCA), anterior cerebral artery (ACA) and terminal internal carotid artery (ICA).

Sickle cell disease, a chronic haemolytic anaemia in which abnormal haemoglobin (HbS) forms with a tendency to cause red blood cells to distort and block small blood vessels, is the most common cause of ischaemic stroke in children worldwide. Even within this single disease entity there are several factors that contribute to

stroke. These include a cerebral vasculopathy known as moya moya disease, an underlying predilection to infection, tissue hypoxia and precipitation of sickling vaso-occlusive crisis resulting from chronic anaemia, high white cell count, adenotonsillar hyperplasia causing obstructive sleep apnoea, cardiomegaly and a generalised procoagulant state.

Stroke in sickle cell disease is clinically apparent in 9% of children with sickle cell disease under the age of 20 years, but silent infarction occurs in as many as 25%. The imaging pattern of infarction is typically of arterial watershed infarction between the major cerebral arterial territories. A fifth of strokes in sickle cell disease may be haemorrhagic. The diploic space of the calvarium may be diffusely thickened due to increased haematopoiesis in order to compensate for the chronic haemolytic anaemia.

The brain MRI and circle of Willis MR angiogram (MRA) may show evidence of a cerebral vasculopathy known as moya moya syndrome. In this there is typically progressive stenosis of the terminal ICA and proximal segments of the major intracranial arteries (Fig. 8-70). There is a predilection for the anterior circulation. As the stenosis progresses, increased flow occurs through proximal collateral vessels, particularly the lenticulostriate and thalamoperforator arteries, resulting in the 'puff of smoke' appearance to which moya moya refers. These are seen as multiple small flow voids within the basal ganglia. Prominent transmedullary veins and pial enhancement may also be seen. Other acquired vascular abnormalities include aneurysms and small arteriovenous malformations.

Referral to a neurosurgical paediatric centre for consideration of external-to-internal carotid (EC–IC) bypass may be indicated. At this point cerebral perfusion imaging to detect 'diffusion–perfusion mismatch' may be helpful in order to assess for critical ischaemia or to select which hemisphere should be revascularised first. This involves a bolus of intravenous contrast medium for MRI perfusion studies and it is important that the child with sickle cell disease is well hydrated for this. Surgical EC–IC bypass may be performed indirectly by mobilisation of part of the temporalis muscle with its blood supply, the superficial temporal artery (STA), and laying it onto the pial surface of the brain, or by direct end-to-side anastomosis between the STA and distal MCA branch. Some centres use multiple calvarial burr holes alone to promote superficial angiogenesis and collateral revascularisation. Postoperative MRA and perfusion imaging after successful EC–IC bypass should show flow through the STA and increased collateral flow within the distal MCA branches. Perfusion imaging will show increased cerebral blood volume and flow to the revascularised hemisphere.

Moya moya accounts for up to 30% of cerebral vasculopathy in paediatric stroke but it is not unique to sickle cell disease, being also idiopathic, secondary to NF1, cranial irradiation, Down's syndrome, human immunodeficiency virus (HIV) and even tuberculous meningitis. Postinfective angiitis associated with varicella zoster, in which the terminal ICA and proximal MCA are usually affected and there is infarction of the basal ganglia, is relatively common (Fig. 8-71). MRA in the majority (but not all) shows evidence of stabilisation or remodelling and improvement of the angiographic appearances at 6-month follow-up.

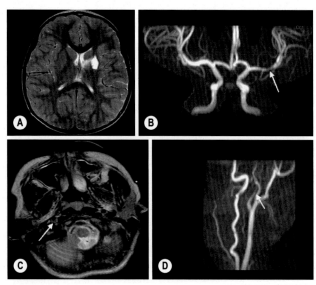

FIGURE 8-71 ■ **Vasculitis.** (A, B) In a child with chicken pox vasculitis, axial T$_2$ and maximum intensity projection (MIP) image of time-of-flight (TOF) circle of Willis MRA show a mature proximal left middle cerebral artery branch infarct with reduced and turbulent flow (arrow) and reduced distal filling. **Arterial dissection.** (C, D) In a 14-year-old girl with acute-onset left hemiplegia, large right middle cerebral artery territory infarct, and internal carotid artery (ICA) dissection is seen. On the axial T$_2$-weighted image there is an eccentric filling defect within the lumen of the right internal carotid artery which is narrowed, confirming the presence of dissection (arrow). The MIP image of the TOF MRA shows a typical rat's tail appearance of a tapering stenosis distal to the right ICA bifurcation (arrow).

Arterial dissection may occur intracranially but is also seen, as it is in young adults especially, not infrequently within the cervical arteries. Vertebral arterial dissection occurs most commonly as the vertebral artery exits the transverse foramen of C2 before passing posterolaterally over the lateral masses of C1 to enter the foramen magnum, and ICA dissection occurs above the bifurcation (Fig. 8-71). Dissections may involve intracranial and extracranial arteries. There may be other rarer causes of cervical arterial disease with more diffuse involvement proximal to the bifurcation, e.g. that seen with the connective tissue disorders such as Marfan's, Ehlers–Danlos type IV, osteogenesis imperfecta type I, autosomal dominant polycystic kidney disease, fibromuscular dysplasia, or other causes of cystic medial necrosis and Menkes' disease. Cervical arterial dissection may occur without an antecedent history of trauma. As this is a potentially treatable cause of stroke,[66] we advocate in all paediatric stroke non-invasive imaging by MRA not only of the intracranial circle of Willis but also of the entire great arteries of the neck from their origins at the aortic arch to their intracranial terminations. Radiological criteria for the diagnosis of dissection are visualisation of an intimal flap or a double lumen in the wall of the artery. These pathognomonic signs are detected in fewer than 10% of adult dissections by catheter angiography, which remains the gold standard for diagnosis. However, tapering arterial occlusion, the 'string sign' or 'rat's tail' appearance (Fig. 8-71), aneurysmal dilatation of the artery and eccentric mural thrombus are other less specific signs. Non-invasive angiographic techniques, CTA and MRA, are less sensitive and less specific than the gold standard of the more invasive DSA. The differences are more marked with the calibre of the vessel under consideration. It may be prudent to consider childhood posterior circulation strokes as caused by vertebral dissection until proven otherwise or cleared by DSA.

Vein of Galen aneurysmal malformations (VGAMs) are a rare cause of paediatric stroke but have a wide range of clinical presentations and account for 30% of vascular malformations in children. Their recognition is important as there is increasing evidence that appropriate endovascular treatment by neuroradiologists with specialist skill in dealing with paediatric high flow AV shunts in a multidisciplinary setting with access to neonatologists, anaesthetists and neurologists is associated with improved outcome. VGAMs are unique congenital malformations of the intracranial circulation characterised by an enlarged midline venous structure, a persistent embryological remnant, with multiple arteriovenous communications leading to aneurysmal dilatation, presumably secondary to high arteriovenous flow. Neonates may present with severe cardiac failure. In infants and children who present with VGAMs the degree of shunting is much smaller and they may have evidence of hydrocephalus with cerebral atrophy. Older children may have headaches and seizures, and also are more likely to develop intracerebral or subarachnoid haemorrhage.

MRI will demonstrate the dilated venous sac, location of fistulous connections and the arteries involved, venous drainage and any evidence of thrombus within the venous sac (Fig. 8-72). MRI can determine the extent of parenchymal damage, including focal infarctions and

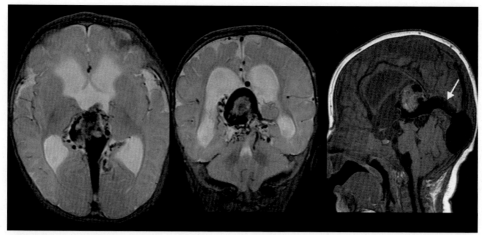

FIGURE 8-72 ■ Vein of Galen malformation (partly occluded by embolisation glue) showing residual flow through the promesencephalic vein, containing a combination of glue and thrombus, via the falcine sinus (arrow) towards the venous confluence. Arterial supply is via a number of choroidal vessels.

generalised cerebral atrophy, although CT is more sensitive for the parenchymal calcification which accompanies chronic venous hypertension. Angiography is the gold standard of diagnosis and ideally should be performed at the time of endovascular treatment. In imaging follow-up, evidence of significant arteriovenous shunting, progressive cerebral damage/atrophy and jugular vein occlusion as a chronic effect of venous hypertension should be sought.

HYPOXIC–ISCHAEMIC INJURY IN THE DEVELOPING BRAIN

Introduction

In the neonatal period brain injury due to hypoxia–ischaemia depends on the degree of brain maturation and on the severity of the event. Babies born preterm (gestational age at birth ≤ 36 weeks) react to hypoxia–ischaemia differently than full-term babies.[1,2] White matter injury is predominant in preterm babies, while grey matter is mostly injured in full-term babies.[3–5] Imaging plays an important role in the diagnostic work-up of these patients, with brain US being the first-line examination performed at bedside, followed by brain MRI. State-of-the-art brain US should be performed using sectorial and high-frequency linear transducers through the anterior, posterior and posterolateral fontanelles.[1,5] The MRI protocols consist of T_2 and T_1 conventional sequences, while diffusion imaging is increasingly becoming part of the routine. Special equipment for monitoring the vital signs, ventilators and, for very premature babies, MR-compatible incubators are necessary for safe and state-of-the-art brain MRI.

Encephalopathy of Premature Neonate—Patterns of Injury

Periventricular leukomalacia and brain haemorrhagic disease are the two main patterns of brain injury associated with hypoxia–ischaemia in the premature neonate.

Periventricular Leukomalacia

There are two forms of periventricular leukomalacia (PVL), the focal form (fPVL) and the diffuse form (dPVL). The pathological substrate of fPVL is necrosis of all cell elements of the brain tissue surrounding the lateral ventricles and that of dPVL is injury of the premyelinating oligodendrocytes (pre-OLs) associated with astrocytosis and microgliosis.[2,6] Long and short penetrating arteries with underdeveloped distal parts vascularise the immature brain.[2] Brain tissue between and at the end of these arteries represents watershed areas that receive deficient blood supply under conditions of hypoxia–ischaemia.[2] fPVL represents a watershed infarct in the periventricular white matter giving rise to micro- and macrocysts.[1] In dPVL, injury of pre-OLs results in decreased numbers of mature oligodendrocytes responsible for myelination and is characterised by hypomyelination and microstructural changes in brain connectivity.[2,7] In fPVL, brain US initially demonstrates hyperechogenic periventricular white matter which progressively (8–25 days) gives rise to the development of coalescent macro- or microcysts[1,5] (Figs. 8-73A, B). On brain MRI areas of impending fPVL appear with restricted diffusion and those with cystic components with increased diffusion.[8] Areas of established PVL are characterised by ventriculomegaly, irregular (in the case of fPVL) or regular (in dPVL) outline of the body of lateral ventricles, thinning of the periventricular white matter and signal abnormalities of the white matter in the peritriginal regions[9] (Figs. 8-73C, D). Cystic lesions of PVL appear with low signal intensity on T_1- and high signal on T_2-weighted sequences.[10] After corrected age of 1 month, the presence of abnormal signal intensity (low on T_1 and high on T_2) in the posterior limb of the internal capsule predicts a poor motor outcome.[5] Brain US is usually normal at the initial stages of dPVL. On brain MRI, dPVL is characterised by ventriculomegaly with regular outlines of the lateral ventricles (Fig. 8-74).

Brain Haemorrhagic Disease

Brain haemorrhagic disease consists of germinal matrix haemorrhage (GMH), intraventricular haemorrhage

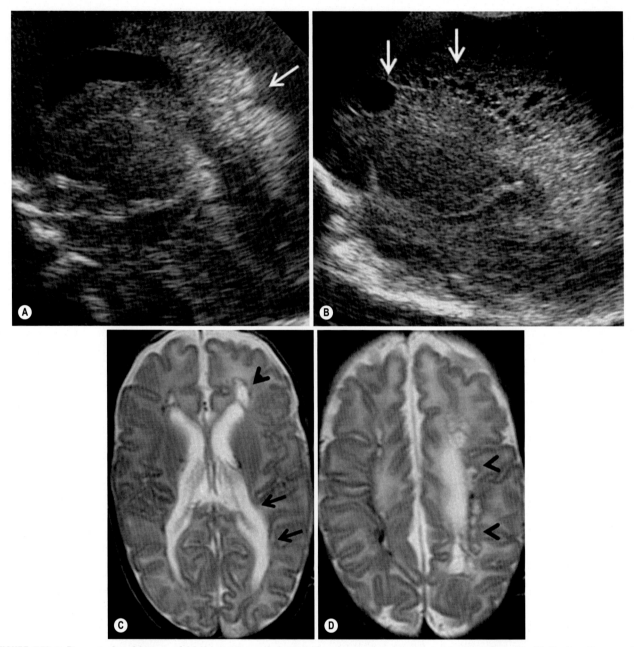

FIGURE 8-73 ■ **Prematurity, history of birth at 32 weeks' gestational age due to placental abruption.** (A, B) Brain ultrasound. Day 10 of life: sagittal (A) image demonstrating increased heterogeneous echogenicity of the periventricular white matter (arrow). Day 25 of life: sagittal (B) images demonstrating multiple cysts of the periventricular white matter (arrows). (C, D) Brain MRI. Chronological age 2.5 months: T_2-weighted axial images (C, D) demonstrating thinning of the periventricular white matter, irregular outline of the lateral ventricles (arrows) and periventricular cysts (arrowheads).

(IVH) and paraventricular haemorrhagic infarct (PHI). GMH may appear 24 h after birth and starts from the germinal matrix, a highly vascular collection of neuroglial precurcor cells located under the ventricular ependymal.[1,5] Regression of the germinal matrix starts at 12–16 gestational weeks and disappears at term. Around 24 gestational weeks, germinal matrix is only present under the frontal horns of the lateral ventricles. Increased vessel fragility and immature autoregulation of the cerebral blood flow are responsible for germinal matrix haemorrhage in premature babies.[5] Haemorrhage may be limited at the germinal matrix or extend into the ventricle with

or without associated ventricular dilatation. Brain US shows an ovoid lesion located anterior to the caudothalamic groove, initially homogeneously hyperechogenic, then heterogeneously hyperechogenic and finally cystic[5] (Figs. 8-75A, B). IVH may result from rupture of GMH into the ventricles or from bleeding at the level of choroid plexuses. Brain US shows echogenic material into the lateral ventricles, sometimes extending into the third ventricle[1] (Fig. 8-76). MRI demonstrates a variety of signal intensities, depending on the age of haemorrhage, with high signal at the subacute stage and signal void at the chronic stage.[5] Post-haemorrhagic hydrocephalus may appear as complication of large IVH. Paraventricular haemorrhagic infarct (PHI) is almost always associated with IVH and results from compression and obstruction of terminal veins lying under the germinal matrix.[5] Brain US shows a frontoparietal hyperechogenic triangular lesion pointing towards the lateral ventricle. A

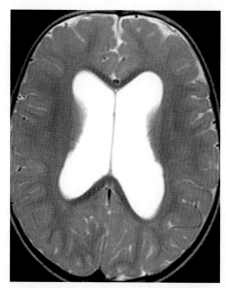

FIGURE 8-74 ■ **Prematurity, history of birth at 30 weeks' gestational age.** Brain MRI. Chronological age 2.5 months: T_2-weighted axial image demonstrating thinning of the periventricular white matter with regular outline of the lateral ventricles.

liquefaction and sometimes communication of the lesion with the lateral ventricle is observed at the latter stages[1] (Fig. 8-77). Lesions lying proximal to the ventricular trigones carry a better neurological outcome.[11] Early MRI demonstrates a haemorrhagic paraventricular lesion associated with IVH; late MRI shows a cystic lesion surrounded by gliosis and communicating with the lateral ventricle.

Encephalopathy of Term Neonate—Patterns of Injury

Depending on the severity of hypoxia–ischaemia, three main types of lesions have been described:[4,12]

1. Parasagittal lesions represent watershed infarcts affecting the cortex and the subcortical white matter at the territories between anterior and middle and posterior and middle cerebral arteries.[3,4] Decreased brain perfusion is the underlying cause. Brain US shows subcortical leukomalacia, initially hyperchogenic and then multicystic. In older children brain atrophy is observed in the affected areas.[13,14] Brain MRI reveals T_1 and T_2 prolongation of the affected areas.[12]

2. Diffuse lesions affecting the cortex, the basal ganglia and the white matter are due to partial prolonged asphyxia (1–3 h). Brain US shows initially increased echogenicity of the cortex and the basal ganglia and later macrocystic encephalomalacia.[4,13,14] Brain MRI reveals heterogeneous signal

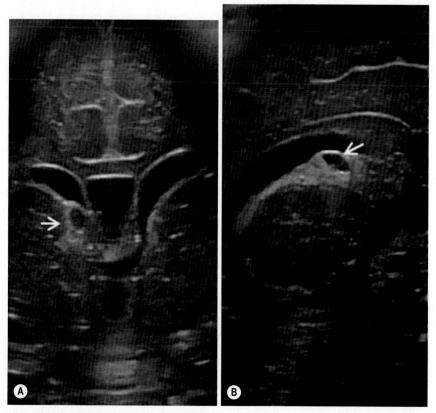

FIGURE 8-75 ■ **Prematurity, history of birth at 31 weeks' gestational age.** Brain ultrasound. Day 7 of life: coronal (A) and sagittal (B) images demonstrating a centrally cystic ovoid lesion located at the right lateral ventricle, anterior to the caudothalamic groove (arrows).

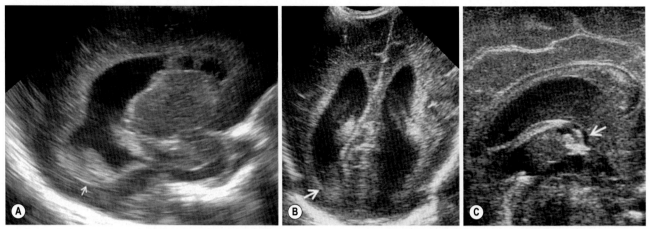

FIGURE 8-76 ■ **Prematurity, history of birth at 29 weeks' gestational age.** Brain ultrasound. Day 8 of life: sagittal (A) and coronal (B) images demonstrating echogenic material into the right lateral ventricle (arrows) compatible with blood. Midline sagittal (C) image demonstrates echogenic clot pending from the foramen of Monro into the third ventricle (arrow).

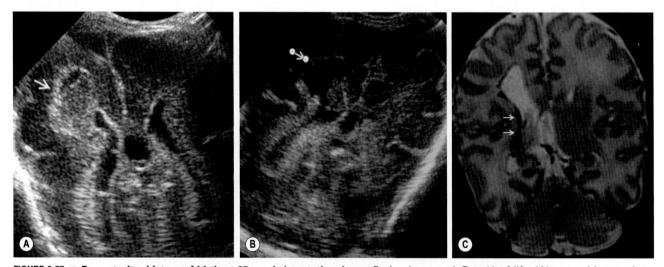

FIGURE 8-77 ■ **Prematurity, history of birth at 25 weeks' gestational age.** Brain ultrasound. Day 10 of life: (A) coronal image demonstrating echogenic venous infarct adjacent to right lateral ventricle (arrow). Day 20 of life: (B) coronal image demonstrating liquefaction of the lesion and the formation of a cavity communicating with the lateral ventricle (arrow). Brain MRI. Day 21 of life: (C) coronal T_2-weighted image shows the cystic infarct communicating with the right lateral ventricle. Signal void at the lateral wall of the ventricle (arrows) represents haemosiderin.

intensity of the white matter and focal loss of the grey–white matter differentiation ('missing cortex' sign). Follow-up MRI demonstrates macrocystic encephalomalacia[3,4] (Fig. 8-78).

3. Lesions of the basal ganglia, the perirolandic cortex and the brainstem may occur after acute total asphyxia (10–15 min).[12–14] Brain US reveals hyperechogenicity of the affected areas, and brain MRI shows heterogeneous increased signal intensity (Fig. 8-79). At later stages, atrophy develops.

MISCELLANEOUS ACQUIRED TOXIC OR METABOLIC DISEASE

Kernicterus is the result of the toxic effect of neonatal unconjugated hyperbilirubinaemia on the brain. The brain regions that have selective susceptibility include the globus pallidi, subthalamic nuclei and hippocampi, as well as cranial nerves VIII, VII and III. Neonates with bilirubin encephalopathy have a depressed conscious level, hypotonia and seizures with opisthotonus. Delayed effects include extrapyramidal signs (athetosis), deafness, gaze palsies and developmental delay. In the acute stage there is signal abnormality with bilateral symmetrical T_2 prolongation and swelling of the globus pallidi. There may be T_1 shortening also. Eventually the pallidal changes will progress to atrophy with variable persistent gliotic change. US and CT are initially normal, although later there may be evidence of calcification.

Hypoglycaemia may also present with a non-specific encephalopathy, subsequently leading to seizures. This is a problem particularly with neonates who have immature enzyme pathways and relatively poor glycogen reserves, particularly in the context of increased requirements due to sepsis or associated hypoxia–ischaemia but may also be

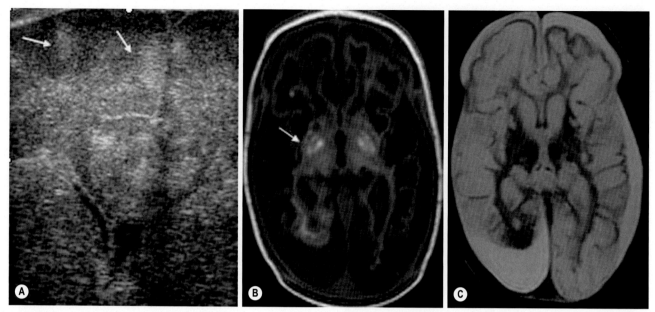

FIGURE 8-78 ■ **Full term, 37 weeks' gestational age severe prolonged perinatal asphyxia.** (A) Brain US. Day 3: coronal image demonstrating, heterogeneity of brain echostructure and increased echogenicity of the cortex (arrows). (B, C) Brain MRI. Day 20: axial T_1- and T_2-weighted images demonstrate extensive macrocystic encephalomalacia in the white matter and hypersignal of the putamen the pallidum (arrows).

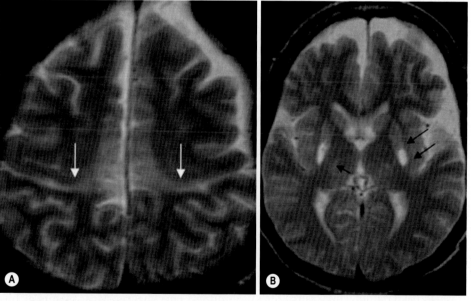

FIGURE 8-79 ■ **Full term, 38 weeks' gestational age severe perinatal asphyxia.** Dyskinetic cerebral palsy epilepsy, mental retardation. Brain MRI. 30 years: (A, B) axial T_2-weighted images demonstrating atrophy of the lentiform nuclei (arrowhead), signal abnormalities in the thalami (black arrows) and abnormal signal intensity in the perirolandic cortex (white arrows).

the end result of some inborn errors of metabolism or hyperinsulinism. Imaging studies may show evidence of a diffuse encephalopathy with brain swelling and oedema, but the findings are typically most severe in the parieto-occipital regions and thalami. There is T_1 and T_2 prolongation with swelling affecting the cortex and subcortical white matter with variable restricted diffusion (Fig. 8-80), progressing to the chronic sequelae of cerebral infarction

with evidence of gliosis, cavitation and atrophy. Pallidal damage may also occur.

Hypernatraemia is most commonly seen in premature infants, particularly if there is additional dehydration, e.g. due to diarrhoea. Affected infants have a depressed conscious level and irritability. There is an osmotic water shift from the intracellular to the extracellular space, resulting in interstitial oedema, manifest by T_1 and T_2

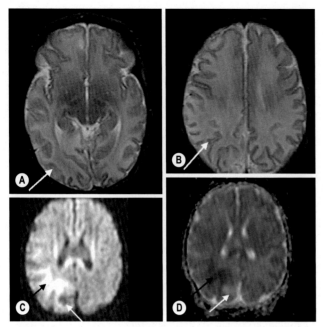

FIGURE 8-80 ■ Neonate with seizures and hypoglycaemia shows (A, B) increased signal within the parieto-occipital cortex and white matter, with patchy loss of the normal cortical low signal (arrows). (C) Diffusion-weighted image and (D) ADC map show that the diffusion changes are a mixture of restricted (black arrows) and increased diffusion (white arrows). *All* of these changes, including the T₂ and restricted areas of diffusion, completely resolved on follow-up.

prolongation with increased diffusion, but also in parenchymal haemorrhage as the brain shrinks and bridging dural veins are torn as they are pulled away from the calvarium.

Toxic exposure should be considered in children, particularly adolescents, with acute neurological symptoms and bilateral symmetrical grey matter involvement. Toxins include toluene or other organic solvents, cyanide and carbon monoxide poisoning, the latter also associated with bilateral symmetrical pallidal signal changes.

INTRACRANIAL AND INTRASPINAL INFECTIONS

Congenital Infections (TORCH)

These infections are acquired in utero or during passage through the birth canal; bacterial infections spread from the cervix to the amniotic fluid while toxoplasmosis, rubella, cytomegalovirus (CMV), syphilis and human immunodeficiency virus (HIV) spread via the transplacental route, and herpes simplex virus (HSV) is acquired from direct exposure to maternal type II herpetic genital lesions during delivery. The stage of brain development judged by the gestational age is more important than the actual organism in determining the pattern of CNS injury. Therefore in utero infections acquired before 16–18 weeks, when neurons are forming within the germinal matrix and migrating to form the cerebral cortex, produce lissencephaly and a small cerebellum. Spontaneous abortion is also a frequent outcome during this time.

Between 18 and 24 weeks, when the cortical neurons are organising but the immature brain is unable to mount an inflammatory response, the infective insult may produce localised dysplastic cortex, polymicrogyria and porencephaly. This is seen as a smooth-walled cavity isointense to CSF on all sequences in continuity with the ventricular system and without evidence of gliosis. From the third trimester onwards the insult results in asymmetrical cerebral damage with gliosis, cystic change and calcification.

CMV is the most common cause of serious viral infection in fetuses and neonates in the West, occurring in up to 1% of all births. It is acquired transplacentally and the vertical transmission rate is 30–40%. The classical manifestations of CMV disease at birth include hepatosplenomegaly, petechiae, thrombocytopenia, microcephaly, chorioretinitis and sensorineural deafness occurring in up to 10% of CMV infection, but there is also an increased risk of developing deafness and other neurological deficits up to 2 years after exposure. The mechanism of injury may be due to a direct insult to the germinal matrix cells leading to periventricular calcification, cortical malformations with microcephaly and cerebellar hypoplasia, or due to the virus causing a vascular insult.

Transfontanelle cranial US may demonstrate branching curvilinear hyperechogenicity in the basal ganglia, or 'lenticulostriate vasculopathy', which may also be seen with other congenital infections, hypoxia–ischaemia and trisomy 13 and 21. Infants affected in the second trimester have lissencephaly with a thin cortex, hypoplastic cerebellum, ventriculomegaly and periventricular calcification, which is more reliably detected on CT than MRI. Those injured later, probably during the period of cortical organisation in the second trimester, have polymicrogyria, with less ventricular dilatation and cerebellar hypoplasia, and later infection produces parenchymal damage, large ventricles, calcification and haemorrhage without an underlying structural brain malformation. Temporal pole cysts are also a feature.

Toxoplasmosis is a protozoan infection caused by ingestion by the mother of *Toxoplasma gondii* oocytes in undercooked meat. The transmission rate is high and increases from 30% at 6 months' gestation to approaching 100% at term. The incidence of congenital infection is approximately 1 in 1000 to 1 in 3400 but it accounts for 1% of all stillbirths. When the CNS is involved the infection may cause a granulomatous meningitis or diffuse encephalitis. Most infants at birth are asymptomatic, although sequelae such as seizures, hydrocephalus and chorioretinitis may appear later. Imaging features of microcephaly and parenchymal calcification are similar to CMV infection, although cerebellar hypoplasia and polymicrogyria are not seen, and the ventriculomegaly may be due to an active ependymitis causing obstructive hydrocephalus rather than diffuse cerebral damage (Fig. 8-81). The severity of brain involvement correlates with earlier maternal infection.

The CNS involvement in HSV is a rapidly disseminating diffuse encephalitis, unlike the pattern of involvement in children or adults in which disease starts within the mesial temporal lobes and spreads within the limbic

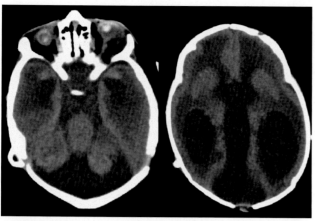

FIGURE 8-81 ■ **CT of a neonate with congenital TORCH infection.** Both the globes are small and calcified (phthisis bulbi). There is a Dandy–Walker malformation and hydrocephalus with transependymal oedema.

system. CT and MRI of neonatal infection show widespread asymmetrical regions of hypodensity or T_2 hyperintensity mainly in the white matter. As the disease progresses there is increasing swelling and cortical involvement (CT cortical hyperdensity and T_1/T_2 shortening on MRI) and meningeal enhancement. Subsequent loss of brain parenchyma occurs early on, often as early as the second week, eventually resulting in profound cerebral atrophy, cystic encephalomalacia and calcification.

Congenital rubella is now very rare in the West following the introduction of mass immunisation programmes, but immigrant populations remain at risk as do populations where uptake of the MMR vaccine is low. In the first 8 weeks, cataracts, glaucoma and cardiac malformations occur, while in the third trimester infection may be asymptomatic. Brain imaging appearances demonstrate similar changes to other congenital infections depending on the timing of the insult.

It is estimated that over 60 million people worldwide are infected with HIV. Almost half are women and vertical transmission of HIV accounts for 90% of newly diagnosed cases. Children with congenitally acquired AIDS usually present between the ages of 2 months and 8 years with non-specific signs such as hepatosplenomegaly and failure to thrive. Neonatal presentation is unusual. Affected children may develop a progressive HIV encephalopathy in which dementia, spasticity and increasing head size occur. A more static form is also seen in which cognitive and motor developmental delay predominate. Global atrophy and bilateral basal ganglia calcification are the most common imaging findings. Diffuse symmetrical periventricular and deep white matter abnormalities are seen in almost half of children with HIV encephalopathy and are usually associated with mild atrophy. HIV may also cause corticospinal tract degeneration.

Meningitis

Meningitis is the most common infection in childhood. The diagnosis is made not on imaging but on the presence of clinical symptoms and signs and the results of lumbar puncture. Indeed, in uncomplicated meningitis, the imaging is usually normal, and the role of neuroimaging is to detect the complications of meningitis. Neuroimaging is indicated when the diagnosis is unclear, if the meningitis is associated with persistent seizures or focal neurological deficits, if symptoms or signs suggest raised intracranial pressure, or when recovery is unduly slow.

Pathophysiology

Organisms reach the meninges by five main routes: direct spread from an adjacent infection, especially otitis media and sinusitis; haematogenous spread; rupture of a superficial cortical abscess; passage through the choroid plexus; or from direct penetrating trauma. Cerebral infarction (venous and arterial) is seen in 30% of neonates with bacterial meningitis. Infection spreads along the adventitia of penetrating cortical vessels within the periventricular spaces. Arterial thrombosis may arise from the resulting arterial wall inflammation and necrosis, or from a similar process affecting the arteries that traverse basal meningitic exudates. Venous thrombosis and subsequent infarction is particularly common in the presence of subdural empyemas due to veins becoming thrombosed as they traverse the infected subdural space. Extension of the infection through thrombosed vessels into the brain parenchyma can result in cerebritis and abscess formation. Fibropurulent exudates in the basal cisterns, ventricular outlet foramina or over the brain convexity result in hydrocephalus due either to the obstruction of CSF flow or failure of resorption. Ventriculitis occurs in about 30% of children with meningitis and is particularly common in neonates with ependymal changes seen in severe or prolonged meningitis. Later on, ventricular enlargement may persist due to damage to the adjacent periventricular white matter and parenchymal loss.

Neonatal meningitis has two distinct clinical presentations. The first presents in the first few days of life with overwhelming generalised sepsis, often in association with complicated labour, such as premature rupture of membranes. The second develops after the first week, with milder systemic sepsis but with more meningitic features.

In older infants and children acute bacterial meningitis has a mortality of 5% in the developed world, which rises to between 12% and 50% in developing countries where there is a high incidence of permanent neurological sequelae.

Uncomplicated Meningitis

Although neuroimaging is not performed for this indication alone and is usually normal, occasionally meningeal enhancement may be seen on CT or MRI. MRI is more sensitive than CT, but the sensitivity of either/both is insufficient to warrant imaging as a diagnostic test for meningitis. Imaging findings are more useful for chronic and granulomatous meningitides where dense enhancing basal exudates may be seen within the cisternal spaces. Recurrent meningitis is unusual and full neuro-axis imaging is often applied to identify underlying risk factors (see below).

Imaging of Complications (Table 8-4)

Hydrocephalus may be detected on CT or MRI and may reflect a combination of obstructed CSF flow and impaired absorption. Ependymitis may cause debris/haemorrhage within the ventricular system, resulting in obstructive hydrocephalus at the foramen of Monro, cerebral aqueduct and fourth ventricular outlet foramina. Purulent exudates may impair CSF absorption within the subarachnoid space, resulting in communicating hydrocephalus.

Sterile subdural effusions are often seen as a complication of meningitis, particularly in neonates with *Streptococcus pneumoniae* or *Haemophilus influenzae*. They are not empyemas, do not need to be surgically treated and will regress as the meningitis is treated. On imaging, the subdural collections have density and signal characteristics similar to CSF on CT and MRI, though they may be slightly hyperintense to CSF on MRI. Enhancement is not usually seen; however, leptomeningeal (pial) enhancement, to be distinguished from pachymeningeal (dural) enhancement, may be seen as a result of underlying brain infarction or due to leptomeningeal inflammation.

Subdural empyemas may require urgent surgical drainage to prevent further cerebritis and cerebral infarction. These appear as more proteinaceous subdural collections (increased density on CT, intermediate T_1 signal intensity relative to CSF, T_2 hyperintensity) with pachymeningeal (dural) and leptomeningeal enhancement (Fig. 8-82).

Imaging evidence for ventriculitis, usually spread via the choroid plexus, comes from the finding of debris layered posteriorly within the ventricular system and ependyma which are hyperdense on CT. Hydrocephalus may be seen and there may be isolation of various components of the ventricular system, resulting in some parts draining adequately while others remain dilated as debris obstructs the CSF outlet foramina. Infection may extend directly into the adjacent brain parenchyma, causing cerebritis.

Thrombosis of deep venous sinuses and cortical veins may occur, particularly in children with dehydration (Fig. 8-83). The symptoms of deep venous sinus thrombosis, such as headache, impaired consciousness and prolonged fitting, cannot be distinguished from the symptoms of the underlying meningitis and neuroimaging is required for confirmation. Cavernous sinus thrombosis is uncommon, is more commonly seen with paranasal sinus, dental or orbital infection, and tends to present with ophthalmoplegia due to involvement of the cranial nerves II, IV and VI as they pass through the cavernous sinus. Direct involvement of the cavernous carotid artery by infection may produce a mycotic aneurysm. In generalised sepsis, the sagittal and transverse sinuses are most commonly involved.

Deep venous sinus thrombosis may be seen as a hyperdense expanded sinus on unenhanced CT. As the thrombus becomes less dense, intravenous enhancement may demonstrate the 'empty delta' sign as a filling defect

TABLE 8-4 Intracranial Complications of Meningitis in Infants

Pathology	Imaging
Cerebritis	Diffuse hypodensity (CT), hyperintensity (T_2-weighted MRI) involving cortex and white matter, gyral swelling, ill-defined enhancement
Abscess formation	Peripheral rim enhancement surrounding central necrotic cavity, adjacent oedema
Subdural effusion	Cerebrospinal fluid density/signal subdural collection, no pathological enhancement
Empyema	Higher density (CT), restricted diffusion (MRI) subdural collection with pachymeningeal/dural enhancement
Deep venous thrombosis	Hyperdense expanded venous sinus (CT), lack of T_2 flow void, expanded sinus (MRI), variable haemorrhagic venous infarction
Cavernous sinus thrombosis	Expanded cavernous sinus, filling defects on CTV, signal drop off MRV
Arterial thrombosis	Large arterial territory infarct, basal ganglia/thalamic small perforating arterial territory infarcts
Ventriculitis	Debris within ventricular system, hyperdense ependyma (pre-contrast), ependymal contrast enhancement, ventricular isolation
Hydrocephalus	Obstructive intraventricular (foramen of Monro, cerebral aqueduct), obstructive extraventricular, communicating
Deafness	CT/MRI evidence of labyrinthitis ossificans

within the sinus lumen. A dense cortical vein may also be seen on CT, but neither CT nor MRI can reliably detect cortical vein thrombosis.

The diagnosis of deep venous sinus thrombosis may be missed in up to 40% of patients at CT; MRI with MR venography (MRV) is more sensitive. In the subacute phase thrombus is seen as T_1 shortening within an expanded sinus and this finding may be sufficient to make the diagnosis. In the acute phase when the thrombus is isointense on T_1-weighted imaging and hypointense on T_2-weighted imaging, it can be mistaken for flowing blood, although the sinus, in the latter, should not be expanded. MRV is useful to confirm absence of flow in the thrombosed sinus.

Venous infarction may occur in up to 40% of children with deep venous sinus thrombosis. Venous infarcts are often bilateral, do not conform to an arterial territory but to the territory of venous drainage, and are frequently haemorrhagic. They are parasagittal when the superior sagittal sinus is involved, thalamic when the internal cerebral veins or straight sinus/vein of Galen is involved and temporal lobe when the transverse or sigmoid sinus or vein of Labbé (one of the deep superficial venous system anastomoses connecting the middle cerebral vein to the transverse sinus) are involved. On diffusion imaging, there is a mixture of restricted and free diffusion even when non-haemorrhagic.

Arterial infarction may be seen as wedge-shaped cortical and white matter hypodensity conforming to a major

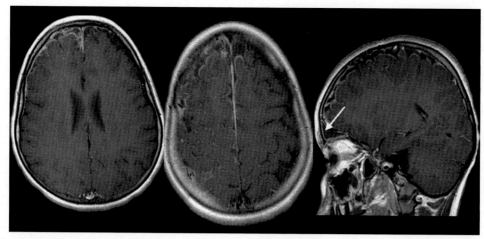

FIGURE 8-82 ■ **Bilateral subdural empyemas.** There is leptomeningeal and pachymeningeal enhancement (arrows) most marked over the right cerebral convexity and extending back to the vertex (on the sagittal view). There is enhancing debris within the subdural space and the signal is slightly increased compared to cerebrospinal fluid. The source of infection was from the frontal sinus (arrow).

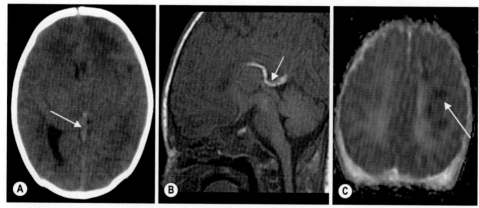

FIGURE 8-83 ■ **Venous sinus thrombosis in a child with recent history of nausea and vomiting.** (A) CT shows hyperdense thrombus within the vein of Galen just reaching the internal cerebral veins (arrow). There is diffuse cerebral swelling with more hypodense change and swelling affecting the left hemisphere and thalami. (B) Sagittal T_1-weighted MRI confirms the diagnosis with T_1 shortening in keeping with methaemoglobin in the internal cerebral veins and vein of Galen (arrow). (C) The ADC map shows patchy restricted diffusion (low signal) (arrow) within the deep white matter in keeping with infarction.

arterial territory on CT or as T_2 hyperintensity and T_1 hypointensity with cortical highlighting on MRI. The basal meningitis may occlude small perforating branches from the circle of Willis, causing small infarcts in the region of the deep grey nuclei (basal ganglia and thalami).

Labyrinthitis ossificans, the most common cause of acquired deafness in childhood, is one of the sequelae of bacterial meningitis resulting from direct spread of infection from the meninges into the inner ear. Faint enhancement of the membranous labyrinth may be seen on enhanced T_1-weighted images in acute infection. In some children inflammation persists; fibrosis and ossification subsequently develop and may be detected on high-resolution CT of the temporal bone, as increased density within the membranous labyrinth. High-resolution T_2-weighted MRI (e.g. performed with 3DFT-CISS imaging) may be more sensitive than CT to the changes of labyrinthitis ossificans, and T_2 signal drop-off may detect the fibrous stage before ossification when children are still suitable for cochlear implantation. Once the typical appearances of diffuse labyrinthitis ossificans develop, cochlear implantation is much more difficult (Fig. 8-84).

Tuberculous Infection

Tuberculosis (TB) has risen in incidence recently, and while it remains a serious problem in children, there does not appear to have been an increase in tuberculous meningitis in children as yet, possibly due to targeted immunisation of at-risk immigrant populations. TB may cause meningitis, cerebritis and abscess formation (tuberculomas). With leptomeningeal disease, which may be seen without evidence of miliary TB elsewhere, thick enhancing purulent soft-tissue exudates may be seen in the subarachnoid space, particularly in the basal cisterns, and associated with hydrocephalus, basal ganglia and thalamic infarcts. Larger major arterial branch cortical infarcts are seen less frequently. Tuberculomas are seen as solid or ring-enhancing lesions, particularly at the grey–white matter junction.

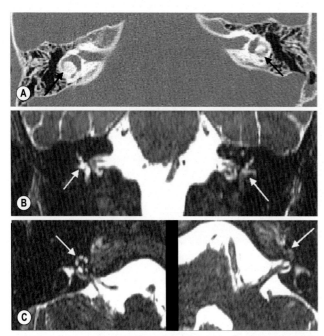

FIGURE 8-84 ■ **Child with recent meningitis and new sensorineural deafness.** (A) High-resolution axial CT through the petrous bones shows increased density in keeping with calcification within the lateral semicircular canals (arrows). (B) Coronal and (C) axial CISS MRI show reduced T_2 signal within all the semicircular canals (arrows), particularly the left, confirmed on the oblique axial views (C). There is reduced signal within the cochlea, again worse on the left (arrows). These are typical features of labyrinthitis ossificans.

Bacterial Infection: Cerebritis and Abscess Formation

Cerebritis is the earliest stage of purulent brain infection, may be focal or multifocal, and may resolve or evolve into frank abscess formation. Predisposing conditions include middle ear, dental and paranasal sinus infection, penetrating injury, postoperative complication or dermal sinus, immune deficiency, and any cause of arteriovenous shunting (e.g. cyanotic congenital heart disease). Fungal infection may also cause brain abscesses, particularly in immunocompromised children, but in this case the lesion may not be able to encapsulate because this requires the ability to mount an adequate immune response. Radiological differentiation between cerebritis and abscess formation is important because cerebritis may respond to antibiotics while an abscess may require surgical drainage as an adjunct. During the cerebritis stage CT and MRI show an ill-defined area of oedema with swelling with or without variable ill-defined enhancement and haemorrhagic transformation. As the infection becomes more established, focal areas may become walled-off and abscess formation occurs. On imaging this appears as a space-occupying lesion with a central region of pus manifest as low density on CT, or T_2 hyperintensity on MRI, surrounded by an enhancing wall. The wall of the cavity may demonstrate T_1/T_2 shortening. Typically there is surrounding oedema. The central region of pus shows restricted diffusion and this may help to differentiate abscesses from necrotic or cystic tumours which usually demonstrate central areas of increased diffusion. Imaging can be used to monitor response to treatment although there may be a lag time between the resolution of imaging findings and clinical response.

Neurocysticercosis

Cysticercosis occurs from ingestion of the encysted form of *Taenia solium* (porcine tapeworm). Humans act as the intermediate host and neurological disease occurs as the host mounts an inflammatory response and the parasites die. In children a typical presentation is with parenchymal cysts associated with seizures, headache and focal neurological deficits. These may occur anywhere within the brain but typically at the grey–white matter interface. Calcification may occur and may be punctate within the solid component or may occur within the wall of the cyst. Perilesional oedema is the result of the inflammatory response to the dying larva. Lesions at various stages of development may be seen. Therefore active lesions seen as regions of oedema may coexist with ring or solid enhancing lesions with or without oedema, and with foci of calcification without oedema or enhancement which are burnt-out lesions following the death of the parasite.

There are also leptomeningeal, intraventricular and racemose forms of neurocysticercosis. Leptomeningeal disease is demonstrated on CT or MRI by soft tissue filling the basal cisterns with marked contrast enhancement. Granulomata with variable calcification may be seen within the subarachnoid space. Hydrocephalus and brain infarcts are also complications. Intraventricular cysticerci are important to detect because of the risk of acute-onset hydrocephalus and sudden death. MRI is more sensitive than CT at identifying the cysts with their scolex. In the racemose form there are multilobular cysts without a scolex within the subarachnoid space, typically in the cerebellopontine angles, suprasellar region and basal cisterns and Sylvian fissures. They may demonstrate enhancement and may coexist with leptomeningitis.

Viral Encephalitis

The typical pattern of viral encephalitis is that of patchy and asymmetrical disease with a predeliction for grey matter. The anterior temporal and inferior frontal cortical regions are a classical location for herpes encephalitis. Another characteristic herpes virus pattern is the involvement of the hippocampi and cingulate gyrus as a limbic encephalitis. More widespread hemispheric involvement is seen with a variety of enteroviruses, echovirus and Coxsackie virus in particular.

A more unusual pattern of deep grey matter and upper brainstem disease is seen with rare types of viral encephalitis. Patchy enhancement with oedema has been seen with Epstein–Barr virus infection and may also be mimicked by mycoplasma infection. Thalamic and upper brainstem involvement, occasionally with haemorrhagic change, is a feature of Japanese encephalitis and the related West Nile virus.

Acute cerebellitis presents infrequently in children with sudden onset of truncal ataxia, dysarthria, involuntary eye movements due to a swollen cerebellum, and nausea, headache and vomiting due to resulting hydrocephalus. Fever and meningism may also be present. The many causes of a swollen cerebellum include infectious (e.g. pertussis), post-infectious (e.g. acute disseminated encephalomyelitis [ADEM]), toxic, such as lead poisoning, and vasculitis. Imaging shows effacement of the cerebellar fissures, enlarged cerebellum, signal abnormality affecting the cortex and white matter, and variable hydrocephalus. Although the cerebellar swelling may resolve spontaneously, surgical CSF diversion may be necessary as a temporary measure.

Infection in Immunocompromised Children

Children with primary, acquired or iatrogenic immuno-deficiencies are vulnerable to opportunistic and unusual organisms. Examples include fungal infections such as aspergillosis, actinomyces and unusual bacterial infections such as atypical mycobacteria. The host's ability to develop an inflammatory response may be limited and the interpretation of images should be considered in this context. Contrast enhancement remains a useful hallmark. A diffuse pattern of nodular leptomeningeal and parenchymal disease may be seen. Conversely, focal large parenchymal abscesses or mycetomas may develop.

Spinal Infections

The patterns of discitis and spondylitis in children are similar to those of young adults and do not need to be discussed in detail in this chapter. However, special mention should be made of congenital spinal abnormalities that may harbour or increase the risk of spinal infection. These children may present with recurrent meningitis. Spinal imaging may reveal a dorsal dermal sinus tract or an intraspinal dermoid.

Brain and Cord Inflammation

Children may develop CNS disease known as acute disseminated encephalomyelitis (ADEM) following an infection, usually viral, or vaccination. This is assumed to be a post-infectious inflammatory immune-mediated phenomenon. Affected children present with focal neurological deficits, headache, fever and altered consciousness following a recent infection. Classically, ADEM is a monophasic disease occurring at multiple sites within the brain and spinal cord. Most children recover completely, although 10–30% will have a permanent neurological deficit. Occasionally ADEM may present with relapses occurring within a few months of the original presentation, but these are still considered as part of a monophasic inflammatory process. When relapses occur that are more disseminated in time or place, the diagnosis of multiple sclerosis (MS) may be made. On follow-up imaging, children with ADEM have no new lesions and complete or partial resolution of the majority of old lesions, while in MS there are new lesions which may or may not be symptomatic.

On MRI, multiple asymmetrical areas of demyelination seen as increased signal intensity on T_2-weighted imaging with swelling occur within the subcortical white matter of both hemispheres and may also involve the cerebellum and spinal cord. Cortical and deep grey matter may also be involved but to a lesser extent (Fig. 8-85). Diffusion-weighted imaging shows increased free diffusion within the lesions. Occasionally, a fulminant haemorrhagic form may develop. Periventricular and callosal lesions (such as Dawson's fingers) are more in keeping with MS lesions, while cortical abnormality is not seen with MS and deep grey matter involvement, though seen in both, is more frequent in ADEM. Other differentials include viral encephalitis, which typically is more cortically based, and vasculitis (the lesions should also show restricted diffusion).

TRAUMA

Birth Trauma

Extracranial haemorrhage may be seen as a consequence of birth trauma and more often with instrumental

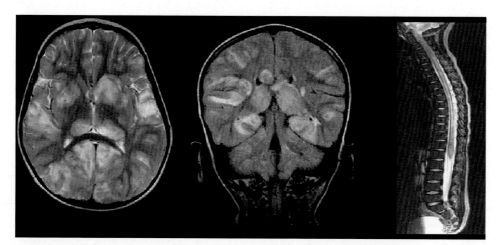

FIGURE 8-85 ■ **Acute disseminated encephalomyelitis in an 11-year-old boy with recent viral illness and acute impaired consciousness.** MRI shows bilateral, asymmetrical, mainly subcortical, cerebral hemisphere white matter lesions but also involving the cortex and deep grey matter. The cerebellum and spinal cord are also involved. There is focal swelling of the involved regions. The imaging features are typical of acute disseminated encephalomyelitis. The child made a full recovery.

delivery. It does not usually require imaging but may be detected on images done for intracranial assessment. Subgaleal haemorrhage may occur deep to the scalp aponeurosis. As there is a large potential space, the extent of haemorrhage may occasionally be severe, requiring transfusion. Cephalhaematoma is a traumatic subperiosteal haemorrhage between the vault and the outer layer of periosteum and is therefore confined by the sutures. It may calcify peripherally where the periosteum calcifies. Very rarely, forceps may cause skull fractures. These may be linear, depressed or 'ping pong' (depressed without a fracture line, but to be distinguished from an asymptomatic parietal depression which is a normal variant) with a cephalhaematoma overlying them. Caput succedaneum is due to diffuse oedema and bleeding under the scalp and is more commonly seen with prolonged vaginal or ventouse delivery.

Birth trauma can result in a subdural haematoma, which may be seen even without instrumental delivery. Most are small, clinically silent and infratentorial, although they may extend above the tentorium cerebelli, and resolve spontaneously within 4 weeks. Occasionally they are large and associated with extensive intracranial haemorrhage and hydrocephalus. However, small posterior fossa subdural bleeds are common incidental findings on MRI when newborn infants are imaged for clinical CNS illness.

The spinal cord may be injured by distraction during a difficult delivery, usually a breech delivery, typically affecting the lower cervical and upper thoracic regions. The cord can be transected while the soft and compliant spine remains undamaged. A more common birth-related neurological injury is brachial plexus damage secondary to traction of the shoulder during a breech delivery of the head. Brachial plexus MRI may show CSF signal pseudomeningoceles around the avulsed nerve roots.

Growing Skull Fractures

Growing skull fractures are seen when there is a dural tear deep to the fracture and usually also when there is localised brain parenchymal damage, which may be associated with a focal neurological deficit or seizures (Fig. 8-86). CSF pulsation may keep the tear open, preventing healing of both the dura and the fracture. The fracture margins become progressively widened on serial radiographs and are bevelled and sclerotic. It usually occurs in children under 1 year with 90% occurring under the age of 3. A leptomeningeal cyst with arachnoid adhesions can cause further pressure erosion.

Spinal Trauma

The investigation of spinal trauma in children requires knowledge of the normal appearances of the developing spine on plain radiographs. The distance between the anterior arch of C1 and the dens can be up to 5 mm in normal children, and there is increased mobility not only between C1 and C2 but also between C3 and C4. The prevertebral soft tissues should not exceed two-thirds of the width of the C2 vertebral body. Increased mobility in many children allows anterior 'pseudoluxation' of C2 on

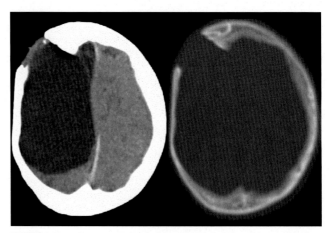

FIGURE 8-86 ■ **Large cerebral parenchymal defect in association with frontal bone defect which increased in size following a frontal bone linear fracture.** Note the well-corticated margins of the fracture.

C3 by up to 4 mm but the posterior elements should always remain correctly aligned and the distance should reduce in extension.

There is generalised ligamentous laxity of the immature spine. This may allow significant injury to the spinal cord in the absence of detectable bony injury causing SCIWORA (spinal cord injury without radiographic abnormality). In the appropriate clinical setting a proper evaluation may therefore require carefully performed flexion and extension views, and MRI to look for soft tissue and cord injury.

Atlanto-Axial Rotatory Fixation

This entity is discussed in this section for convenience, although there is often little or no history of trauma in these cases. Torticollis is common in children. Most cases are acute and the symptoms disappear without treatment within a week. Rarely it may be caused by rotatory fixation between C1 and C2, and with variable degrees of subluxation, and may occur within a normal range of movement and without subluxation. Atlanto-axial rotatory fixation should be suspected if the symptoms of torticollis persist for more than 2 weeks. The diagnostic test (CT is best) must prove that there is a fixed relationship between C1 and C2 in all positions, and in particular, on turning the head to the opposite side of the clinical presentation. Atlanto-axial rotatory fixation is present if there is rotation between C1 and C2 which remains constant throughout all positions. The treatment is aggressive with traction; if it is unsuccessful, the atlanto-axial rotatory fixation will result in a permanent rotatory malalignment requiring surgery. Secondary degenerative changes and eventually fusion may occur.

Non-Accidental Head Injury

Imaging of the brain is particularly important for the diagnosis of the so-called 'shaken baby syndrome' (see also Chapter 6). The triad of retinal haemorrhages, subdural haemorrhages and encephalopathy is accepted as a useful marker for this condition. The mechanism for injury is thought to be that of vigorous or violent shaking or such shaking followed by an impact injury. The emphasis is on rapid and alternating forces of acceleration and deceleration acting on an unsupported head. The strength of force required to cause these injuries is unknown and not easy to study scientifically. However, experienced workers would agree that such injuries cannot occur from the normal handling of an infant or young child. Subarachnoid haemorrhage, cerebral contusions, lacerations or 'splits' in the brain parenchyma and diffuse cerebral oedema with little evidence of external impact injury are supportive hallmarks of the shaken baby syndrome.

During shaking, the brain also comes into contact with the inner surface of the skull, and there may also be a final impact, and cerebral contusions are seen. The mechanism behind the repeated trauma also causes shearing injuries in the brain, often located in the subcortical region at the junction of white and grey matter. MRI detects these injuries more frequently than CT. Brain oedema is a very important feature of the shaken baby syndrome, the mechanism of which is hypothesised to be due to hypoxic–ischaemic injury. The oedema is usually massive, with reduced or absent grey–white matter differentiation, and is worst in the parieto-occipital regions. The basal ganglia, brainstem and cerebellum are, in turn, relatively preserved. The outcome of brain injury caused by shaking when severe brain oedema is present is usually grim. There is rapid destruction of brain tissue and significant atrophy becomes obvious after 2–3 weeks. In severe cases the end result is multicystic encephalomalacia, and microcephaly with marked mental and motor disability (Fig. 8-87).

HYDROCEPHALUS

The term 'hydrocephalus', literally 'water on the brain', is unfortunately a non-specific term which refers to any condition in which the ventricles are enlarged, including cerebral atrophy. The clinical and radiological challenge is to identify those forms that are likely to benefit from intervention. Some qualifying terms have been used to distinguish some of these entities. The terms communicating and non-communicating hydrocephalus are used to indicate extraventricular obstructive hydrocephalus and intraventricular obstructive hydrocephalus, respectively. These need to be distinguished from ventriculomegaly due to underlying lack of brain parenchyma, through atrophy or primary lack of brain development; some authors have suggested avoiding the use of the term hydrocephalus altogether for these cases. The concepts fail to hold true in a sizeable minority of cases, where the changes following intervention may not appear to follow expectations. For these, an appreciation of the complexities of CSF physiology may be helpful. Although it is generally accepted that those forms of hydrocephalus that are likely to benefit from interventions are caused by an imbalance between CSF production and absorption, the exact pathophysiology of these mechanisms remains incompletely understood. CSF is produced by the choroid

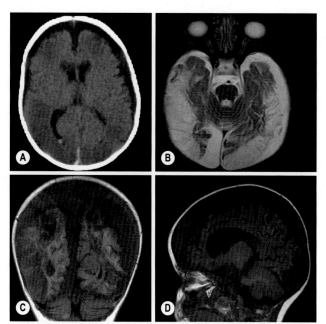

FIGURE 8-87 ■ **Brain injury in 'shaken baby syndrome'.** (A) The initial CT shows posterior interhemispheric subdural and intraventricular blood. There are bilateral hypodense subdural collections overlying both hemispheres. Extensive bilateral hypodense parenchymal lesions consistent with contusions or infarction are seen. (B) Follow-up MRI shows evolution of the parenchymal damage with marked atrophy and large chronic subdural collections. (C) Coronal and (D) sagittal T_1-weighted sequence shows the subdural collections have signal slightly greater than cerebrospinal fluid in keeping with proteinaceous contents from previous haemorrhage. There is cortical T_1 shortening suggesting the parenchymal lesions are regions of cerebral infarction.

plexuses and is mostly absorbed through the brain and cord with a lesser contribution from the arachnoid granulations. There is a net flow of CSF through the ventricular system, from lateral to third to fourth ventricles, which is influenced by cerebrovascular pulsations.

Post-haemorrhagic and post-infective hydrocephalus account for a significant proportion of hydrocephalus presenting in neonates and infants. Apart from these, congenital causes include aqueductal stenosis/gliosis, Chiari II malformation (usually occurring after repair of the associated lumbosacral myelomeningocele) and other malformations such as the Dandy–Walker malformation. Rarer causes include congenital midline tumours and vascular (e.g. vein of Galen) malformations. Before closure of the fontanelles (i.e. up to 2 years), the most reliable clinical sign is progressive macrocephaly documented by serial head circumference measurements. Caution should be exercised in the case of an asymmetrical skull or preferential growth in one direction due to craniosynostosis, which may give a spuriously enlarged head circumference without hydrocephalus. Alongside an increasingly disproportionate head circumference which crosses centiles on growth charts, other features of hydrocephalus in this age group include frontal bossing, calvarial thinning, presence of a tense, bulging anterior fontanelle, sutural diastasis and enlargement of scalp veins. Sunsetting eyes with failure of upward gaze, lateral rectus palsies and leg spasticity due to stretching of the corticospinal tracts as they descend from the motor strip around the ventricles are also seen.

In older children posterior fossa neoplasms and aqueduct stenosis are the most common causes of hydrocephalus. Early morning headache, nausea, vomiting, papilloedema, leg spasticity, cranial palsies and alterations in conscious level are the dominant clinical features as the skull is rigid. The fontanelles have fused and the sutures are fusing, and therefore increasing head circumference, fontanelle bulging and sutural diastasis are not features.

Imaging indicators of intraventricular obstructive (non-communicating) hydrocephalus include dilatation of the temporal horns disproportionate to lateral ventricular dilatation, enlargement of the anterior and posterior recesses of the third ventricle with inferior convexity of the floor of the third ventricle, transependymal (periventricular interstitial) oedema and bulging of fontanelles The sulcal spaces, major fissures and basal cisterns are small or obliterated. A careful survey of the regional ventricular dilatation may reveal the location as well as the cause of obstruction. Other features, such as changes in the configuration of the frontal horns of the lateral ventricles, specifically widening of the radius of the frontal horn, and a decrease in the angle it makes with the midline plane, are less useful. Further features classically described in chronic hydrocephalus, such as erosion of the dorsum sellae and copper-beaten skull, are even less reliable.

Extraventricular obstructive (communicating) hydrocephalus, however, may reveal a range of findings from ventricular and sulcal prominence to 'normal' CT/MRI appearances. It may have a variety of causes, ranging from haemorrhage and proteinaceous cellular debris with infection and disseminated malignancy to venous hypertension from impaired venous drainage to impaired arterial compliance from diffuse arteriopathies. In some cases, a combination of both forms of obstructive hydrocephalus would be expected.

Assessment of the cortical sulci for effacement disproportionate to ventricular size in children can be difficult and it requires some knowledge of the normal appearances for age; in normal younger children, under 2, the ventricles and subarachnoid spaces are more prominent, and should not be misinterpreted as 'atrophic' or due to hydrocephalus. Knowledge of the head size is important in making this distinction, being large in hydrocephalus and benign enlargement of the subarachnoid spaces, or small if there is cerebral atrophy. Again it may not be possible to be certain about the findings in the absence of serial measurements documenting trends. In benign enlargement of the subarachnoid spaces, there is believed to be a mismatch between the rate of skull growth and rate of growth of the developing brain. The child is neurologically normal. There is rapid skull growth, often to above the 95th centile by the time of presentation, but this then stabilises and both the size of the subarachnoid spaces and head size have usually normalised by age 2 years. The extra space anterior to the cerebral convexities is distinguishable from subdural collections by lack of mass effect on the adjacent brain and the presence of crossing veins within the subarachnoid space. The

importance of its recognition is to indicate that no intervention is required, with the expectation that the situation will normalise with age.

In the second decade the hemispheric cortical sulci become much less conspicuous and the ventricles less prominent, which should equally not be misinterpreted as due to cerebral oedema or the presence of a 'tight' brain. In this case in the normal child the basal cisterns should not be effaced.

An attempt should be made to identify a structural cause for the hydrocephalus. The narrowest parts of the ventricular system are the most susceptible to mechanical obstruction, i.e. the foramina of Monro, cerebral aqueduct and fourth ventricular outflow foramina. Masses causing obstructive hydrocephalus at the foramina of Monro include superior extension of suprasellar tumours and arachnoid cysts, colloid cysts, which may cause sudden acute and life-threatening hydrocephalus, and giant cell astrocytomas in tuberous sclerosis. Masses effacing the cerebral aqueduct include tectal plate gliomas, superior extension of midline posterior fossa tumours and brainstem diffuse astrocytomas and inferior extension of pineal region tumours. Atrial diverticula from dilated lateral ventricles may herniate into the quadrigeminal and supracerebellar cisterns and may also compress the tectum. These may be distinguished from large arachnoid cysts using multiplanar MRI to confirm continuity with the ventricular system.

More diffuse patterns of obstruction, including isolation of pockets of CSF, may be caused by haemorrhage, infection, disseminated tumour and reparative fibrosis. Clues to the underlying cause include evidence of haemosiderin staining or superficial siderosis in previous haemorrhage; focal atrophy or porencephaly from previous haematomas; the presence of hyperdense exudates in the basal cisterns, subarachnoid space and pial enhancement with infection or pial neoplastic dissemination.

Aqueduct stenosis is one of the most common causes of hydrocephalus in children but may present at any time from birth to adulthood. It may be developmental or acquired gliosis secondary to infection or intraventricular haemorrhage. Classically, the lateral and third ventricles are dilated and the fourth ventricle is of normal size, and there is no evidence of a tectal plate tumour. On sagittal MRI there is focal narrowing of the cerebral aqueduct, normally proximally at the level of the superior colliculi or at the intercollicular sulcus with posterior displacement of the tectal plate. Proximal to this, the aqueduct is dilated. Occasionally a congenital web may be seen as a very thin sheet of tissue across the distal aqueduct.

Overproduction of CSF is a very rare cause of hydrocephalus, most often seen with choroid plexus papillomas. These tumours may cause hydrocephalus by other mechanisms, e.g. obstructive hydrocephalus of the lateral ventricle due to mass effect at the body/trigone or foramen of Monro of the lateral ventricle, and haemorrhage within the ventricular system. A highly proteinaceous exudate produced by the tumour can cause communicating hydrocephalus due to impaired extraventricular drainage of CSF. Spinal cord tumours may be associated with hydrocephalus due to proteinaceous exudates or pial dissemination of disease, both causing impaired absorption of CSF. Indeed, in the cases of unexplained hydrocephalus, spinal imaging is recommended to exclude a possible occult intraspinal lesion.

Chiari II malformation is a common cause of hydrocephalus presenting early in life. The underlying aetiology is disputed; it may not be due to simple craniocervical junction obstruction but due to the displacement of the fourth ventricular outlet foramina within the spinal canal inferior to the foramen magnum, i.e. within the spinal canal, where the capacity for CSF absorption is reduced. Some specific features should be looked for when assessing these children for hydrocephalus or shunt malfunction. Children with occipital headaches at night probably have some degree of shunt malfunction which may present with potentially fatal signs of brainstem compression and apnoeic attacks. Also, the fourth ventricle should be slit-like, so the presence of a normal-sized or enlarged fourth ventricle suggests a shunt malfunction or isolation of the fourth ventricle requiring diversion.

Finally, hydrocephalus may be seen as a consequence of raised intracranial venous pressure. Examples include syndromic skull base abnormalities in craniosynostosis(es) and leading to stenosis of the jugular outflow foramina. Vascular causes include venous thrombosis, the vein of Galen aneurysmal malformation and dural arteriovenous shunts. Persistent untreated raised intraventricular pressure may result in secondary parenchymal damage affecting adjacent white matter and resulting in impaired cognitive function, permanent spasticity and blindness.

As well as by removing the obstructive lesion, hydrocephalus can be treated by CSF diversion. This can be performed initially by external ventricular drainage, or more permanently by ventriculoperitoneal, ventriculoatrial shunting, or third ventriculostomy. Here a surgical defect is made in the floor of the third ventricle, allowing CSF drainage into the suprasellar cistern.

Shunt malfunction from obstruction of the shunt by choroid plexus or glial tissue and subsequent ventricular dilatation is best assessed by comparison with baseline or previous imaging. In addition to a recurrence of the signs of hydrocephalus, there may be the appearance of fluid tracking along the length of the shunt tubing. Assessment of shunt tubing integrity may be made by plain radiograph imaging of the tube from the skull to the abdomen/pelvis. The scout view of a brain CT may also be useful to pick up disrupted shunt tubing or disconnection of the valve. As well as separation of the fragments, calcification may be seen at either end of the shunt disruption due to inflammation and fibrotic change where the shunt has become tethered and then distracted. Knowledge of the type of shunt inserted, or discussion with the neurosurgeon who inserted it, should allow distinction of the normal radiolucent components of the shunt (often as it exits the calvarium) from shunt distraction.

Patency of a third ventriculostomy can be inferred on MRI by visualising the surgical defect and detecting rapid CSF flow through it into the suprasellar cistern, manifest as large hypointense flow voids on T_2-weighted imaging. This may be aided by imaging without any flow compensation.

The incidence of shunt infection has declined over the years and in most neurosurgical centres runs at around 1–5%, being slightly higher in infants. Imaging may detect evidence of ventriculitis: enlarged ventricles with hyperdense ependyma on CT, ependymal enhancement and debris within the ventricular system. This may progress to cerebritis with devastating consequences for the developing brain parenchyma. Other shunt complications include the development of abdominal ascites, pseudocyst formation and perforated abdominal viscus. Rarely, shunted hydrocephalic patients may become symptomatic without ventricular dilatation and develop the 'slit ventricle' syndrome. This has a number of potential causes which include overdrainage of CSF, stiff, poorly compliant ventricles which allow raised intraventricular pressure without ventricular dilatation, intermittent shunt malfunction and headaches unrelated to the shunt.

SUMMARY

Paediatric neuroradiology is a subspecialist field drawing from knowledge and expertise in neuroimaging, neuropathology, paediatrics, embryology and genetics. Some skill is required in adapting neuroimaging techniques to suit the paediatric population, especially in terms of sedation/general anaesthesia and image optimisation. The range of conditions encountered is very different from that seen in adults. The management aims and options are also often different from adult cases.

REFERENCES

1. Barkovich AJ. Concepts of myelin and myelination in neuroradiology. Am J Neuroradiol 2000;21:1099–109.
2. Wimberger DM, Roberts TP, Barkovich AJ, et al. Identification of 'premyelination' by diffusion weighted MRI. J Comput Assist Tomogr 1995;19:28–33.
3. Huppi PS, Maier SE, Peded S, et al. Microstructural development of human newborn cerebral white matter assessed in vivo by diffusion tensor magnetic resonance imaging. Pediatr Res 1998;44:584–90.
4. Engelbrecht V, Rassek M, Preiss S, et al. Age-dependent changes in magnetization transfer contrast of white matter in the pediatric brain. Am J Neuroradiol 1998;19:1923–9.
5. Barkovich AJ. MR of the normal neonatal brain: assessment of deep structures. Am J Neuroradiol 1998;19:1397–403.
6. Barkovich AJ, Kjos BO, Jackson DE, et al. Normal maturation of the neonatal and infant brain: MR imaging at 1.5T. Radiology 1988;166:173–80.
7. Yakovlev PI, Lecours AR. The myelogenetic cycles of regional maturation of the brain. In: Minkowski A, editor. Regional Development of the Brain in Early Life. Oxford: Blackwell; 1967. pp. 3–70.
8. Van der Knaap MS, Van Wezel-Miejler G, Barth PG, et al. Normal gyration and sulcation in preterm and term neonates: appearance on MR images. Radiology 1996;200:389–96.
9. Martin E, Kikinis R, Zuerrer M, et al. Developmental stages of human brain: an MR study. J Comput Assist Tomogr 1988;12:917–22.
10. Barkovich AJ, Kjos BO. Normal postnatal development of the corpus callosum as demonstrated by MR imaging. Am J Neuroradiol 1988;9:487–91.
11. Aoki S, Okada Y, Nishimura K, et al. Normal deposition of brain iron in childhood and adolescence: MR imaging at 1.5T. Radiology 1989;172:381–5.
12. Cox TD, Elster AD. Normal pituitary gland: changes in shape, size and signal intensity during the first year of life at MR imaging. Radiology 1991;179:721–4.
13. Tortori-Donati P, Fondelli M, Rossi A, et al. Cystic malformations of the posterior cranial fossa originating from a defect of the posterior membranous area. Mega cisterna magna and persisting

Blake's pouch: two separate entities. Childs Nerv Syst 1996;12: 303–308.

14. Hart MN, Malamud N, Ellis WG. The Dandy–Walker syndrome. A clinicopathological study based on 28 cases. Neurology 1972; 22:771–80.

15. Joubert M, Eisenring JJ, Robb JP, et al. Familial agenesis of the cerbellar vermis. A syndrome of episodic hyperpnea, abnormal eye movements, ataxia and retardation. Neurology 1969;19:813–25.

16. Kendall B, Kingsley D, Lambert SR, et al. Joubert syndrome: a clinical–radiological study. Neuroradiology 1990;31:502–6.

17. Toelle SP, Yalcinkaya C, Kocer N, et al. Rhombencephalosynapsis: clinical findings and neuroimaging in 9 children. Neuropediatrics 2002;33:209–14.

18. Meltzer CC, Smirniotopoulos JG, Jones RV. The striated cerebellum: an MR imaging sign in Lhermitte-Duclos disease (dysplastic gangliocytoma). Radiology 1995;194:699–703.

19. Naidich TP, McLone DG, Fulling KH. The Chiari II malformation: Part IV. The hindbrain deformity. Neuroradiology 1983;25: 179–97.

20. Wolpert SM, Anderson M, Scott RM, et al. Chiari II malformation: MR imaging evaluation. Am J Roentgenol 1987;149:1033–42.

21. Hetts SW, Sherr EH, Chao S, et al. Anomalies of the corpus callosum: an MR analysis of the phenotypic spectrum of associated malformations. Am J Roentgenol 2006;187:1343–8.

22. Barkovich AJ, Kuzniecki RI, Jackson GD, et al. Developmental and genetic classification for malformations of cortical development. Neurology 2005;65:1873–87.

23. Blumcke I, Thom M, Aronica E, et al. The clinicopathological spectrum of focal cortical dysplasias: a consensus classification proposed by an ad hoc Task Force of the ILAE Diagnostic Methods Commission. Epilepsia 2010;52(1):158–74.

24. Barkovich AJ. The phakomatoses. In: Paediatric Neuroimaging. 3rd ed. Philadelphia: Lippincott, Williams & Wilkins; 2005. pp. 440–504.

25. Herron J, Darrah R, Quaghebeur G. Intra-cranial manifestations of the neurocutaneous syndromes. Clin Radiol 2000;55:82–98.

26. Neurofibromatosis. In: National Institutes of Health Consensus Development Conference. Arch Neurol 1988;575–8.

27. Balcer LJ, Liu GT, Heller G, et al. Visual loss in children with neurofibromatosis type 1 and optic pathway gliomas: relation to tumor location by magnetic resonance imaging. Am J Ophthalmol 2001;131:442–5.

28. Goh WH, Khong PL, Leung CS, et al. T2-weighted hyperintensities (unidentified bright objects) in children with neurofibromatosis 1: their impact on cognitive function. J Child Neurol 2004;19: 853–8.

29. Roach ES, Gomez MR, Northrup H. Tuberous sclerosis complex consensus conference: revised clinical diagnostic criteria. J Child Neurol 1998;13:624–8.

30. Kingsley D, Kendall B, Fitz C. Tuberous sclerosis: a clinicoradiological evaluation of 110 cases with particular reference to atypical presentation. Neuroradiology 1986;28:171–90.

31. Baron Y, Barkovich AJ. MR imaging of tuberous sclerosis in neonates and young infants. Am J Neuroradiol 1999;20:907–16.

32. Braffman B, Naidich TP. The phakomatoses: Part II. von Hippel–Lindau disease, Sturge–Weber syndrome, and less common conditions. Neuroimaging Clin N Am 1994;4:325–48.

33. Marti-Bonmarti L, Menor F, Mulas F. The Sturge–Weber syndrome: correlation between the clinical status and radiological CT and MRI findings. Childs Nerv Syst 1993;9:107–9.

34. Naidich TP, Blaser SI, Delman BN, et al. 2002 Embryology of the spine and spinal cord, in Proceedings of the 40th Annual Meeting of the American Society of Neuroradiology, Vancouver, BC, May 13–17, pp. 3–13.

35. Barkovich AJ. Congenital anomalies of the spine. In: Barkovich AJ, editor. Pediatric Neuroimaging. 4th ed. Philadelphia: Lippincott Williams & Wilkins; 2005.

36. Rossi A, Gandolfo C, Morana G, et al. Current classification and imaging of congenital spinal abnormalities. Semin Roentgenol 2006;41:250–73.

37. Rowland Hill CA, Gibson PJ. Ultrasound determination of the normal location of the conus medullaris in neonates. Am J Neonat Radiol 1995;16:469–72.

38. Beek FJ, de Vries LS, Gerards LJ, Mali WP. Sonographic determination of the position of the conus medullaris in premature and term infants. Neuroradiology 1996;38 (Suppl. 1):S174–7.

39. McLone DG, Dias MS. Complications of myelomeningocele closure. Pediatr Neurosurg 1991–1992;17:267–73.

40. Drolet B. Birthmarks to worry about. Cutaneous markers of dysraphism. Dermatol Clin 1998;16:447–53.

41. Thompson D. Hairy backs, tails and dimples. Curr Paediatr 2000;10:177–83.

42. Pang D, Zovickian J, Oviedo A. Long-term outcome of total and near-total spinal cord lipomas and radical reconstruction of the neural placode: part 1—surgical technique. Neurosurgery 2009;65:511–29.

43. Hughes JA, De Bruyn R, Patel K, Thompson D. Evaluation of spinal ultrasound in spinal dysraphism. Clin Radiol 2003;58: 227–33.

44. Pang D, Dias MS, Ahab-Barmada M. Split cord malformation. Part I: a unified theory of embryogenesis for double spinal cord malformations. Neurosurgery 1992;31:451–80.

45. Pang D. Split cord malformation. Part II: clinical syndrome. Neurosurgery 1992;31:481–500.

46. Faris JC, Crowe JE. The split notochord syndrome. J Pediatr Surg 1975;10:467–72.

47. Duhamel B. From the mermaid to anal imperforation: the syndrome of caudal regression. Arch Dis Child 1961;36:152–5.

48. Carey JC, Greenbaum B, Hall BD. The OEIS complex (omphalocele, exstrophy, imperforate anus, spinal defects). Birth Defects Orig Artic Ser 1978;14:253–63.

49. Currarino G, Coln D, Votteler T. Triad of anorectal, sacral, and presacral anomalies. Am J Roentgenol 1981;137:395–8.

50. Pang D. Sacral agenesis and caudal spinal cord malformations. Neurosurgery 1993;32:755–79.

51. Van Der Knaap MS, Valk J. Magnetic Resonance Imaging of Myelination and Myelination Disorders. 3rd ed. Berlin: Springer Verlag; 2005.

52. Patay Z. Metabolic disorders. In: Carty H, et al, editors. Imaging Children. 2nd ed, vol 2. Edinburgh: Churchill Livingstone; 2005. pp. 1899–956.

53. Hayward R, Jones B, Dunaway D, Evans R, editors. The clinical management of craniosynostosis. Clin Dev Med 2004;163.

54. World Health Organization. Classification of tumours. Pathology and genetics. In: Kleihues P, Cavenee W, editors. Tumours of the Nervous System. Cambridge: IARC Press; 2000.

55. Jaspan T. CCLG brain tumour imaging protocol. Available at <http://www.cclg.org.uk>; Jan 2009.

56. Saunders DE, Phipps KP, Wade AM, et al. Surveillance imaging strategies following surgery and/or radiotherapy for childhood cerebellar low-grade astrocytoma. J Neurosurg 2005;102(Suppl. 2): 172–8.

57. Saunders DE, Hayward RD, Phipps KP, et al. Surveillance neuroimaging of intracranial medulloblastoma in children: how effective, how often, and for how long? J Neurosurg 2003;99: 280–6.

58. Good CD, Wade AM, Hayward RD, et al. Surveillance neuroimaging in childhood intracranial ependymoma: how effective, how often, and for how long? J Neurosurg 2001;94:27–32.

59. Rumboldt Z, Camacho DL, Lake D, et al. Apparent diffusion coefficients for differentiation of cerebellar tumors in children. Am J Neuroradiol 2006;27:1362–9.

60. Arai K, Sato N, Aoki J, et al. MR signal of the solid portion of pilocytic astrocytoma on T2-weighted images: is it useful for differentiation from medulloblastoma? Neuroradiology 2006;48:233–7.

61. Fischbein NJ, Prados MD, Wara W, et al. Radiologic classification of brain stem tumors: correlation of magnetic resonance imaging appearance with clinical outcome. Pediatr Neurosurg 1996;24: 9–23.

62. Bowers DC, Georgiades C, Aronson LJ. Tectal gliomas: natural history of an indolent lesion in pediatric patients. Pediatr Neurosurg 2000;32:24–9.

63. Chong WK, Saunders DS, Ganesan V. Stroke is an important paediatric illness. Pediatr Radiol 2004;34:2–4.

64. Paediatric Stroke Working Group. Stroke in childhood. Clinical guidelines for diagnosis, management and rehabilitation. London: Clinical Effectiveness and Evaluation Unit, Royal College of Physicians; 2004.

65. Ganesan V, Prengler M, McShane MA, et al. Investigation of risk factors in children with arterial ischemic stroke. Ann Neurol 2003;53:167–73.

66. DeVeber G. In pursuit of evidence-based treatments for paediatric stroke: the UK and Chest guidelines. Lancet Neurol 2005;4:432–6.

SUBJECT INDEX

Page numbers followed by '*f*' indicate figures, '*t*' indicate tables, and '*b*' indicate boxes.

Printed in the United States
By Bookmasters